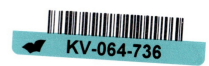

M1200S033
SoS

Amit S. Kalgutkar, Deepak Dalvie,
R. Scott Obach, and Dennis A. Smith

Reactive Drug Metabolites

Methods and Principles in Medicinal Chemistry

Previous Volumes of this Series:

Amit S. Kalgutkar, Deepak Dalvie, R. Scott Obach, and Dennis A. Smith

Reactive Drug Metabolites

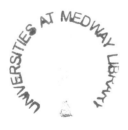

WILEY-VCH

WILEY-VCH Verlag GmbH & Co. KGaA

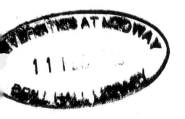

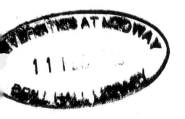

Series Editors

Prof. Dr. Raimund Mannhold
Molecular Drug Research Group
Heinrich-Heine-Universität
Universitätsstrasse 1
40225 Düsseldorf
Germany
mannhold@uni-duesseldorf.de

Prof. Dr. Hugo Kubinyi
Donnersbergstrasse 9
67256 Weisenheim am Sand
Germany
kubinyi@t-online.de

Prof. Dr. Gerd Folkers
Collegium Helveticum
STW/ETH Zurich
8092 Zurich
Switzerland
folkers@collegium.ethz.ch

Authors

Dr. Amit S. Kalgutkar
Pfizer Global R&D
Pharmacokinetics, Metabolism
MS 8220-3529
Groton CT 06340
USA

Dr. Deepak Dalvie
Pfizer Global R&D
Pharmacokinetics, Metabolism
10628 Science Center Drive
La Jolla CA 06340
USA

Dr. R. Scott Obach
Pfizer Global R&D
Pharmacokinetics, Metabolism
MS 8118D-2008
Groton CT06340
USA

Dr. Dennis A. Smith
Pfizer Inc.
IPC475
Ramsgate Road
Sandwich, Kent CT13 9NJ
United Kingdom

■ All books published by **Wiley-VCH** are carefully produced. Nevertheless, authors, editors, and publisher do not warrant the information contained in these books, including this book, to be free of errors. Readers are advised to keep in mind that statements, data, illustrations, procedural details or other items may inadvertently be inaccurate.

Library of Congress Card No.: applied for

British Library Cataloguing-in-Publication Data
A catalogue record for this book is available from the British Library.

Bibliographic information published by the Deutsche Nationalbibliothek
The Deutsche Nationalbibliothek lists this publication in the Deutsche Nationalbibliografie; detailed bibliographic data are available on the Internet at http://dnb.d-nb.de.

© 2012 Wiley-VCH Verlag & Co. KGaA, Boschstr. 12, 69469 Weinheim, Germany

Composition   Thomson Digital, Noida, India
Printing and Binding   Markono Print Media Pte Ltd, Singapore
Cover Design   Schulz Grafik-Design, Fußgönheim

Print ISBN: 978-3-527-33085-0
ePDF ISBN: 978-3-527-65577-9
ePub ISBN: 978-3-527-65576-2
mobi ISBN: 978-3-527-65575-5
oBook ISBN: 978-3-527-65574-8

Printed in Singapore
Printed on acid-free paper

Contents

Preface

The most common reasons for clinical failure and the withdrawal of already marketed drugs are insufficient efficacy and unexpected human toxicity [1, 2]. To some extent, both reasons are inherently related: low doses generate fewer side effects but often lack activity, whereas higher doses are effective but may be toxic. Target-related side effects, such as hERG channel inhibition, were the reason for several drug failures in past decades. Nowadays, such antitarget activities are already discovered during preclinical profiling. More critical is idiosyncratic toxicity, not detectable in clinical phase II studies, sometimes not even in phase III studies, because it occurs only in a very minor percentage of the population. Most often such rare toxic events are not related to the drug itself but to the generation of reactive metabolites. Correspondingly, it is of utmost importance to know the structural features that are responsible for the production of such toxic metabolites and to understand the underlying mechanisms of action. By eliminating or modifying these partial structures, the risk of idiosyncratic toxicity can be avoided or at least reduced. However, as discussed in this book, about 50% of the most prescribed drugs show a structural alert for potential toxicity; at least most of them must be considered to be "false positives." Sometimes very minor differences determine whether a compound forms a toxic metabolite or not.

A lesson that is told to every young medicinal chemist is to stay away from irreversible inhibitors. Whereas this indeed is good advice, we have to accept that some of the most important drugs either are irreversible inhibitors themselves, such as acetylsalicylic acid, the penicillins, cephalosporins, and related lactam antibiotics, or produce reactive metabolites, such as omeprazole, clopidogrel, isoniazid, and several others. However, these drugs or their reactive metabolites either have sufficient specificity for their therapeutic target or react with it directly at their site of generation. As a consequence, these drugs are sufficiently safe for human use. Despite the many examples of successful covalent drugs, interest in their role as drug candidates has emerged only recently.

This book by Amit Kalgutkar and his colleagues Deepak Dalvie, Scott Obach, and Dennis Smith discusses all relevant aspects of reactive drug metabolites, especially under the perspective of their relevance for drug toxicity. Numerous examples illustrate their generation and the various mechanisms of toxic action. Introductory chapters present a historical perspective of reactive drug metabolites, their role in genotoxicity, and the role of various drug-metabolizing enzymes, especially the cytochrome P450 enzymes, as well as the role of reactive metabolites in drug-induced toxicity. The following two chapters describe structural alerts that indicate the potential formation of reactive metabolites. The next two chapters are dedicated to the role of reactive metabolites in pharmacological action and to the analysis of structure–toxicity relationships. The common misunderstanding that natural products *per se* are nontoxic is discussed in a chapter on their bioactivation, followed by a chapter on experimental approaches for the detection of reactive metabolite formation. Highly valuable for medicinal chemists is a chapter on case studies that describe the elimination or reduction of reactive metabolite formation in lead optimization. Structural alerts give a warning, but almost all of the most-prescribed drugs have a structural toxicity alert, in contrast to the excellent safety records of (most of) these drugs, as discussed in the following chapter; especially the dose range is responsible, whether toxic effects are observed. The last three chapters discuss reversible and irreversible inhibitors as drug candidates and the important issue of risk–benefit analysis, ending in a section on "More questions than answers."

The series editors would like to thank Amit Kalgutkar and his colleagues for their enthusiasm to write this book, which is another important contribution to our series "Methods and Principles in Medicinal Chemistry." Due to its content, it will be of utmost importance for all scientists involved in drug research, medicinal chemists, as well as biochemists and biologists. Last but not least, we thank the publisher Wiley-VCH, in particular Frank Weinreich and Heike Nöthe, for their engagement in this project and their ongoing support of the entire book series.

September 2012
Düsseldorf
Weisenheim am Sand
Zürich

Raimund Mannhold
Hugo Kubinyi
Gerd Folkers

References

1 Kennedy, T. (1997) Managing the drug discovery/development interface. *Drug Discovery Today*, **3**, 436–444.

2 Schuster, D., Laggner, C., and Langer, T. (2005) Why drugs fail – a study on side effects in new chemical entities. *Current Pharmaceutical Design*, **11**, 3545–3559.

A Personal Foreword

Throughout our careers in drug research, we have tried to understand the role of metabolites in drug efficacy and safety. Oxidative processes invariably yield reactive intermediates that are part of the process of drug metabolism. In most cases, these processes are extremely rapid and confined to the catalytic active site of the drug-metabolizing enzyme (e.g., cytochrome P450) concerned with metabolism; the resultant stable metabolite is the only evidence that such a process has occurred. Occasionally, some reactive species are quasi-stable and escape this environment to interact with other enzymes, tissue macromolecules, and/or DNA. The possible outcomes of this escape have consumed the past 50 years of dedicated research.

The science of reactive intermediates formed as metabolites of drugs developed from the pioneering work on the carcinogenicity of polycyclic aromatic hydrocarbons and other planar heterocyclic aromatic compounds. This early work demonstrated how epidemiological studies (e.g., high rates of cancer in chimney sweeps and shoe manufacturers) could be biochemically linked to the irreversible reaction of small organic molecules with macromolecules such as DNA. These important advances also contributed to the understanding of oxidative enzymes present in liver and other organs. Detoxification and activation processes were seen as a vital balance to the health of individuals. The association of some oxidative processes leading to reactive metabolites rather than the more abundant stable forms was embraced in the search to understand drug toxicity. By the 1970s, a strong body of opinion had formed that cellular necrosis, hypersensitivity, and blood dyscrasias induced by drugs could result from the formation of reactive metabolites. The hepatotoxicity of certain drugs such as acetaminophen could be linked to an overdose, leading to the formation of an overwhelming amount of a reactive metabolite. However, the field was vastly more complicated since many drugs showed these toxicities in only a small percentage of patients. Clues to an immunological component through drugs such as halothane and tienilic acid that had circulating antibodies to drug or modified proteins moved the science into new fields. The metabolism of drugs, such as the sulfonamide antibiotics, which cause severe skin toxicities (Stevens–Johnson syndrome), to metabolites that produced specific T cell responses is a more recent finding in this context.

With this long history, the question could be asked why now publish a work dedicated to the field? The answer lies in the multiple directions the research has taken us and in the increasing focus on drug safety. An area that was researched mainly in academic centers (of undoubted excellence), drug toxicity is now being researched, in varying degrees, in every drug discovery and development organization. There is no recipe, no standard protocol, and no regulatory mandates. Best practice is a distillation of all the knowledge and an application to each institutions research and disease area interests. This volume tries to provide that knowledge.

The research on reactive metabolites already has major influences on drug discovery, development, and prescribing to the patient population. For instance, certain functional groups are associated with a high risk of reactive metabolite formation and their inclusion should always be subject to scrutiny. Despite earlier findings, there is emerging evidence that toxicities produced by reactive metabolites show a dose–response relationship. This directly influences the design of future agents in terms of their pharmacological potency, intrinsic clearance, and so on. The possibility to predict which patients will undergo toxicity is becoming more practical. Human leukocyte antigen (HLA) class I alleles process reactive metabolite adducts. The protein adduct is attached to specific HLA molecules on the antigen-presenting cells and recognized by effector T cells via the T cell receptor to cause T cell activation. HLA-B*5701 is carried by 100% of patients who are patch test positive for abacavir hypersensitivity and screening for this HLA is highly predictive of the toxicity. Similar diagnostics are gradually emerging for other toxicities. Drugs may in future include this information and testing as part of individualized medicine.

In this book, we have tried to distill the knowledge gained during our careers and our passion for this subject into a single volume that takes the reader through all aspects of reactive metabolites and drug toxicity: the history, the chemistry, the way to search for reactive metabolites, which structures and which drugs form them, why natural products may not be as benign as their devotees think, and also the central debate on benefit risk and the imprecise sources of information on which judgments are made. The authors hope that this volume will contribute to safer and better drugs; if so, their efforts will be repaid many folds.

Amit S. Kalgutkar
Deepak Dalvie
R. Scott Obach
Dennis A. Smith

1
Origin and Historical Perspective on Reactive Metabolites

Abbreviations

AFB$_1$	Aflatoxin B$_1$
BQ	Benzoquinone
BSA	Bovine serum albumin
CYP	Cytochrome P450
GSH	Glutathione
GSSG	Glutathione disulfide
NAPQI	*N*-Acetyl-*p*-benzoquinoneimine
TCPO	1,2-Epoxy-3,3,3-trichloropropane
TFA	Trifluoroacetic acid
TFAC	Trifluoroacetyl chloride

1.1
Mutagenesis and Carcinogenesis

The concept that chemicals, including drugs, could exert harmful effects on living organisms by their conversion into reactive metabolites probably dates back to the 1950s. The most compelling evidence began to be drawn in the 1960s from the area of carcinogenicity and studies looking at processing by metabolism of compounds to unstable, reactive metabolites. These studies drew from the human occupational exposure and animal experiments, which linked polycyclic aromatic hydrocarbons and certain other planar heterocyclic aromatic compounds, containing one or more nitrogen, sulfur, or oxygen atoms, to carcinogenic effects in humans. Human exposure was via coal tars, soot, pitch, dyes, adhesives, oil products, and tobacco smoke. Detailed examination showed that these compounds required bioactivation to electrophilic metabolites to exert their mutagenic or carcinogenic effects [1, 2]. In most cases, oxidation by cytochrome P450 (CYP) enzymes was seen as the rate-limiting step in the activation process to produce the reactive electrophilic species. Among the metabolic pathways identified for polycyclic aromatic hydrocarbons was the bay-region dihydrodiol epoxide pathway [3]. It involves three enzyme-mediated

Reactive Drug Metabolites, First Edition. Amit S. Kalgutkar, Deepak Dalvie, R. Scott Obach, and Dennis A. Smith.
© 2012 Wiley-VCH Verlag GmbH & Co. KGaA. Published 2012 by Wiley-VCH Verlag GmbH & Co. KGaA.

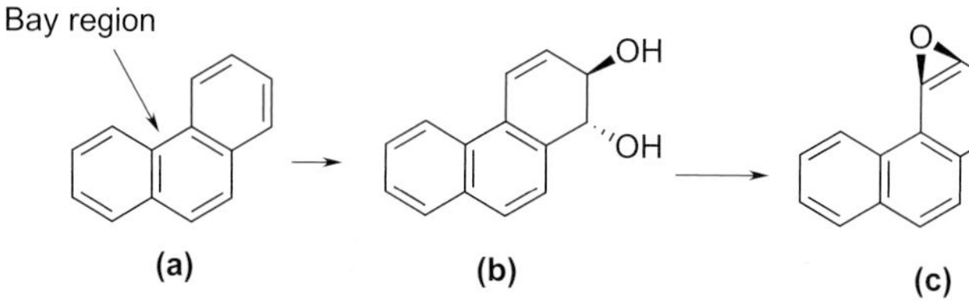

Bay region

(a)   (b)   (c)

Figure 1.1 Conversion of phenanthrene (a) to its diol (b) by cytochrome P450 and epoxide hydrolase and its ultimate carcinogen/mutagen (c) bay-region diol epoxide by cytochrome P450.

reactions (Figure 1.1): first, oxidation of a double bond catalyzed by CYP enzymes to unstable arene oxides; second, hydrolysis of the arene oxides by microsomal epoxide hydrolase to dihydrodiols; and, finally, a second CYP-catalyzed oxidation at the double bond adjacent to the diol function to generate a vicinal diol epoxide [3]. The vicinal diol epoxide was formed in the sterically hindered bay region. The bay-region diol epoxides are electrophiles capable of covalently binding to DNA. The formation of bay-region diol epoxides has been demonstrated with several polycyclic aromatics such as benzo[a]pyrene, chrysene, 5-methylchrysene, benzo[c] phenanthrene, benz[a]anthracene, and phenanthrene. Other potentially reactive metabolites with possible mutagenic and carcinogenic activity were being discovered at the same time via studies on known carcinogens (e.g., N-hydroxylation of 2-acetylaminoflourene) [4].

Functional *in vitro* tests for mutagens (and ultimately carcinogens) were pioneered in the 1970s by Ames and coworkers (see Chapter 2 for utility of the Ames test in drug discovery). Their work examined a set of carcinogens, including aflatoxin B_1 (AFB$_1$), benzo[a]pyrene, acetylaminofluorene, benzidine, and N,N-dimethylamino-*trans*-stilbene, and used a rat or human liver homogenate to form reactive metabolites and colonies of *Salmonella* histidine mutants for mutagen detection. These experiments demonstrated that for the set of carcinogens there was a ring system sufficiently planar for a stacking interaction with DNA base pairs and a chemical functionality capable of being metabolized to a reactive species [5].

The work on mutagenesis and carcinogenesis has evolved continuously so that the effects of DNA binding are far more understood. For instance, AFB$_1$ is present in certain foodstuffs, particularly in developing mold, and is recognized as a major contributor to liver cancer in parts of the developing world (also see Chapter 9) (Figure 1.2).

AFB$_1$ forms an epoxide (the *exo* isomer is ~1000 times more genotoxic than the *endo* form) that reacts with DNA to form a guanine–AFB$_1$ DNA conjugate [6].

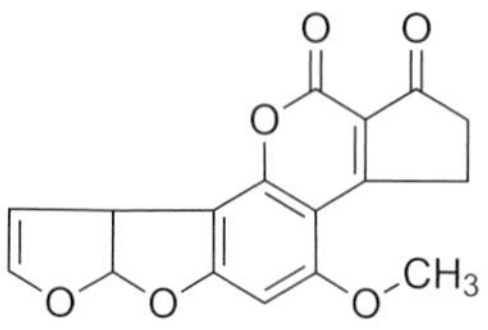

Figure 1.2 Structure of aflatoxin (AFB$_1$).

This difference in DNA reactivity and toxicity is believed to be due to DNA intercalation (affinity) and reactivity via an S_N2 pathway. The *exo* epoxide has an aqueous half-life of 1 s but is still stable enough to migrate into the cell nucleus and modify DNA [6]. Different CYPs produce different amounts of the *exo* and *endo* forms, but the major human CYP isozyme, that is, CYP3A4, produces exclusively the *exo* form. The damage caused to DNA is specific and the effects on the ultimate protein coded for have been researched. The activation of proto-oncogenes and inactivation of tumor suppressor genes in cells are considered as major events in the multistep process of carcinogenesis. p53 is a tumor suppressor gene, which is mutated in about half of all human cancers. About 80% of these mutations are missense mutations that lead to amino acid substitution and alter the protein conformation and stability of p53. These changes can also alter the sequence-specific DNA binding and transcription factor activity of p53. Thus, the role of p53 in DNA repair, cell cycle control, and programmed cell death can be substantially altered. AFB_1 exposure is correlated with a G:C to T:A transversion that leads to a serine substitution at residue 249 of p53, resultant altered activity, and ultimately hepatocellular carcinoma [7].

1.2
Detection of Reactive Metabolites

Reactive metabolites exist in aqueous solution for a short finite time. Their detection *per se* is difficult. The work in carcinogenicity established ways through which the problem could be tackled. Urinary products may reflect the presence of a reactive metabolite in downstream products (see Section 1.4) with stable metabolites formed by conjugation, hydration, or rearrangement of the reactive species. Sometimes, the conjugates include hydrolysis products of proteins (or genetic material), which are the target for covalent modification by the reactive metabolite. Often, *in vitro* systems such as liver microsomes with exogenously added nucleophilic trapping agents such as the endogenous antioxidant glutathione (GSH) provide further substantive chemical clues. Some form of functional tests (such as the *Salmonella* Ames test in Section 1.1) is invaluable, but broader toxicity findings are usually unavailable. Benzene is a toxin carcinogen that also causes certain blood dyscrasias including acute myeloid leukemia and aplastic anemia. It is thus carcinogenic and also myelotoxic. The principal site of toxicity is the bone marrow. The toxicity of the chemical was recognized by epidemiology and associated with, among others, the shoe industry, where it was a major constituent of glues used to bond the soles to the shoe upper. While metabolism of benzene to phenol was known before the nineteenth century, detailed investigations into the bioactivation mechanism revealed the existence of the electrophilic benzene oxide as the putative carcinogenic entity (similar to examples of polycyclic hydrocarbons in Section 1.1). The identification of the epoxide was through the isolation of the stable dihydrodiol metabolite of benzene [8]. It would be tempting to conclude that the toxicity could be explained with this finding.

In vivo studies [9] sampling urine have over the years revealed different evidence for reactive metabolite formation. These include

I) ring-hydroxylated metabolites including phenol, catechol, hydroquinone, and 1,2,4-trihydroxybenzene;
II) *trans,trans*-muconic acid, a ring-opened metabolite formed from muconaldehydes;
III) *N*-acetyl-5-(2,5-dihydroxyphenyl)-L-cysteine, a downstream conjugate of benzene, phenol, and hydroquinone;
IV) *S*-phenylmercapturic acid, a GSH-derived metabolite.

Detailed *in vitro* studies [8] have indicated that the complex pathway derives from a single enzymatic step involving the formation of benzene oxide primarily by CYP2E1 in the liver. Benzene oxide equilibrates spontaneously with the corresponding oxepine valence tautomer, which can open the ring to yield a reactive α,β-unsaturated aldehyde, *trans,trans*-muconaldehyde. Reduction or oxidation of *trans,trans*-muconaldehyde gives rise to 6-hydroxy-*trans,trans*-2,4-hexadienal and *trans,trans*-muconic acid. Both *trans,trans*-muconaldehyde and the hexadienal metabolites are myelotoxic in animal models. Alternatively, benzene oxide can undergo conjugation with GSH, resulting in the eventual formation and urinary excretion of *S*-phenylmercapturic acid. Benzene oxide is also a substrate for epoxide hydrolase, which catalyzes the formation of benzene dihydrodiol, itself a substrate for dihydrodiol dehydrogenase, producing catechol. Finally, benzene oxide spontaneously rearranges to form phenol, which subsequently undergoes conjugation (glucuronic acid or sulfate) or oxidation to hydroquinone and 1,2,4-trihydroxybenzene. The two diphenolic metabolites of benzene, catechol and hydroxyquinone, undergo further oxidation to the corresponding *ortho*-(1,2)- or *para*-(1,4)-benzoquinones (BQs) that can by myelotoxic. The 1,2- and 1,4-BQs are highly electrophilic and capable of reacting with DNA.

Benzene oxide is surprisingly stable and has a half-life of around 8 min when added to rat blood and 34 min in aqueous buffer. The metabolite therefore can perfuse out the liver to reach all the organs of the body. The toxicity of benzene in bone marrow may be due to benzene oxide formed in the liver being further oxidized in the bone marrow [8]. Benzene illustrated the complex nature of many investigations, revealing multiple possible chemical alternatives that may contribute to the toxicity in different ways.

1.3

Induction and Inhibition: Early Probes for Reactive Metabolites and Hepatotoxicants

Undoubtedly this focus on chemically reactive metabolites and cancer helped scientists to postulate and experimentally test if drug toxicity could also be initiated by such metabolites. Gillette [10] in the 1970s, among others, suggested cellular necrosis, hypersensitivity, blood dyscrasias, and fetotoxicities could be the result of reactive metabolites. Much of the early work focused on rodent toxicants at high doses and used metabolic inducers and inhibitors. Thus, bromobenzene was shown to be metabolized via a reactive metabolite pathway (epoxide) and was recovered as mercapturic acid (GSH conjugate) and dihydrodiol derivatives in the excreta. In studies utilizing identical doses of bromobenzene, pretreatment of rats with phenobarbital, which induced the metabolism of bromobenzene, increased liver cell necrosis, while SKF525A, which inhibited bromobenzene metabolism, decreased liver cell necrosis. Similar studies implicated reactive metabolites in the hepatotoxicity of acetaminophen and furosemide. Acetaminophen research helped define a number of important areas of reactive metabolite research as detailed below. Acetaminophen has remained a focus because the drug when given or ingested in large doses causes hepatotoxicity in all species, albeit with different sensitivities (in humans the toxic dose is around 20–40 g), although some changes in hepatic function have been observed in daily doses as low as 2 g. The toxicity is related to dose size, and *in vitro* and *in vivo* models can be readily established.

1.4
Covalent Binding and Oxidative Stress: Possible Mechanisms of Reactive Metabolite Cytotoxicity

Early investigations lacked many of the physicochemical measures available today, but the 1980s were critical in the identification of covalent binding *per se* and/or redox recycling and oxidative stress as possible toxic outcomes of reactive metabolite formation. Identifying the reactive species actually binding was problematic. Different target proteins were often added to incubations and synthetic metabolites used. Acetaminophen was a major focus. The compound when radiolabeled bound to hepatic microsomes from phenobarbital-pretreated mice [11]. Cysteine and GSH inhibited this binding, whereas several non-thiol amino acids did not. Bovine serum albumin (BSA), when used as an alternative target protein, inhibited covalent binding to microsomal protein in a concentration-dependent manner. BSA has a single thiol group and the binding now occurred to BSA. When α-s1-casein was substituted (a nonfree protein), little binding to the protein occurred. In duplicate experiments synthetic *N*-acetyl-*p*-benzoquinoneimine (NAPQI) (the two-electron oxidation product of acetaminophen) reproduced the results, identifying it as the reactive arylating metabolite of acetaminophen and suggesting that downstream effects of interactions with thiol groups may be responsible for the toxicity.

The reaction with thiol groups may be important but other aspects of reactive metabolite formation began to be examined [12]. The reaction of NAPQI with GSH in aqueous solution forms an acetaminophen–GSH conjugate and acetaminophen and glutathione disulfide (GSSG). Similar reactions occur in hepatocytes, but the GSSG is rapidly converted back to GSH by the NADPH-dependent glutathione reductase and a rapid oxidation of NADPH. Inhibitors of glutathione reductase prevent this and enhance cytotoxicity without changing the extent of covalent binding. Dithiothreitol added to isolated hepatocytes after maximal covalent binding of NAPQI, but preceding cell death protects cells from cytotoxicity and regenerates protein thiols. Thus, the toxicity of NAPQI to isolated hepatocytes may not result simply from covalent binding but from its oxidative effects on cellular proteins.

1.5
Activation and Deactivation: Intoxication and Detoxification

As work on reactive metabolites has progressed, so the balance between competing pathways, detoxifying reactions (such as GSH conjugate formation), and actual inherent species or individual sensitivity has become progressively more important. Without this knowledge it is tempting to conclude that it is the formation rate and amount of a particular metabolite that is important.

Acetaminophen showed varying toxicity when tested in different species. The drug and its toxic reactive metabolite, NAPQI, were, therefore, investigated in hepatocytes from different species [13]. Clear conclusions were drawn from these early studies in which acetaminophen triggered cell blebbing and loss of viability in the cells from mouse and hamster in contrast to human and rat hepatocytes, which were much more resistant to these effects. When NAPQI itself was tested, there were no significant differences in the sensitivity of the cells, from any species, to the toxic effects. The conclusion reached in these studies was that species differences in sensitivity to the hepatotoxicity of acetaminophen were due to differences in the rate of formation of NAPQI and not due to any intrinsic differences in sensitivity or any difference in the fate of NAPQI once formed. Later studies [14] have seen some correlations but without such clear-cut conclusions, observations often concluded that the actual test system, or conditions, produced significant variation. In these studies all the metabolites were quantified. These were separated into those downstream of NAPQI (GSH, cysteinylglycine, cysteine, and mercapturate conjugates) and alternative pathways (metabolites, such as the glucuronide and sulfate conjugates). The ratio of downstream NAPQI/alternative pathway metabolites excreted was 2.2, 1.0, 0.25, 0.1, and 0.08 for hamsters, mice, rabbits, rats, and guinea pigs, respectively, and inversely related to the hepatotoxic dose reported for these species. This is supportive of species sensitivity being determined by the balance between toxification and detoxification metabolic pathways [15].

It is likely that species differences in acetaminophen toxicity are due to a combination of pharmacokinetic (metabolism) differences and other biological variations. There is a natural inclination to believe that metabolism differences explain different responses, but the evidence in many cases is lacking. This is particularly true when the products of metabolism differ along with species responses.

1.6
Genetic Influences on Reactive Metabolite Formation

Early focus, even in the 1980s, was to look for at-risk populations. Understanding of enzymology and genetic variation was at an early stage but some links were

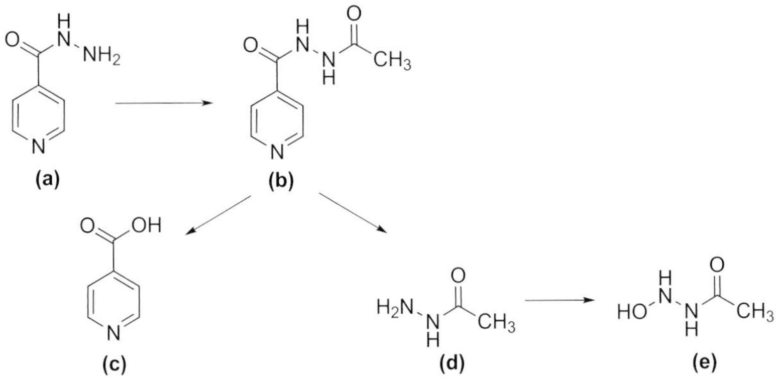

Figure 1.3 Pathway of isoniazid (a) metabolism forming *N*-acetylisoniazid (b) by acetylation, hydrolysis to isonicotinic acid (c) and *N*-acetylhydrazine (d), and subsequent *N*-hydroxylation (e).

established. Isoniazid, an antitubercular drug, caused hepatotoxicity in around 1% of the population. Increased risk was observed in fast acetylators of the drug that formed comparatively more of the metabolite *N*-acetylisoniazid. This hepatotoxicity could also be observed in animal studies together with covalent binding of radio-activity in the liver. Radiolabeled (^{14}C) versions of the metabolite bound covalently only when the acetyl group was labeled and not when the ^{14}C was incorporated into the pyridine ring [16]. Pathways suggested involved the formation of an *N*-hydroxy derivative, which dehydrated to a diazene that could fragment in the presence of oxygen to radical species (Figure 1.3).

1.7
Halothane: the Role of Reactive Metabolites in Immune-Mediated Toxicity

Halothane anesthesia may be followed by changes in liver function. For 25–30% of patients there is a minor degree of disturbance of liver function shown by increased serum transaminases or glutathione-*S*-transferase. With this mild change subsequent reexposure to halothane is not necessarily associated with evidence of liver damage. In 1 in 20 000 patients normally having past experience of halothane anesthesia, massive liver cell necrosis can occur, frequently leading to fulminant hepatic failure. This type of liver damage has clinical, serological, and immunological features strongly indicating an immune-mediated idiosyncratic reaction [17].

Halothane metabolism [18] produces three main excreted metabolites: trifluoro-acetic acid (TFA), *N*-triflouroacetyl-2-aminoethanol, and, to a lesser extent, *N*-acetyl-*S*-(2-bromo-2-chloro-1,1-difluoroethyl)-L-cysteine. The last two metabolites are downstream products of reactive metabolites. They are formed by hydroxylation of halothane with spontaneous loss of hydrogen bromide to form trifluoroacetyl chloride (TFAC), which would form TFA by hydrolysis or *N*-triflouroacetyl-2-aminoethanol by reaction with intracellular products. TFAC is also known to acylate lysine residues on proteins. Dehydrofluorination to 2-bromo-2-chloro-1,1-difluroethylene is the likely route to the cysteine conjugate.

CYP2E1 is the major catalyst in conversion of halothane to the reactive metabolite TFAC [19] and formation of trifluoroacetylated proteins. Trifluoroacetylated CYP2E1 was detected immunochemically in livers of rats treated with halothane and high levels of autoantibodies that recognized purified rat CYP2E1 but not purified rat CYP3A were detected by enzyme-linked immunosorbent assay in 14 of 20 (70%) sera from patients with halothane hepatitis. In contrast, only very low levels of such antibodies were detected in sera from healthy controls, from patients anesthetized with halothane without developing hepatitis, or from patients with other liver diseases. The intracellular location of trifluoroacetyl adducts was predominantly in the endoplasmic reticulum and also, to a lesser extent, on the cell surface. Thus, halothane metabolism by CYP2E1 results in the cell surface expression of acetylated CYP2E1 that could be important as an antigen in halothane hepatotoxicity.

1.8
Formation of Reactive Metabolites, Amount Formed, and Removal of Liability

Other inhaled anesthetics such as isoflurane and desflurane [20] also have TFAC as a metabolic product as evidenced by recoveries of TFA. However, the degree of biotransformation of these anesthetics is much less than that of halothane. This lower degree of exposure to the reactive metabolite may be an important factor in a much lower immune response and hepatotoxic risk. A later gaseous anesthetic sevoflurane [20] is biotransformed to a lesser degree than halothane (3–5% versus 18–25%), and much less total mass of metabolites is formed. The primary organic metabolite of sevoflurane is hexafluoroisopropanol, not TFAC. This metabolite is not chemically reactive in comparison to TFAC. Hexafluoroisopropanol does not accumulate, being rapidly cleared by glucuronidation that in turn is rapidly excreted in the urine. This is in contrast to halothane, where TFA (from TFAC) is detectable in urine for up to 12 days after 75 min of anesthesia (Figure 1.4).

1.9
Antibodies: Possible Clues but Inconclusive

Similar to halothane, tienilic acid forms antibodies that are associated with hepatotoxicity. In this case the circulating antibodies recognize CYP2C9, the principal CYP isozyme in the metabolism of tienilic acid. Moreover, tienilic acid is a very potent mechanism-based inhibitor of CYP2C9. Again the haptenized protein appears on the surface of the hepatocyte [21]. Other covalently altered enzymes are apparently the hapten for antibody production. For instance, iproniazid, an irreversible monoamine oxidase-B inhibitor, causes antibodies to be formed against monoamine oxidase-B. While it is enticing to link outcome to an immunological

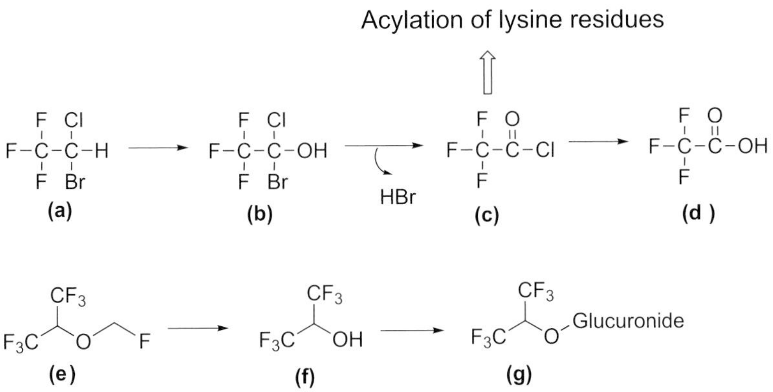

Acylation of lysine residues

Figure 1.4 Structure of halothane (a), its hydroxylated metabolite (b), the reactive trifluoroacetyl chloride (c, TFAC) formed by HBr loss, and the downstream product trifluoroacetic acid (d, TFA). The metabolism of sevoflurane (e) is shown in comparison, where the principal stable metabolite is hexafluoroisopropanol (f), rapidly converted to a glucuronic acid conjugate (g).

mechanism, many patients have circulating antibodies with no sign of toxicity. Practolol, a β-adrenoceptor antagonist with an acetylated aniline template, was responsible for oculomucocutaneous syndrome. An antibody specific to a practolol-reactive metabolite, most probably formed by oxidation of the aniline nitrogen, was found in the plasma of practolol-treated patients with or without a history of adverse reaction to the drug. No antibodies were detected in patients treated with other β-blocking drugs. Titer of the antibody was highly variable [22].

1.10
Parent Drug and Not Reactive Metabolites, Complications in Immune-Mediated Toxicity

Sulfonamide antibacterials are one of the earliest examples of chemotherapy against infection and are inhibitors of tetrahydropteroic acid synthetase. The natural substrate for this enzyme is *para*-aminobenzoic acid. Sulfonamides mimic the natural substrate with the *para*-aminobenzene (aniline) being retained but with the carboxylic acid being replaced by the isostere sulfonamide. The drugs cause serious skin toxicities including erythema multiforme, Stevens–Johnson syndrome, and toxic epidermal necrolysis. The *N*-4-hydroxylamine metabolite of these drugs, which can be formed in the skin, was initially identified and a rationale of covalent binding to proteins and induction of specific adverse immune response was developed. Anilines can be oxidized to more than one reactive metabolite and the nitroso intermediate has been shown to be a potent antigenic determinant [23, 24]. Surprisingly and contrary to the theories on reactive metabolites, T cell responses against the parent drug have also been detected. These T cells are low in proportion and highly selective, being responsive only to the particular drug used in the treatment such as sulfamethoxazole. Thus, they do not react to related sulfonamide antibacterial agents such as sulfapyridine or sulfadiazine. In contrast, those generated from reactive metabolites of sulfamethoxazole can be stimulated by other structurally related drugs such as sulfapyridine and sulfadiazine.

1.11
Reversible Pharmacology Should not be Ignored as a Primary Cause of Side Effects

Phenytoin is responsible for "fetal hydantoin syndrome," a defined set of side effects on the embryo, which include embryonic death, intrauterine growth retardation, mild central nervous system dysfunction, and craniofacial abnormalities. Original theories as causes included reactive metabolite formation. Phenytoin teratogenesis was postulated to result from epoxide formation [25] and covalent binding of the epoxide, the ultimate teratogen, to constituents of gestational tissue. Some experimental evidence was obtained in which Swiss mice were given teratogenic doses of phenytoin with and without a nonteratogenic dose of 1,2-epoxy-3,3,3-trichloropropane (TCPO), an epoxide hydrolase inhibitor. TCPO significantly increased the incidence of I-induced cleft lip and palate and enhanced the embryolethality twofold compared to phenytoin alone. The covalent binding of phenytoin-derived radioactivity in fetuses and placenta was enhanced by TCPO.

Further experiments looking at other causes have shown that the syndrome is unequivocally linked to phenytoin's reversible secondary pharmacology, namely, its blockade of the IKr delayed rectifier K^+ channel. In rodents the expression of this channel is age-specific, making the fetal heart especially sensitive compared to the mature animal. IKr blockers (which include phenytoin) initiate concentration-dependent embryonic bradycardia/arrhythmia resulting in hypoxia, explaining embryonic death and growth retardation, and episodes of severe hypoxia, followed by generation of reactive oxygen species within the embryo during reoxygenation, causing orofacial clefts and distal digital reductions and alterations in embryonic blood flow and blood pressure, inducing cardiovascular defects [26].

1.12
Conclusions: Key Points in the Introduction

This historical review serves as a stepwise introduction to the book. The important topics that have been introduced in this chapter will be explored in much greater detail in subsequent chapters and include the following:

1) Genotoxicity of many carcinogenic compounds could be linked to reactive metabolites.
2) These reactive metabolites covalently bind to DNA and lead to misreading of the message.
3) The genotoxins have a shape determined by their receptor (DNA) being planar and able to intercalate.

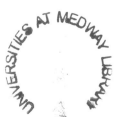

4) Similar reactive metabolites could also interact with proteins and cause other forms of toxicity.
5) Effects such as cellular necrosis, hypersensitivity, blood dyscrasias, and fetotoxicities could be due to reactive metabolites.
6) Cell necrosis, such as hepatotoxicity, could be caused by interaction with protein targets and alteration of protein function or by redox recycling and oxidative stress.
7) Other toxicity mechanisms could be triggered by generation of antigens and an autoimmune response.
8) The amount of metabolite formed may be critical in determining the outcome; moreover, structural changes that limit or prevent metabolite formation mitigate the risk.
9) Compounds can produce multiple reactive metabolites, the effects of which could be accumulative.
10) The identification of reactive metabolites may disguise other toxicity mechanisms such as reversible pharmacology or even autoimmune roles of the parent compound.

References

1 Miller, E.C. and Miller, J.A. (1966) Mechanism of chemical carcinogenesis: nature of proximate carcinogens and interactions with macromolecules. *Pharmacology Reviews*, **18** (1), 805–838.

2 Miller, E.C. and Miller, J.A. (1981) Searches for ultimate chemical carcinogens and their reactions with cellular macromolecules. *Cancer*, **47** (10), 2327–2345.

3 Xue, W. and Warshawsky, D. (2005) Metabolic activation of polycyclic and heterocyclic aromatic hydrocarbons and DNA damage. *Toxicology and Applied Pharmacology*, **206** (1), 73–93.

4 Cramer, J.W., Miller, J.A., and Miller, E.C. (1960) N-Hydroxylation: a new metabolic reaction observed in the rat with the carcinogen 2-acetylaminofluorene. *Journal of Biological Chemistry*, **235** (3), 885–888.

5 Ames, B.N., Durston, W.E., Yamasaki, E., and Lee, F.D. (1973) Carcinogens are mutagens: a simple test system combining liver homogenates for activation and bacteria for detection. *Proceedings of the National Academy of Sciences of the United States of America*, **70** (8), 2281–2285.

6 Guengerich, F.P. (2001) Forging the links between metabolism and carcinogenesis. *Mutation Research*, **488** (3), 195–209.

7 Hussain, S.P., Schwank, J., Staib, F., Wang, X.W., and Harris, C.C. (2007) P53 mutations and hepatocellular carcinoma: insights into the etiology and pathogenesis of liver cancer. *Oncogene*, **26** (15), 2166–2176.

8 Monks, T.J., Butterworth, M., and Lau, S.S. (2010) The fate of benzene-oxide. *Chemico-Biological Interactions*, **184** (1–2), 201–206.

9 Medeiros, A.M., Bird, M.G., and Witz, G. (1997) Potential biomarkers of benzene exposure. *Journal of Toxicology and Environmental Health*, **51** (6), 519–539.

10 Gillette, J.R. (1974) A perspective on the role of chemically reactive metabolites of foreign compounds in toxicity. I. Correlation of changes in covalent binding of reactivity metabolites with changes in the incidence and severity of toxicity. *Biochemical Pharmacology*, **23** (21), 2785–2794.

11 Streeter, A.J., Dahlin, D.C., Nelson, S.D., and Baillie, T.A. (1984) The covalent binding of acetaminophen to protein.

Evidence for cysteine residues as major sites of arylation *in vitro*. *Chemico-Biological Interactions*, **48** (3), 349–366.

12 Albano, E., Rundgren, M., Harvison, P.J., Nelson, S.D., and Moldeus, P. (1985) Mechanisms of *N*-acetyl-*p*-benzoquinone imine cytotoxicity. *Molecular Pharmacology*, **28** (3), 306–311.

13 Tee, L.B., Davies, D.S., Seddon, C.E., and Boobis, A.R. (1987) Species differences in the hepatotoxicity of paracetamol are due to differences in the rate of conversion to its cytotoxic metabolite. *Biochemical Pharmacology*, **36** (7), 1041–1052.

14 Jemnitz, K., Veres, Z., Monostory, K., Kobori, L., and Vereczkey, L. (2008) Interspecies differences in acetaminophen sensitivity of human, rat, and mouse primary hepatocytes. *Toxicology In Vitro*, **22** (4), 961–967.

15 Gregus, Z., Madhu, C., and Klaassen, C.D. (1988) Species variation in toxication and detoxication of acetaminophen *in vivo*: a comparative study of biliary and urinary excretion of acetaminophen metabolites. *Journal of Pharmacology and Experimental Therapeutics*, **244** (1), 91–99.

16 Timbrell, J.A., Mitchell, J.R., Snodgrass, W.R., and Nelson, S.D. (1980) Isoniazid hepatotoxicity: the relationship between covalent binding and metabolism *in vivo*. *Journal of Pharmacology and Experimental Therapeutics*, **213** (20), 364–369.

17 Neuberger, J.M. (1990) Halothane and hepatitis. Incidence, predisposing factors and exposure guidelines. *Drug Safety*, **5** (1), 28–38.

18 Cohen, E.N., Trudell, J.R., Edmunds, H.N., and Watson, E. (1975) Urinary metabolites of halothane in man. *Anesthesiology*, **43** (4), 392–401.

19 Eliasson, E. and Kenna, J.G. (1996) Cytochrome P450 2E1 is a cell surface autoantigen in halothane hepatitis. *Molecular Pharmacology*, **50** (3), 573–582.

20 Frink, E.J. (1995) The hepatic effects of sevoflurane. *Anesthesia and Analgesia*, **81** (6S), S46–S50.

21 Dansette, P.M., Bonierbale, E., Minoletti, C., Beaune, P.H., Pessayre, D., and Mansuy, D. (1998) Drug-induced immunotoxicity. *European Journal of Drug Metabolism and Pharmacokinetics*, **23** (4), 443–451.

22 Amos, H.E., Lake, B.G., and Artis, J. (1978) Possible role of antibody specific for a practolol metabolite in the pathogenesis of oculomucocutaneous syndrome. *British Medical Journal*, **1** (6110), 402–404.

23 Sanderson, J.P., Naisbitt, D.J., Farrell, J., Ashby, C.A., Tucker, M.J., Rieder, M.J., Pirmohamed, M., Clarke, S.E., and Park, B.K. (2007) Sulfamethoxazole and its metabolite nitroso sulfamethoxazole stimulate dendritic cell costimulatory signaling. *Journal of Immunology*, **178** (9), 5533–5542.

24 Castrejon, J.L., Berry, N., El-Ghaiesh, S., Gerber, B., Pichler, W.J., Park, B.K., and Naisbitt, D.J. (2010) Stimulation of human T cells with sulfonamides and sulfonamide metabolites. *Journal of Allergy and Clinical Immunology*, **125** (2), 411–418.

25 Martz, F., Failinger, C., and Blake, D.A. (1977) Phenytoin teratogenesis: correlation between embryopathic effect and covalent binding of putative arene oxide metabolite in gestational tissue. *Journal of Pharmacology and Experimental Therapeutics*, **203** (1), 231–239.

26 Danielsson, B.R., Skold., A.C., and Azarbayjani, F. (2001) Class III antiarrhythmics and phenytoin: teratogenicity due to embryonic cardiac dysrhythmia and reoxygenation damage. *Current Pharmaceutical Design*, **7** (9), 787–802.

2
Role of Reactive Metabolites in Genotoxicity

Abbreviations

CYP	Cytochrome P450
GSH	Glutathione
HPB	4-Hydroxy-1-(3-pyridyl)-1-butanone
NAT	*N*-Acetyltransferase
NNAL	4-(Methylnitrosamino)-1-(3-pyridyl)-1-butanol
NNK	4-(Methylnitrosamino)-1-(3-pyridyl)-1-butanone
NNN	*N'*-Nitrosonornicotine
SULT	Sulfotransferases

2.1
Introduction

The role of metabolism in the generation of reactive metabolites that are responsible for forming covalent bonds to nucleic acids and causing mutagenic lesions is now well established for many endogenous and exogenous xenobiotics. Approximately half of the chemicals listed as "known" human carcinogens and "probable" human carcinogens (Table 2.1) by the International Agency for Research on Cancer require metabolic activation to reactive species that are ultimately responsible for the carcinogenic activity of the parent compound. Virtually, any molecule that forms reactive metabolites possesses the propensity to modify DNA and elicit a genotoxic/carcinogenic response. However, there are certain commonalities in carcinogenic substances with respect to functional groups capable of generating DNA-reactive metabolites.

2.2
Carcinogenicity of Aromatic and Heteroaromatic Amines

Several aromatic amines (e.g., benzidine, 2-naphthylamine, and 4-aminobiphenyl, Figure 2.1) are of industrial importance because of their applications in the dyestuff

Reactive Drug Metabolites, First Edition. Amit S. Kalgutkar, Deepak Dalvie, R. Scott Obach, and Dennis A. Smith.
© 2012 Wiley-VCH Verlag GmbH & Co. KGaA. Published 2012 by Wiley-VCH Verlag GmbH & Co. KGaA.

Table 2.1 Examples of carcinogenic substances that require metabolic activation to reactive intermediates for their carcinogenic activities.

Human Carcinogens	Probable Human Carcinogens	
Aflatoxins	Acrylamide	*para*-Cresidine
4-Aminobiphenyl	Adriamycin (doxorubicin)	Dacarbazine
Aristolochic acid	Bischloroethyl nitrosourea	2,4-Diaminoanisole sulfate
Benzene	Chloramphenicol	Dibenz[a,h]acridine
Benzidine (and dyes metabolized to benzidine)	1-(2-Chloroethyl)-3-cyclohexyl-1-nitrosourea	Ethylene dibromide
Benzo[*a*]pyrene	4-Chloro-*ortho*-toluidine	Diepoxybutane
Bis(chloromethyl)ether and chloromethylether	Cyclopenta[cd]pyrene	1,1-Dimethylhydrazine
1,3-Butadiene	Dibenz[a,h]anthracene	1,6-Dinitropyrene
Chlorambucil	Dibenzo[a,l]pyrene	Furan
Cyclophosphamide	Diethyl sulfate	Hydrazobenzene
Diethylstilbestrol	5-Methoxypsoralen	5-Methylchrysene
Ethylene oxide	*N*-Methyl-*N*-nitrosourea	Methyleugenol
Melphalan	Nitrogen mustard	Metronidazole
8-Methoxypsoralen	*N*-Nitrosodiethylamine	Nitrobenzene
2-Naphthylamine	2-Nitrotoluene	1-Nitropyrene
N'-Nitrosonornicotine	Trichloroethylene	Ochratoxin A
4-*N*-(Nitrosomethylamino)-1-(3-pyridyl)-1-butanone	1,2,3-Trichloropropane	Propylthiouracil
Phenacetin	Vinylbromide	Safrole
Sulfur mustards	Vinylfluoride	Styrene
Tamoxifen	2-Acetylaminofluorene	Thiourea
Thiotepa	2-Aminoanthraquinone	
ortho-Toluidine	*ortho*-Aminoazotoluene	
Vinyl chloride	2-Amino-3,4-dimethylimidazo[4,5-f]quinoline (MeIQ)	
	2-Amino-3,4-dimethylimidazo[4,5-f]quinoxaline (MeIQx)	
	2-Amino-3-methylimidazo[4,5-f]quinoline (IQ)	
	2-Amino-1-methyl-6-phenylimidazo[4,5-b]pyridine (phIP)	
	ortho-Anisidine	
	Benz[*a*]anthracene	
	Bromodichloromethane	
	4-Chloro-*ortho*-phenylenediamine	

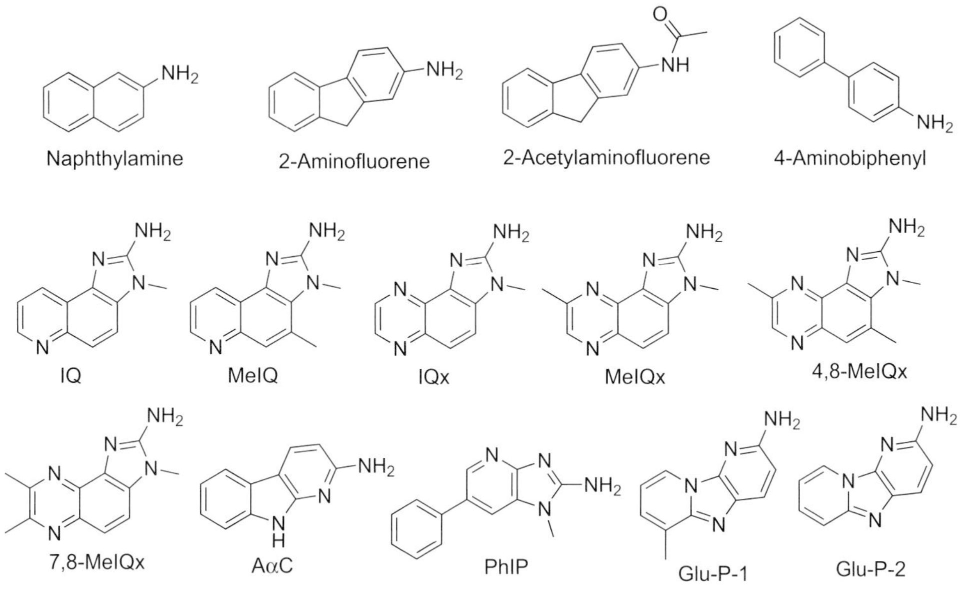

Figure 2.1 Examples of carcinogenic aromatic amines and heteroaromatic amines found in food.

industry and as antioxidants in rubber and other commercial products. The carcinogenic properties of aromatic amines were evident in the late 1800s from epidemiological reports on the appearance of urinary bladder tumors among workers employed in the German aniline dyestuff industry in the production of "fuchsin" (magenta). This workplace was subsequently associated with frequent occurrence of cancer of the urinary tract, referred to as "aniline cancer" [1]. Although aniline and other aromatic amines failed to produce tumors in rabbits, Hueper *et al.* showed that 2-naphthylamine induced bladder tumors in dogs when administered to the stomach and skin [2]. Likewise, hepatocarcinogenicity of aminoazo dyes such as *ortho*-aminoazotoluene and *N,N*-dimethyl-4-azobenzene ("butter yellow") was also demonstrated in rats [3]. In 1941, the first report on tumorigenesis in bladder, liver, kidney, pancreas, and lung of rats induced by 2-acetylaminofluorene, an aromatic amine intended to be used as a pesticide, was published [4]. Around the same time, Swedish chemist Widmark demonstrated that extracts of fried horse meat induced cancer when applied to mouse skin [5]. Sugimura and coworkers investigated the smoke produced by broiling fish and meat; they demonstrated that the smoke condensate and charred surfaces of broiled fish and meat were highly mutagenic in *Salmonella typhimurium* test systems [6]. Subsequently, heteroaromatic amine derivatives formed as a consequence of pyrolysis of amino acids or protein-containing foods were isolated, their structures were determined, and their biological effects were examined, specifically mutagenicity and carcinogenicity in animals [7, 8] (also see Chapter 9 for additional discussions on bioactivation pathways of natural products). The formation of heteroaromatic amines is the result of a

Maillard reaction, which occurs when amino acids and reducing sugars are heated together [9]. More than 20 such compounds have been identified (see Figure 2.1). Heterocyclic arylamines have also been identified in cigarette smoke condensate and have been shown to be genotoxic [10]. Aromatic amines are also formed in commercial hair dyes, and their contributions to an increased risk of bladder, breast, colon, and lymphatic cancer have been investigated [11].

The mechanism of carcinogenicity of aromatic and heteroaromatic amines involves bioactivation to reactive metabolites [12, 13]. The rate-limiting step is the *N*-oxidation of the amine nitrogen, which is mediated primarily by cytochrome P450 (CYP) enzymes, although flavin-containing monooxygenases and peroxidases are also known to play a role in the bioactivation pathway (Figure 2.2) [14–16]. Studies on aromatic amine oxidation go back to the 1940s, with early work on aminoazo dyes by Mueller and Miller [17]. *N*-Hydroxylation by CYP enzymes was first demonstrated with the acetamide derivative of 2-aminofluorene [18, 19], and further studies extended the work to unsubstituted aromatic amines [20]. CYP1A1 and 1A2 have been generally recognized to be the major enzymes involved in the bioactivation of aromatic and heterocyclic amines in human liver and lung microsomes [21, 22]. The findings with CYP1A2 have been confirmed *in vivo* in human studies, at least with the heteroaromatic amines PhIP and MeIQx (see Figure 2.1). The CYP1A2-selective inhibitor furafylline blocked most of the *in vivo* elimination of these compounds in studies in which the human volunteers consumed burned meat [23]. The *N*-hydroxy products of some heteroaromatic amines can be further oxidized to produce the nitroso intermediates (Figure 2.2). This reaction seems to be selective among the heteroaromatic amines substrates and may contribute to toxicity, through covalent binding to either proteins or DNA. The nitroso derivatives of heteroaromatic amines have been shown to react with DNA, proteins, as well as the endogenous antioxidant glutathione (GSH) [24].

N-Hydroxylamine metabolites are also prone to bioactivation via a phase II conjugation reaction to produce highly reactive ester derivatives that bind covalently to DNA (also see Chapter 9). Among the phase II enzyme systems responsible for the secondary activation step in mammals, *N*-acetyltransferases (NAT) and sulfotransferases (SULT) are most prominent and lead to the formation of reactive *N*-acetoxy and *N*-sulfonyloxy esters, respectively [25–27]. NAT-catalyzed acetylation of *N*-

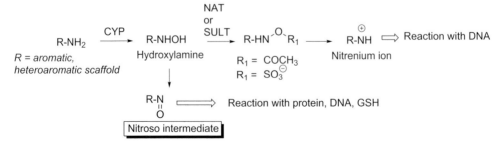

Figure 2.2 Bioactivation of aromatic and heteroaromatic amines via phase I (oxidative) and phase II (conjugation) pathways.

hydroxy aromatic and heteroaromatic amines enhances the genotoxic activity and DNA adduct levels via the generation of reactive N-acetoxyl esters [25–28]. In a similar way, the sulfur esters formed by the action of SULT enzymes are unstable and react readily with DNA [26]. Aromatic and heteroaromatic amines yield DNA adducts primarily through covalent adduction with guanine residues [29], reacting at the N2 and C8 atoms. The finding that photoactivated azide derivatives of IQ, MeIQx, and PhIP bind to DNA to form the same adducts as the N-acetoxy species indicates that the nitrenium ion may be a common intermediate for both reactive intermediates [30]. The N-hydroxy heteroaromatic amines can react directly with DNA, but the reaction is facilitated when reactive ester derivatives undergo heterocyclic cleavage to yield reactive aryl nitrenium ion species, which preferentially react to form DNA adducts (Figure 2.2).

2.3
Carcinogenicity of Nitrosamines

Tobacco-specific nitrosamines have emerged as one of the most important groups of carcinogens in tobacco products (also see Chapter 9 for additional discussions) [31]. Seven tobacco-specific nitrosamines have been identified in tobacco products, but two of these – 4-(methylnitrosamino)-1-(3-pyridyl)-1-butanone (NNK) and N'-nitrosonornicotine (NNN) (Figure 2.3) – are most important because of their carcinogenic activities and their consistent presence in both unburned tobacco and its smoke, frequently in considerable amounts. NNK selectively induces lung tumors in all species tested and is a particularly potent carcinogen in the rat [32]. It also causes tumors of the pancreas, nasal mucosa, and liver [32]. NNN produces esophageal and nasal cavity tumors in rats and respiratory tract tumors in mice and hamsters [32]. Both NNK and NNN are considered carcinogenic to humans by the International Agency for Research on Cancer (Table 2.1).

Dialkylnitrosamines such as NNK require metabolic activation via CYP-catalyzed α-hydroxylation to exert their carcinogenic properties. Figure 2.3 illustrates the α-hydroxylation pathways of NNK and its major metabolite 4-(methylnitrosamino)-1-(3-pyridyl)-1-butanol (NNAL), as well as the $2'$-α-hydroxylation pathway for NNN. α-Hydroxylation of the NNK methyl group leads to the carbinolamine species **1**, which spontaneously loses formaldehyde yielding 4-(3-pyridyl)-4-oxobutanediazo-hydroxide **2**. The same intermediate is formed by $2'$-hydroxylation of NNN. α-Hydroxylation at the methylene group of NNK produces the secondary alcohol metabolite **3**, which spontaneously decomposes to methanediazohydroxide. Similar intermediates are produced by α-hydroxylation of NNAL. Methanediazohydroxide, formed in these reactions from NNK and NNAL, reacts with DNA bases (guanosine, thymidine, cytosine and adenosine) to produce the well-known DNA adducts, O^6-methyl-dGuo, 7-methyl-dGuo, and O^4-methyl-dThd, which are common to many methylating carcinogens [32]. Subsequently, it was demonstrated that neutral thermal or acid hydrolysis of DNA from NNK-, NNN-, or NNAL-treated animals produced 4-hydroxy-1-(3-pyridyl)-1-butanone (HPB), confirming the pathway of

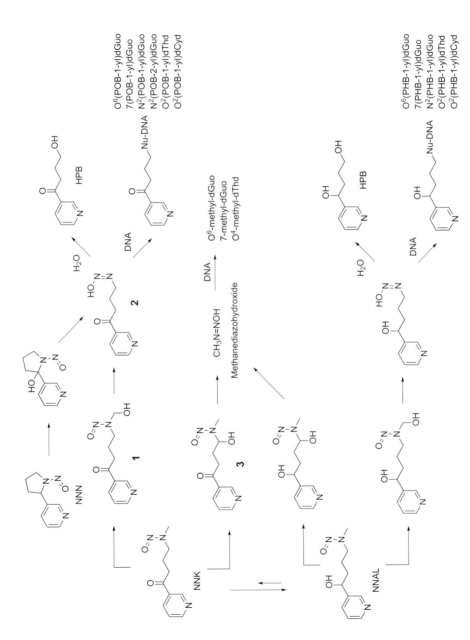

Figure 2.3 Bioactivation pathways of nitrosamines leading to DNA-reactive metabolites.

DNA alkylation involving the diazo intermediate resulting in pyridyloxobutyl (POB)–DNA adducts [33, 34]. Released HPB could be quantified by mass spectrometry, and its presence was established in the lung DNA of smokers, as well as in NNK-treated rodents [35].

2.4
Carcinogenicity of Quinones and Related Compounds

Quinones are ubiquitous in nature and constitute an important class of naturally occurring compounds found in plants, fungi, and bacteria. Naturally occurring quinones are synthesized via the shikimate or polyketide pathways, which are absent in animals. Humans are exposed to endogenous quinones primarily via the oxidative metabolism of catecholamines and estrogens. Human exposure to quinones also occurs via the diet, clinically, or via airborne pollutants such as quinone derivatives of polycyclic aromatic hydrocarbons. From a toxicological perspective, quinones are oxidants and electrophiles. They possess the soft (α,β-unsaturated carbonyl) and hard (carbonyl) electrophilic centers capable of reacting with GSH in a classic 1,4-Michael fashion or with DNA bases in a 1,2- and/or 1,4-Michael fashion [36]. Since nucleophilic 1,4-Michael addition to quinone represents a formal two-electron reduction resulting in a catechol–nucleophile conjugate, their oxidant and electrophilic properties are intimately related.

The carcinogenic activity of estrogens used as replacement therapy is thought to be mediated through CYP-mediated metabolism to the corresponding electrophilic/redox-active quinones (via the intermediate catechol metabolites) [37]. Once formed, the catechol estrogen metabolites can be oxidized by virtually any oxidative enzyme or metal ions affording the reactive *ortho*-quinone metabolites. *ortho*-Quinones and quinone methides (the products of isomerization) are known estrogen metabolites, which cause alkylation and/or oxidative damage to cellular proteins and DNA with estradiol, as illustrated in Figure 2.4 [38]. *ortho*-Quinones are also redox-active compounds and can undergo redox cycling with the semiquinone radical, generating superoxide radicals mediated through CYP/CYP reductase (see Figure 2.4). The reaction of superoxide anion radicals with hydrogen peroxide formed by the enzymatic or spontaneous dismutation of superoxide anion radical, in the presence of trace amounts of iron or other transition metals, gives hydroxyl radicals, which are powerful oxidants responsible for damage to essential macromolecules and DNA [39]. It is noteworthy to point out that the quinone-containing anticancer drugs such as mitomycin C, adriamycin, and daunorubicin (Figure 2.5) exert their pharmacological action via such a quinone–hydroquinone redox cycling, leading to reactive oxygen species [40].

An additional illustration on the carcinogenicity of quinones is evident with tamoxifen, which is used to treat hormone-dependent breast cancer. The increased risk of endometrial cancer associated with tamoxifen therapy has been associated with its bioactivation potential to reactive quinone species (Figure 2.6) [41, 42]. One of the suggested bioactivation pathways involves aromatic ring oxidation to

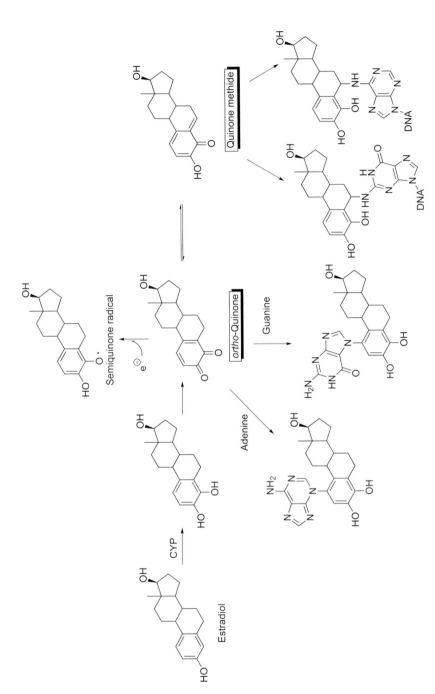

Figure 2.4 Metabolism of estradiol into DNA-reactive *ortho*-quinone and quinone methide metabolites.

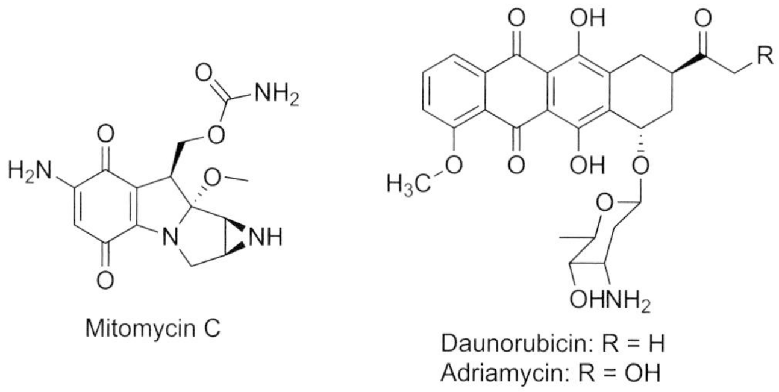

Figure 2.5 Structures of quinone-containing anticancer drugs.

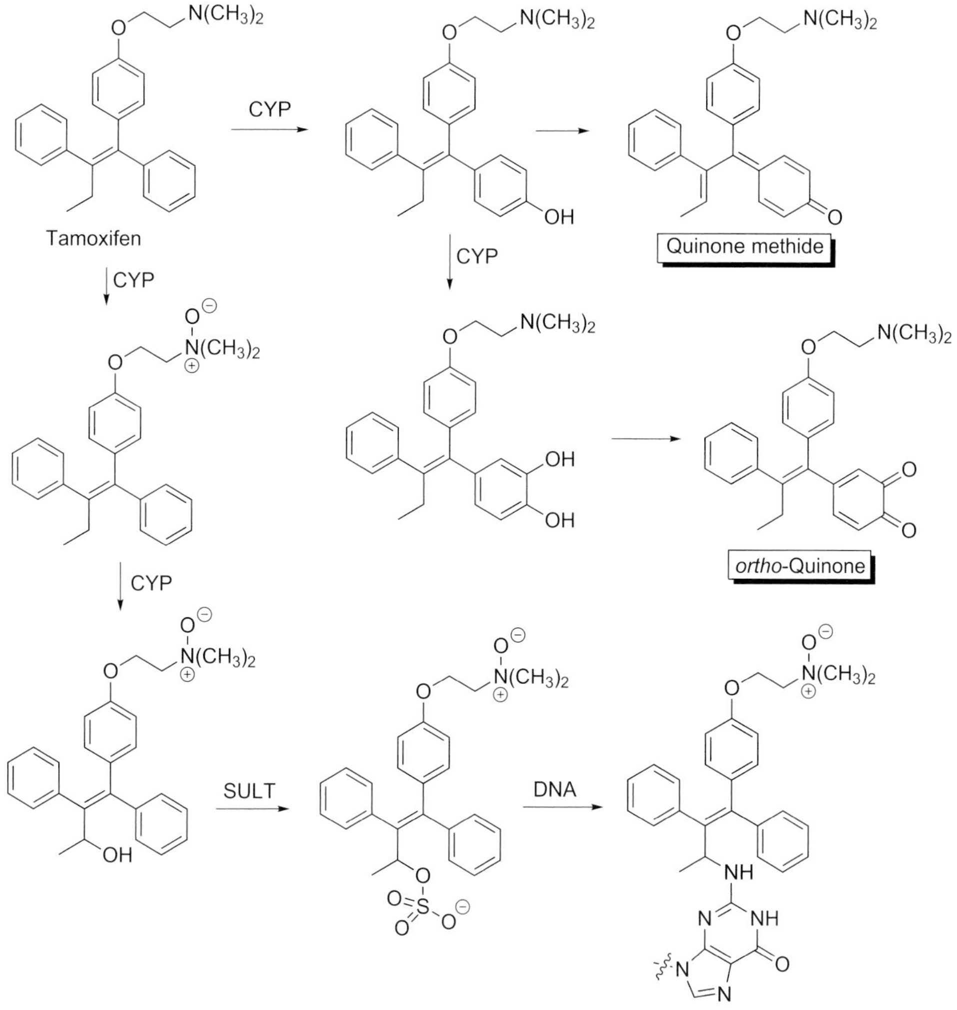

Figure 2.6 Bioactivation pathways of tamoxifen leading to protein- and DNA-reactive metabolites.

4-hydroxytamoxifen, which on a two-electron oxidation can generate the electrophilic quinone methide species. The resulting quinone methide has the potential to alkylate DNA and may initiate the carcinogenic process. Interestingly, the quinone methide is unusually stable; its half-life under physiological conditions is ~3 min and its half-life in the presence of GSH is ~4 min [43]. In addition, tamoxifen can also be metabolized to a catechol intermediate followed by further two-electron oxidation to the *ortho*-quinone, which is capable of reacting with DNA [44]. Apart from bioactivation pathways arising from aromatic ring hydroxylation to quinones, Shibutani *et al.* [41, 42] have characterized tamoxifen–DNA adducts in the endometrium of women treated with tamoxifen, which presumably arise from the α-hydroxylation (on the pendant ethyl group) of a tamoxifen N-oxide metabolite. α-Hydroxytamoxifen undergoes sulfation and loss of sulfate group to a carbocation species, which reacts with 2'-deoxyguanosine (Figure 2.6).

The final example in this category is that of safrole, the main constituent of sassafras oil, which is also present in a number of herbs and spices, such as nutmeg, mace, cinnamon, anise, black pepper, and sweet basil. Sassafras oil is extracted from the root bark of the tree *Sassafras albidum* and was widely used as a natural diuretic, as well as a remedy against urinary tract disorders, until safrole was discovered to be hepatotoxic and weakly carcinogenic [45]. In 1960 the US Food and Drug Administration banned the use of sassafras oil as a food and flavoring additive because of the high content of safrole and its proven carcinogenic effects. Two bioactivation pathways of safrole to potentially hepatotoxic and carcinogenic intermediates have been reported (Figure 2.7) [46–48]. The first one involves CYP-catalyzed hydroxylation of the benzyl carbon producing 1'-hydroxysafrole and conjugation with sulfate generating a reactive sulfate ester. This ester undergoes an

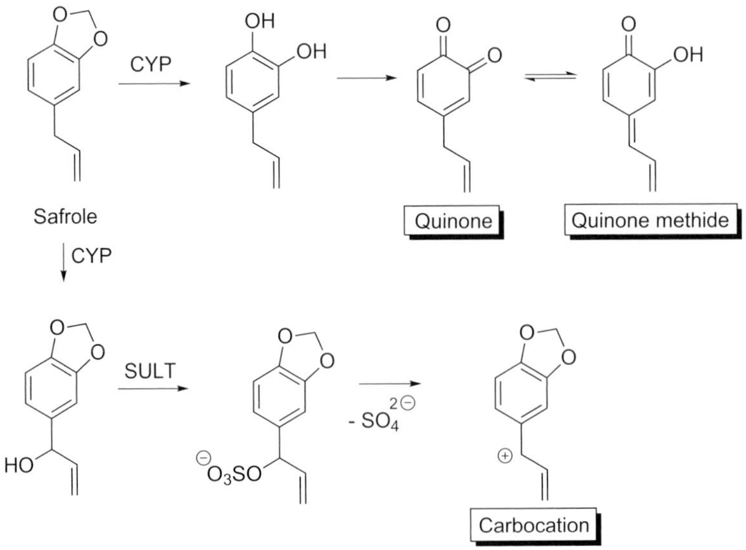

Figure 2.7 Bioactivation pathways of safrole leading to DNA-reactive metabolites.

S_N1 displacement reaction creating a highly reactive carbocation, which alkylates DNA [49]. The second pathway involves methylenedioxy ring scission leading to the formation of the catechol derivative, hydroxychavicol, which is a natural product found in betel leaf [50, 51]. Hydroxychavicol can easily be oxidized to the *ortho*-quinone, which isomerizes nonenzymatically to the more electrophilic *para*-quinone methide. Both pathways could explain the genotoxic effects of safrole, and DNA adducts consistent with the carbocation pathway have been identified *in vitro* and *in vivo* [52–54]. Recently, studies with betel quid chewers demonstrated that betel quid containing safrole-induced DNA adducts is highly associated with the development of oral squamous cell carcinoma in Taiwan [55].

2.5
Carcinogenicity of Furan

Furan is an important industrial intermediate and solvent. It is also an environment contaminant, present in wood smoke, tobacco smoke, and car exhaust. Furan is a liver and kidney toxicant in laboratory animals [56]. It induces hepatocellular adenomas and carcinomas in rats and mice and hepatic cholangiocarcinomas in rats. Based on these results and the large potential for human exposure, furan has been listed as a possible human carcinogen (see Table 2.1) by the National Toxicology Program and the International Agency for Research on Cancer.

The rate-limiting step in furan toxicity appears to be its metabolism to reactive species. The metabolism of furan is initiated by a CYP-catalyzed oxidation to the reactive α,β-unsaturated dialdehyde *cis*-2-butene-1,4-dial presumably via the epoxide intermediate (Figure 2.8) [57, 58]. The dicarbonyl metabolite can be trapped either as a bis-semicarbazone derivative or as GSH conjugate [57–59]. *cis*-2-Butene-1,4-dial also possesses the propensity to alkylate cellular nucleophiles such as amino acids and DNA [60–64]. Products of these reactions have been observed in the urine of furan-treated rats including the mono-GSH reaction product, *N*-[4-carboxy-4-(3-mercapto-1*H*-pyrrol-1-yl)-1-oxobutyl]-L-cysteinylglycine cyclic sulfide (**4**), and a downstream metabolite of this product, *S*-[1-(1,3-dicarboxypropyl)-1*H*-pyrrol-3-yl]methylthiol (**5**) [60, 65]. Three additional urinary metabolites of furan have also been identified as follows: (*R*)-2-acetylamino-6-(2,5-dihydro-2-oxo-1*H*-pyrrol-1-yl)-1-hexanoic acid (**6**), *N*-acetyl-*S*-[1-(5-acetylamino-5-carboxypentyl)-1*H*-pyrrol-3-yl]-L-cysteine (**7**), and its sulfoxide (**8**) [65]. Metabolite **6** results from the reaction of the dicarbonyl metabolite with lysine, whereas metabolites **7** and **8** result from the cross-linking of cysteine and lysine by *cis*-2-butene-1,4-dial (intermediate 9).

cis-2-Butene-1,4-dial reacts readily with 2′-deoxycytidine, 2′-deoxyadenosine, and 2′-deoxyguanosine to form diastereomeric oxadiazabicyclo(3.3.0)octaimine adducts (Figure 2.9) [61, 62]. A general reaction mechanism has been proposed in which the exocyclic nitrogen atom of the nucleoside reacts with the C1 position of *cis*-2-butene-1,4-dial, followed by 1,4-addition of the adjacent endocyclic nucleosidic nitrogen to the remaining α,β-unsaturated aldehyde. The second ring is formed by condensation of the C1 alcohol with the C4 aldehyde, forming a cyclic hemiacetal.

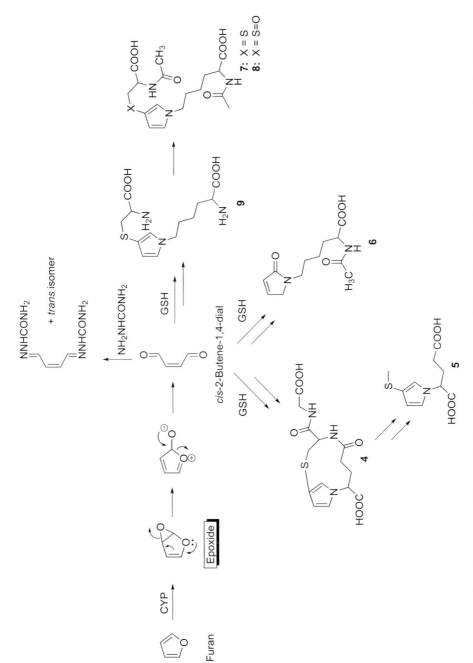

Figure 2.8 Oxidative bioactivation of furan to the electrophilic *cis*-2-butene-1,4-dial metabolite and its downstream adduction with nucleophiles.

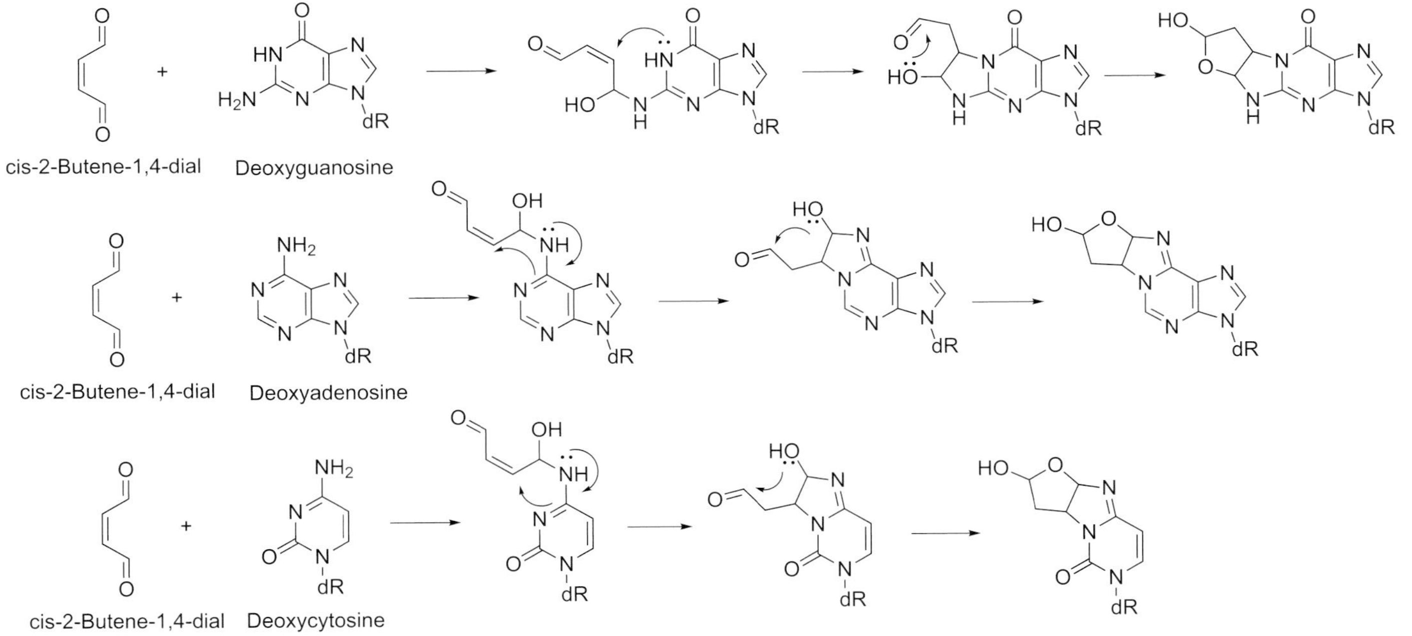

Figure 2.9 Reaction of *cis*-2-butene-1,4-dial, a reactive metabolite of furan, with nucleosides.

cis-2-Butene-1,4-dial   Deoxyguanosine

cis-2-Butene-1,4-dial   Deoxyadenosine

cis-2-Butene-1,4-dial   Deoxycytosine

The cyclic hemiacetal is in rapid equilibrium with the ring-opened aldehyde, with the hemiacetal form dominating under neutral conditions.

For additional examples of furan derivatives associated with toxicity (e.g., aflatoxins, teucrin A, menthofuran), the reader is advised to refer to Chapter 9.

2.6
Carcinogenicity of Vinyl Halides

Vinyl halide derivatives are of interest because of their extensive use as industrial solvents and monomers for polymerization coupled with concerns about carcinogenicity. The evidence for carcinogenicity is most unequivocal in the case of vinyl chloride (the simplest vinyl halide), because of the particular tumor (liver hemangiosarcoma) associated with exposure in industrial workers [66]. The epoxides of vinyl halides (referred to as halooxiranes) are all highly unstable and reactive (Figure 2.10). For example, the epoxide of vinyl chloride, that is, 2-chlorooxirane, has a half-life of ~90 s under physiological conditions, rearranging to 2-chloroacetaldehyde (and hydrolyzing to glycoaldehyde). Both vinyl chloride epoxide and 2-chloroacetaldehyde can react with DNA and proteins; however, kinetically, the DNA reactions are favored with the epoxide and the protein reactions are favored with 2-chloroacetaldehyde (see Figure 2.10) [67, 68]. This is due to the tendency of protein thiols (as "soft" nucleophiles) to undergo facile S_N2 Michael-type reactions with 2-halocarbonyls such as 2-chloroacetaldehyde; vinyl chloride epoxide reactions with nucleic acids are dominated by the attack of ring nitrogens on the unsubstituted methylene of 2-halooxiranes [67]. Reaction with aldehydes is driven by initial Schiff base formation of a carbonyl with an exocyclic nitrogen. Even though vinyl chloride epoxide and 2-chloroacetaldehyde yield the same DNA adduct (e.g., 1,N^2-ethenoguanine, Figure 2.10), the different carbon labeling patterns (using stable-labeled analogues) define the two alternate reactions. The relevance of the haloacyl halides and the epoxides to genotoxicity remains to be firmly established.

2.7
Carcinogenicity of Ethyl Carbamate

Ethyl carbamate (also known as urethane) has been known for some time to produce lung tumors in mice, but its human carcinogenicity is relatively less clear. Much of the interest in ethyl carbamate stems from its presence in products of fermentation, for example, breads, beer, wine, and particularly stone brandies. Miller and coworkers demonstrated that the desaturated analogue vinyl carbamate was carcinogenic and much more effective in the generation of etheno adducts with nucleosides [69–71]. These studies led Miller and coworkers to suggest the basic pathway shown in Figure 2.11, in which the ethyl group was desaturated by CYP enzymes and then yielded a reactive epoxide [69]. This pathway is now generally considered to be the most relevant to the tumorigenicity of ethyl

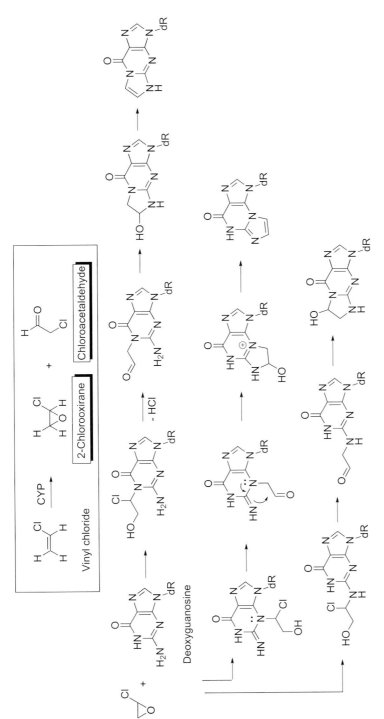

Figure 2.10 Bioactivation of vinyl chloride into DNA- and protein-reactive metabolites by CYP enzymes.

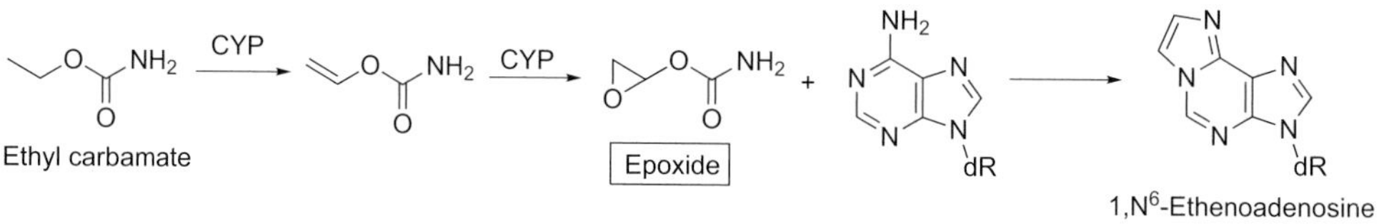

Figure 2.11 Oxidative bioactivation of ethyl carbamate into an electrophilic epoxide.

carbamate [72], although only limited *in vivo* studies have been done with the etheno-DNA adducts that have been characterized with this compound [73].

2.8
Carcinogenicity of Dihaloalkanes

Although the role of glutathione transferases is to detoxify reactive metabolites, studies in the 1970s first documented the ability of these detoxicating enzymes to catalyze the bioactivation of dihaloalkanes such as 1,2-dichloroethane to mutagens [74–76]. The mechanisms were demonstrated to involve the production of the unstable mono-GSH adducts and a subsequent reaction with DNA to form adducts containing the thiol nucleophile (Figure 2.12) [77–80]. The chemistry of the dihaloethane reactions is understood in the context of an episulfonium ion intermediate [79–82].

2.9
Assays to Detect Metabolism-Dependent Genotoxicity in Drug Discovery

Genetic toxicology testing is conducted in the early stages of drug development with the intent of identifying hazards associated with both the parent molecule and its metabolites. Identification of genotoxic metabolites in *in vitro* test systems is

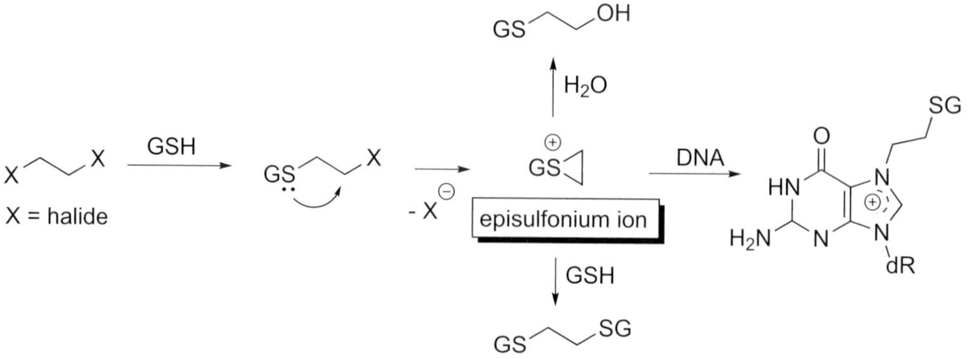

Figure 2.12 Bioactivation of dihaloalkanes by glutathione transferases.

accomplished by employing metabolic activation systems (e.g., Aroclor 1254–induced rat liver S9). According to the International Conference on Harmonization M3, all pharmaceutical sponsors must conduct *in vitro* genetic toxicology hazard identification studies prior to initiation of clinical investigations.

The *Salmonella* reverse mutation assay [83–85] has become an integral part of the safety evaluation of drug candidates and is required by regulatory agencies for drug approvals worldwide. The mutagenic potential of small molecule drug candidates is generally evaluated in genetically different strains of *S. typhimurium*, such as TA98, TA100, TA1535, and TA1537. These test strains all carry some type of defective (mutant) gene that prevents them from synthesizing the amino acid histidine in a minimal bacterial culture medium. In the presence of mutagenic chemicals, the defective gene may be mutated back to the functional state that allows the bacterium to grow in the medium. Because positive findings in the *Salmonella* reverse mutation assay have a good correlation with the outcome of rodent carcinogenicity testing, a positive result leads to the discontinuation of development, particularly for drugs intended for non-life-threatening indications [86, 87].

In addition to the *Salmonella* Ames assay, the micronucleus test is used in toxicological screening for potential genotoxic compounds. Micronuclei induction can result from clastogens (agents that induce chromosomal breaks mainly through interaction with the DNA) or aneugens (agents that induce chromosomal gain/loss mainly through interference with the spindle apparatus), and they can represent pieces of DNA or even whole chromosomes that did not migrate properly during anaphase [88]. The *in vitro* micronucleus assay is routinely used as a screening test for rapid assessment of the *in vitro* chromosomal aberration assay, which is part of several recommended regulatory test batteries for genotoxicity. Micronuclei were first used to quantify chromosomal damage in root tips of the Broad bean, *Vicia faba* [88]. The *in vivo* test normally uses mouse bone marrow or mouse peripheral blood [89]. The *in vivo* micronucleus study is required prior to initiation of phase 2 clinical trials. Identification of a genetic hazard may lead to further investigations to understand the relevance of genotoxic response or the termination of the development of the drug candidate. As in the case of the *Salmonella* assay, the *in vitro* micronucleus test relies on a metabolic activation system (Aroclor 1254–induced rat liver S9/NADPH) to identify indirect clastogens (i.e., metabolites of parent drugs).

2.10
Case Studies in Eliminating Metabolism-Based Mutagenicity in Drug Discovery Programs

Reactive metabolite trapping/covalent binding studies have proven useful in elucidating the biochemical basis of mutagenicity with new chemical entities and the mechanistic insights gathered from such studies have been used in the rational design of compounds, which are devoid of genotoxic liabilities. A case study on the antiobesity agent and 5-hydroxytryptamine 2C agonist 10 (Figure 2.13), which was

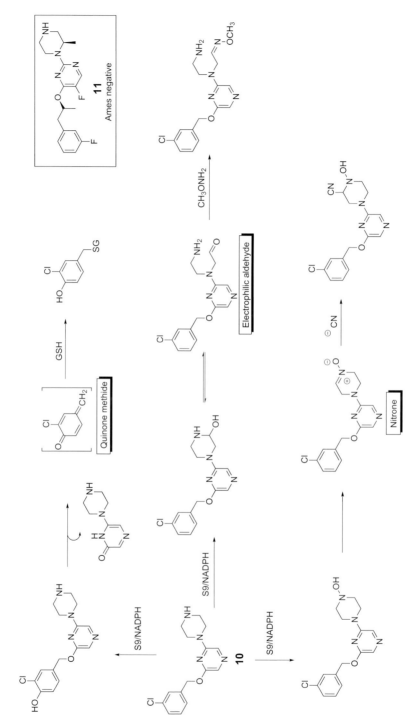

Figure 2.13 Utility of reactive metabolite trapping/covalent binding studies in elucidating the mechanism(s) of S9/NADPH-dependent mutagenic response with the 5-hydroxytryptamine 2C agonist **10**.

mutagenic in the bacterial *Salmonella* Ames assay in an Aroclor 1254–induced rat liver S9/NADPH-dependent fashion, was recently highlighted [90, 91]. In the *Salmonella* assay, **10** produced a significant increase of mutations only in strains TA100 and TA1537 that are known to be sensitive to mainly base-pair and frameshift mutagens. This suggests that the putative mutagenic metabolite exhibits a structural DNA specificity. Studies with [^{14}C]-**10** revealed the irreversible and concentration-dependent incorporation of radioactivity in calf thymus DNA in an S9/NADPH-dependent fashion confirming that **10** was bioactivated to a DNA-reactive metabolite. Reactive metabolite trapping studies in S9/NADPH incubations supplemented with GSH, methoxyl amine, and/or cyanide led to the detection of corresponding thiol, amine, and cyano conjugates of **10** and its downstream metabolites. Structural elucidation of these conjugates allowed an insight into the mechanism leading to the formation of DNA-reactive metabolites. The mass spectrum of the methoxylamine conjugate of **10** was consistent with condensation of amine with an electrophilic, aldehyde metabolite derived from piperazine ring scission in **10**, whereas the mass spectrum of the GSH conjugate suggested a bioactivation pathway involving initial aromatic ring hydroxylation on the 3-chlorobenzyl motif in **10** followed by β-elimination to a quinone methide species that reacted with GSH. Mass spectral data on the cyanide conjugate suggested that metabolism had occurred on the piperazine ring in **10** to an electrophilic nitrone derivative. The observation that methoxylamine and GSH reduced mutagenicity suggested that the trapping agents competed with DNA toward reaction with the reactive metabolites. Overall, the exercise provided indirect information on the structure of DNA-reactive intermediates leading to mutagenic response with **10** and hence a rationale on which to base subsequent chemical intervention strategy for designing nongenotoxic 5-HT$_{2C}$ agonists such as compound **11** (Figure 2.13) [91].

Mutlib and coworkers [92] demonstrated the mutagenicity of a 3-indazolylpiperazine derivative **12** (Figure 2.14) to *S. typhimurium* TA98 in the presence of Aroclor 1254–induced rat liver S9 subcellular fraction and NADPH cofactor. In rat liver S9 or microsomes, **12** underwent a CYP-mediated *N*-deindazolation (loss of indazole ring) as a predominant metabolic pathway. It was speculated that an oxaziridine intermediate, which is an oxidant and a hard electrophile capable of oxidizing or covalently binding to DNA molecules, was formed prior to metabolic cleavage leading to the loss of indazole (Figure 2.14). Attempts to trap the reactive oxaziridine using exogenous GSH, however, were unsuccessful. Failure to detect sulfydryl conjugate(s) is consistent with the fact that the oxaziridine is a hard electrophile and will not react easily with a soft nucleophile such as GSH. As such, the detection of benzoic acid, the product of hydrolysis of the unstable 3-indazolone intermediate, in microsomal incubations of **12** indirectly indicated the existence of an oxaziridine intermediate (see Figure 2.14).

Based on these findings, a structural analogue **13** was prepared, wherein the piperazine ring was replaced with a piperidine ring. The replacement of piperazine with piperidine in **13** would not lead to *N*-deindazolation via the intermediate

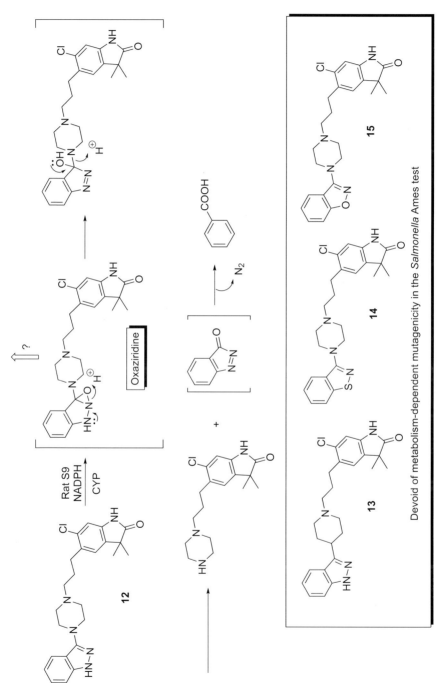

Figure 2.14 Proposed mechanism of S9/NADPH-dependent mutagenic effects of the 3-indazolylpiperazine derivative **12** in the *Salmonella* reverse mutation assay.

oxaziridine. Even though an oxaziridine could be formed, the overall reaction would not proceed favorably because piperidine, in contrast to piperazine, is not a good leaving group. Consistent with this hypothesis, compound **13** was not mutagenic to *S. typhimurium* TA98 in the absence or presence of a metabolic activating system. In contrast to **12**, **13** did not undergo the metabolic cleavage (loss of indazole ring). Furthermore, the structurally related heterocyclic analogues possessing piperazinyl isothiazole (**14**, Figure 2.14) and piperazinyl isoxazole (**15**, Figure 2.14) were not mutagenic to TA98 and TA100 in the absence or presence of metabolic activation. It was subsequently shown that the major route of *in vitro* metabolism for **14** and **15** involved *S*-oxidation and hydroxylation, respectively. These apparent differences in the metabolism of the heterocyclic derivatives (indazole, isothiazole, and isoxazole) are suggestive of a possible link between the metabolism and mutagenicity of compounds bearing a 3-piperazinyl indazole group.

Yet another account of potential medicinal chemistry strategies to resolve metabolism-dependent mutagenicity is evident with the arylindenopyrimidine series of selective dual A_{2A}/A_1 adenosine receptor antagonists exemplified by 2-amino-4-phenyl-8-pyrrolidin-1-ylmethyl-indeno[1,2-d]pyrimidin-5-one **(16)** (Figure 2.93) [93]. Compound **16**, a representative lead compound, was shown to be genotoxic in both the Ames and mouse lymphoma L5178Y assays in a rat liver S9/NADPH-dependent fashion. In the *S. typhimurium* assay, **16** was a frameshift mutagen against tester strain TA1537. Compound **16** also demonstrated irreversible covalent binding to calf thymus DNA in the presence of Aroclor 1254–induced rat liver S9 and NADPH. As such, the recovery of **16** and its enamine metabolite (see Figure 2.15) from acid hydrolysis of covalently modified DNA and protection of covalent binding to DNA by both cyanide ion and methoxylamine suggest that the frameshift mutation in TA1537 strain involved covalent binding via a reactive intermediate instead of simple intercalation to DNA.

Profiling for reactive metabolite formation in rat liver S9 indicated that **16** was bioactivated to several electrophilic species that included endocyclic iminium ion, amino aldehyde, epoxide, and α,β-unsaturated carbonyl intermediates as judged from the detection of corresponding cyano, oxime, and GSH conjugates (Figure 2.15). Mass spectral data indicated that all reactive species arose from the bioactivation of the pyrrolidine ring of **16**. The endocyclic iminium ion and amino aldehyde species appear to be the likely candidates responsible for genotoxicity based on, first, the protection afforded by both cyanide ion and methoxylamine, which reduced the potential to form covalent adducts with DNA, and, second, the fact that the analogues of **16** (e.g., compounds **17** and **18**) designed with low probability to form these reactive intermediates were not genotoxic. It was concluded that **16** also had the potential to be mutagenic in humans based on the formation of the endocyclic iminium ion following incubation with a human liver S9 preparation and the commensurate detection of DNA adducts.

Attempting to understand the relevance of a positive result that is dependent on rat liver S9/NADPH is not a simple task because the known *in vivo* metabolic profiles in rats and humans may not be directly related to *in vitro* metabolism in the presence of S9. In the review by Ku *et al.* [94], an example of the biochemical

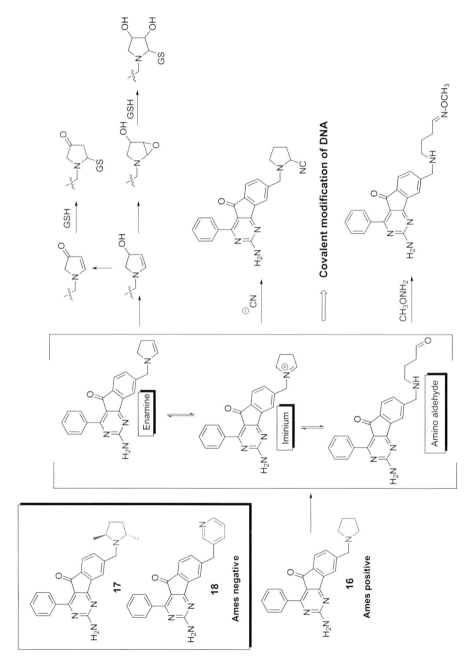

Figure 2.15 Circumventing metabolism-dependent genotoxicity of a pyrrolidine-substituted arylindenopyrimidine derivative **16**.

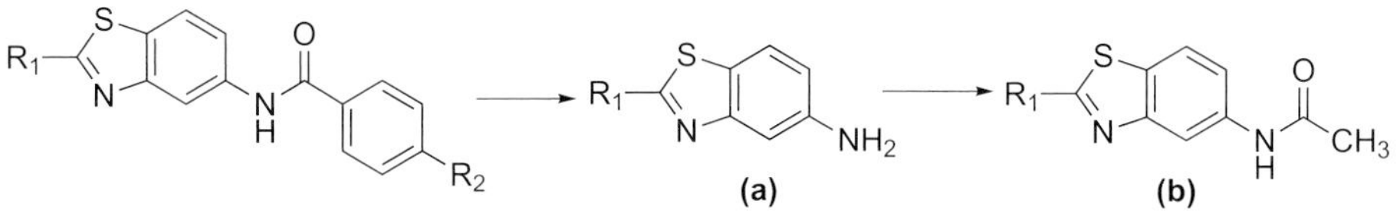

Figure 2.16 Hydrolysis of aromatic carboxamide derivatives into potentially genotoxic metabolites. Heterocyclic amines (a) were found to be positive in genotoxicity assays in the presence of rat S9, whereas the *N*-acetylated metabolites (b) were negative with or without S9.

complexity associated with interpretation of the *in vitro* genotoxicity data becomes apparent with a series of aromatic carboxamide derivatives, which on hydrolytic cleavage yield potentially genotoxic aniline-type metabolites, a finding that is also noted with a limited number of aromatic sulfonamides (Figure 2.16). For reasons that are not fully understood, amide/sulfonamide hydrolytic cleavage is negligible in S9 or microsomal systems. In some cases, cleavage occurs *in vivo* and in hepatocytes *in vitro*, but in others, it is clearly demonstrable only *in vivo*. Although some of the aromatic amine hydrolytic products were tested and showed no evidence of bacterial mutagenicity, others (Figure 2.16) exhibited a genotoxic response. Five different compounds in the series were tested in a bacterial DNA repair test with negative results. Subsequently, metabolism was shown to occur in rat hepatocytes via amide hydrolysis and then *N*-acetylation followed by GSH conjugation. Hydrolysis, but not GSH conjugation, was seen in dog, minipig, and human hepatocytes; it could not be demonstrated in rat S9 or microsomal systems. The heterocyclic amines (products of hydrolysis) from three different parent molecules were found to be positive in the bacterial DNA repair test in the presence of S9, but, interestingly, the *N*-acetylated derivatives were negative with or without S9. Finally, one of the parent molecules was also found to be positive using hepatocytes *in vitro*; the second was negative, but solubility limited the maximum testable concentration. No *in vivo* genotoxicity data are available for the chemical series. The series was dropped from development.

In another example, some of the phenol-based human calcium receptor antagonists (e.g., compound **19** in Figure 2.17) for the potential treatment of osteoporosis were noted to be positive in the *in vitro* micronucleus assay in a rat S9/NADPH fashion. Omission of NADPH abrogated the positive finding in the *in vitro* micronucleus assay suggesting that the compounds were prone to CYP-mediated bioactivation to a reactive metabolite(s). Consistent with this finding, reactive metabolite trapping studies on numerous phenol-based derivatives in rat and human liver microsomes supplemented with NADPH and GSH revealed the formation of GSH adducts derived from addition of the thiol to an *ortho*-quinone-reactive species (Figure 2.17) [95]. Likewise, removal of the phenol motif (e.g., compounds **22** and **23**) abolished both reactive metabolite formation and *in vitro* micronuclei formation. For reasons that remain unclear, most phenol-based analogues in the series formed reactive *ortho*-quinone species, but not all demonstrated a positive response in *in vitro* micronucleus assay. This attribute was crucial in the identification of

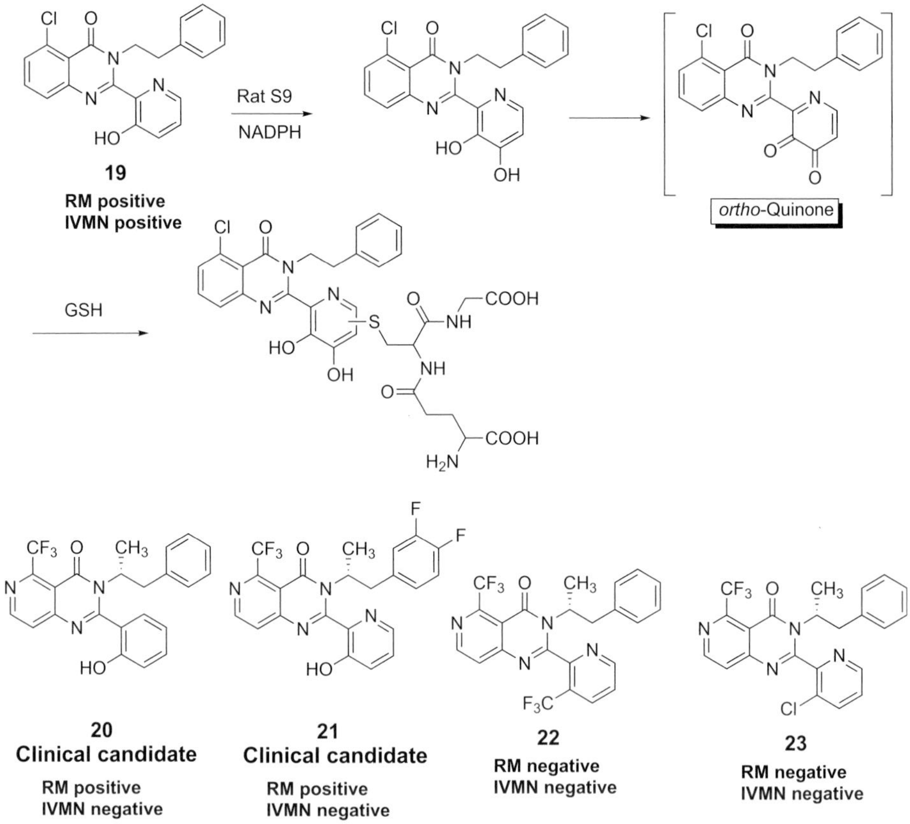

Figure 2.17 Phenol-based human calcium receptor antagonists, some of which display metabolism-dependent positive response in the *in vitro* micronucleus assay.

clinical candidates (e.g., compounds **20** and **21**). Finally, it is noteworthy to point out that the generation of both false-positive and false-negative results in genotoxicity tests is possible; the issues and potential shortcomings of induced rat liver S9 have been reviewed by Dobo *et al.* [96].

References

1 Luch, A. (2005) Nature and nurture – lessons from chemical carcinogenesis. *Nature Reviews*, **5** (2), 113–125.

2 Hueper, W.C., Wiley, F.H., and Wolfe, H.D. (1938) Experimental production of bladder tumors in dogs by administration of beta-naphthylamine.

Journal of Industrial Hygiene and Toxicology, **20**, 46–84.

3 Kinosita, R. (1936) Researches on the carcinogenesis of the various chemical substances. *Gann*, **30**, 423–426.

4 Wilson, R.H., DeEds, F., and Cox, A.J. Jr. (1941) The toxicity and carcinogenic

activity of 2-acetylaminofluorene. *Cancer Research*, **1**, 595–608.

5 Widmark, E.M.P. (1939) Presence of cancer-producing substances in roasted food. *Nature*, **143**, 984.

6 Nagao, M., Honda, M., Seino, Y., Yahagi, T., and Sugimura, T. (1977) Mutagenicities of smoke condensates and the charred surface of fish and meat. *Cancer Letters*, **2** (4–5), 221–226.

7 Sugimura, T. (1978) Let's be scientific about the problem of mutagens in cooked food. *Mutation Research*, **55** (3–4), 149–152.

8 Hatch, F.T. and Felton, J.S. (1986) Toxicologic strategy for mutagens formed in foods during cooking: status and needs. *Progress in Clinical Biological Research*, **206**, 109–131.

9 Jägerstad, M., Grivas, S., Olsson, K., Laser Reutersward, A., Negishi, C., and Sato, S. (1986) Formation of food mutagens via Maillard reactions. *Progress in Clinical Biological Research*, **206**, 155–167.

10 Shimada, T. and Guengerich, F.P. (1991) Activation of amino-α-carboline, 2-amino-1-methyl-6 phenylimidazo[4,5-*b*]pyridine, and a copper phthalocyanine cellulose extract of cigarette smoke condensate by cytochrome P-450 enzymes in rat and human liver microsomes. *Cancer Research*, **51** (19), 5284–5291.

11 Gago-Dominguez, M., Bell, D.A., Watson, M.A., Yuan, J.M., Castelao, J.E., Hein, D. W., Chan, K.K., Coetzee, G.A., Ross, R.K., and Yu, M.C. (2003) Permanent hair dyes and bladder cancer: risk modification by cytochrome P4501A2 and *N*-acetyltransferases 1 and 2. *Carcinogenesis*, **24** (3), 483–489.

12 Ames, B.N., Durston, W.E., Yamasaki, E., and Lee, F.D. (1973) Carcinogens are mutagens: a simple test system combining liver homogenates for activation and bacteria for detection. *Proceedings from the National Academy of Sciences of the United States of America*, **70** (8), 2281–2285.

13 Kim, D. and Guengerich, F.P. (2005) Cytochrome P450 activation of arylamines and heterocyclic amines. *Annual Reviews in Pharmacology and Toxicology*, **45**, 27–49.

14 Frederick, C.B., Mays, J.B., Ziegler, D.M., Guengerich, F.P., and Kadlubar, F.F.

(1982) Cytochrome P-450 and flavin-containing monooxygenase-catalyzed formation of the carcinogen *N*-hydroxy-2-aminofluorene, and its covalent binding to nuclear DNA. *Cancer Research*, **42** (7), 2671–2677.

15 Hammons, G.J., Guengerich, F.P., Weis, C.C., Beland, F.A., and Kadlubar, F.F. (1985) Metabolic oxidation of carcinogenic arylamines by rat, dog, and human hepatic microsomes and by purified flavin-containing and cytochrome P-450 monooxygenases. *Cancer Research*, **45** (8), 3578–3585.

16 Yamazoe, Y., Miller, D.W., Weis, C.C., Dooley, K.L., Zenser, T.V., Beland, F.A., and Kadlubar, F.F. (1985) DNA adducts formed by ring-oxidation of the carcinogen 2-naphthylamine with prostaglandin H synthase in vitro and in the dog urothelium in vivo. *Carcinogenesis*, **6** (9), 1379–1387.

17 Mueller, G.C. and Miller, J.A. (1948) The metabolism of 4-dimethylaminoazobenzene by rat liver homogenates. *Journal of Biological Chemistry*, **176**, 535–544.

18 Cramer, J.W., Miller, J.A., and Miller, E.C. (1960) *N*-Hydroxylation: a new metabolic reaction observed in the rat with the carcinogen 2-acetylaminofluorene. *Journal of Biological Chemistry*, **235**, 885–888.

19 Thorgeirsson, S.S., Jollow, D.J., Sasame, H.A., Green, I., and Mitchell, J.R. (1973) The role of cytochrome P-450 in *N*-hydroxylation of 2-acetylaminofluorene. *Molecular Pharmacology*, **9** (3), 398–404.

20 Kadlubar, F.F., Miller, J.A., and Miller, E.C. (1976) Microsomal *N*-oxidation of the hepatocarcinogen *N*-methyl-4-aminoazobenzene and the reactivity of *N*-hydroxy-*N*-methyl-4-aminoazobenzene. *Cancer Research*, **36** (3), 1196–1206.

21 Guengerich, F.P. and Shimada, T. (1991) Oxidation of toxic and carcinogenic chemicals by human cytochrome P-450 enzymes. *Chemical Research in Toxicology*, **4** (4), 391–407.

22 Shimada, T., Gillam, E.M.J., Sandhu, P., Guo, Z., Tukey, R.H., and Guengerich, F.P. (1994) Activation of procarcinogens by human cytochrome P450 enzymes expressed in *Escherichia coli*. Simplified

bacterial systems for genotoxicity assays. *Carcinogenesis*, **15** (11), 2523–2529.

23 Boobis, A.R., Lynch, A.M., Murray, S., de la Toore, R., Solans, A., Farre, M., Segura, J., Gooderham, N.J., and Davies, D.S. (1994) CYP1A2-catalyzed conversion of dietary heterocyclic amines to their proximate carcinogens is their major route of metabolism in humans. *Cancer Research*, **54** (1), 89–94.

24 Kim, D., Kadlubar, F.F., Teitel, C.H., and Guengerich, F.P. (2004) Formation and reduction of aryl and heterocyclic nitroso compounds and significance in the flux of hydroxylamines. *Chemical Research in Toxicology*, **17** (4), 529–536.

25 Kato, R. (1986) Metabolic activation of mutagenic heterocyclic aromatic amines from protein pyrolysates. *Critical Reviews in Toxicology*, **16**, 307–348.

26 Chou, H.C., Lang, N.P., and Kadlubar, F.F. (1995) Metabolic activation of the *N*-hydroxy derivative of the carcinogen 4-aminobiphenyl by human tissue sulfotransferases. *Carcinogenesis*, **16** (2), 413–417.

27 Schut, H.A.J. and Snyderwine, E.G. (1999) DNA adducts of heterocyclic amine food mutagens: implications for mutagenesis and carcinogenesis. *Carcinogenesis*, **20** (3), 353–368.

28 Oda, Y., Yamazaki, H., Watanabe, M., Nohmi, T., and Shimada, T. (1995) Development of high sensitive umu test system: rapid detection of genotoxicity of promutagenic aromatic amines by *Salmonella typhimurium* strain NM2009 possessing high *O*-acetyltransferase activity. *Mutation Research*, **334** (2), 145–156.

29 Kadlubar, F.F., Unruh, L.E., Beland, F.A., Straub, K.M., and Evans, F.E. (1980) In vitro reaction of the carcinogen *N*-hydroxy-2-naphthylamine with DNA at the C-8 and N^2 atoms of guanine and at the N6 atom of adenine. *Carcinogenesis*, **1** (1), 139–150.

30 Wild, D., Dirr, A., Fasshauer, I., and Henschler, D. (1989) Photolysis of arylazides and generation of highly electrophilic DNA-binding and mutagenic intermediates. *Carcinogenesis*, **10** (2), 335–341.

31 Hecht, S.S. (2008) Progress and challenges in selected areas of tobacco carcinogenesis. *Chemical Research in Toxicology*, **21** (1), 160–171.

32 Hecht, S.S. (1998) Biochemistry, biology, and carcinogenicity of tobacco-specific *N*-nitrosamines. *Chemical Research in Toxicology*, **11** (6), 559–603.

33 Hecht, S.S., Spratt, T.E., and Trushin, N. (1988) Evidence for 4-(3-pyridyl)-4-oxobutylation of DNA in F344 rats treated with the tobacco specific nitrosamines 4-(methylnitrosamino)-1-(3-pyridyl)-1-butanone and *N*'-nitrosonornicotine. *Carcinogenesis*, **9** (1), 161–165.

34 Murphy, S.E., Palomino, A., Hecht, S.S., and Hoffmann, D. (1990) Dose response study of DNA and hemoglobin adduct formation by 4-(methylnitrosamino)-1-(3-pyridyl)-1-butanone in F344 rats. *Cancer Research*, **50** (17), 5446–5452.

35 Holze, D., Schlobe, D., Tricker, A.R., and Richter, E. (2007) Mass spectrometric analysis of 4-hydroxy-1-(3-pyridyl)-1-butanone-releasing DNA adducts in human lung. *Toxicology*, **232** (3), 277–285.

36 Monks, T.J. and Jones, D.C. (2002) The metabolism and toxicity of quinones, quinoneimines, quinonemethides, and quinone-thioethers. *Current Drug Metabolism*, **3** (4), 425–538.

37 Bolton, J.L. and Thatcher, G.R.J. (2008) Potential mechanisms of estrogen quinone carcinogenesis. *Chemical Research in Toxicology*, **21** (1), 93–101.

38 Cavalieri, E., Chakravarti, D., Guttenplan, J., Hart, E., Ingle, J., Jankowiak, R., Muti, P., Rogan, E., Russo, J., Santen, R., and Sutter, T. (2006) Catechol estrogen quinones as initiators of breast and other human cancers: implications for biomarkers of susceptibility and cancer prevention. *Biochimica et Biophysica Acta*, **1766** (1), 63–78.

39 Rajapakse, N., Butterworth, M., and Kortenkamp, A. (2005) Detection of DNA strand breaks and oxidized DNA bases at the single-cell level resulting from exposure to estradiol and hydroxylated metabolites. *Environmental and Molecular Mutagenesis*, **45** (4), 397–404.

40 Asche, C. (2005) Antitumor quinones. *Mini Reviews in Medicinal Chemistry*, **5** (5), 449–467.

41 Terashima, I., Suzuki, N., and Shibutani, S. (1999) Mutagenic potential of alpha-(*N2*-deoxyguanosinyl)tamoxifen lesions, the major DNA adducts detected in endometrial tissues of patients treated with tamoxifen. *Cancer Research*, **59** (9), 2091–2095.

42 Shibutani, S., Ravindernath, A., Suzuki, N., Terashima, I., Sugarman, S.M., Grollman, A.P., and Pearl, M.L. (2000) Identification of tamoxifen–DNA adducts in the endometrium of women treated with tamoxifen. *Carcinogenesis*, **21** (8), 1461–1467.

43 Fan, P., Zhang, F., and Bolton, J.L. (2000) 4-Hydroxylated metabolites of the antiestrogens tamoxifen and toremifene are metabolized to unusually stable quinone methides. *Chemical Research in Toxicology*, **13** (1), 45–52.

44 Zhang, F., Fan, P., Liu, X., Shen, L., van Breemen, R.B., and Bolton, J.L. (2000) Synthesis and reactivity of a potential carcinogenic metabolite of tamoxifen: 3,4-dihydroxytamoxifen-*o*-quinone. *Chemical Research in Toxicology*, **13** (1), 53–62.

45 Fennell, T.R., Miller, J.A., and Miller, E.C. (1984) Characterization of the biliary and urinary glutathione and *N*-acetylcysteine metabolites of the hepatic carcinogen 1′-hydroxysafrole and its 1′-oxo metabolite in rats and mice. *Cancer Research*, **44** (8), 3231–3240.

46 Bolton, J.L., Acay, N.M., and Vukomanovic, V. (1994) Evidence that 4-allyl-*o*-quinones spontaneously rearrange to their more electrophilic quinone methides: potential bioactivation mechanism for the hepatocarcinogen safrole. *Chemical Research in Toxicology*, **7** (3), 443–450.

47 Miller, E.C., Swanson, A.B., Phillips, D.H., Fletcher, T.L., Liem, A., and Miller, J.A. (1983) Structure–activity studies of the carcinogenicities in the mouse and rat of some naturally occurring and synthetic alkenylbenzene derivatives related to safrole and estragole. *Cancer Research*, **43** (3), 1124–1134.

48 Rietjens, I.M., Boersma, M.G., van der Woude, H., Jeurissen, S.M., Schutte, M.E., and Alink, G.M. (2005) Flavonoids and alkenylbenzenes: mechanisms of mutagenic action and carcinogenic risk. *Mutation Research*, **574** (1–2), 124–138.

49 Miller, E.C., Miller, J.A., Boberg, E.W., Delclos, K.B., Lai, C.C., Fennell, T.R., Wiseman, R.W., and Liem, A. (1985) Sulfuric acid esters as ultimate electrophilic and carcinogenic metabolites of some alkenylbenzenes and aromatic amines in mouse liver. *Carcinogenesis: A Comprehensive Survey*, **10**, 93–107.

50 Nakagawa, Y., Suzuki, T., Nakajima, K., Ishii, H., and Ogata, A. (2009) Biotransformation and cytotoxic effects of hydroxychavicol, an intermediate of safrole metabolism, in isolated rat hepatocytes. *Chemico-Biological Interactions*, **180** (1), 89–97.

51 Dietz, B.M. and Bolton, J.L. (2011) Biological reactive intermediates (BRIs) formed from botanical dietary supplements. *Chemico-Biological Interactions*, **192** (1–2), 72–80.

52 Luo, G. and Guenthner, T.M. (1996) Covalent binding to DNA in vitro of 2′,3′-oxides derived from allylbenzene analogs. *Drug Metabolism and Disposition*, **24** (9), 1020–1027.

53 Gupta, K.P., van Golen, K.L., Putman, K.L., and Randerath, K. (1993) Formation and persistence of safrole–DNA adducts over a 10,000-fold dose range in mouse liver. *Carcinogenesis*, **14** (8), 1517–1521.

54 Daimon, H., Sawada, S., Asakura, S., and Sagami, F. (1998) In vivo genotoxicity and DNA adduct levels in the liver of rats treated with safrole. *Carcinogenesis*, **19** (1), 141–146.

55 Chung, Y.T., Hsieh, L.L., Chen, I.H., Liao, C.T., Liou, S.H., Chi, C.W., Ueng, Y.F., and Liu, T.Y. (2009) Sulfotransferase 1A1 haplotypes associated with oral squamous cell carcinoma susceptibility in male Taiwanese. *Carcinogenesis*, **30** (2), 286–294.

56 Wiley, R.A., Traiger, G.J., Baraban, S., and Gammal, L.M. (1984) Toxicity–distribution relationships among 3-alkylfurans in mouse liver and kidney. *Toxicology and Applied Pharmacology*, **74** (1), 1–9.

57 Chen, L.J., Hecht, S.S., and Peterson, L.A. (1995) Identification of *cis*-2-butene-1,4-dial as a microsomal metabolite of furan.

Chemical Research in Toxicology, **8** (7), 903–906.

58 Peterson, L.A., Cummings, M.E., Vu, C.C., and Matter, B.A. (2005) Glutathione trapping to measure microsomal oxidation of furan to *cis*-2-butene-1,4-dial. *Drug Metabolism and Disposition,* **33** (10), 1453–1458.

59 Chen, L.J., Hecht, S.S., and Peterson, L.A. (1997) Characterization of amino acid and glutathione adducts of *cis*-2-butene-1,4-dial, a reactive metabolite of furan. *Chemical Research in Toxicology,* **10** (8), 866–874.

60 Lu, D., Sullivan, M.M., Phillips, M.B., and Peterson, L.A. (2009) Degraded protein adducts of *cis*-2-butene-1,4-dial are urinary and hepatocyte metabolites of furan. *Chemical Research in Toxicology,* **22** (6), 997–1007.

61 Gingipalli, L. and Dedon, P.C. (2001) Reaction of *cis*- and *trans*-2-butene-1,4-dial with 2′-deoxycytidine to form stable oxadiazabicyclooctaimine adducts. *Journal of the American Chemical Society,* **123**, 2664–2665.

62 Byrns, M.C., Predecki, D.P., and Peterson, L.A. (2002) Characterization of nucleoside adducts of *cis*-2-butene-1,4-dial, a reactive metabolite of furan. *Chemical Research in Toxicology,* **15** (3), 373–379.

63 Byrns, M.C., Vu, C.C., and Peterson, L.A. (2004) The formation of substituted 1,N2-etheno-2′-deoxyadenosine and 1,N2-etheno-2′-deoxyguanosine adducts by *cis*-2-butene-1,4-dial, a reactive metabolite of furan. *Chemical Research in Toxicology,* **17** (12), 1607–1613.

64 Byrns, M.C., Vu, C.C., Neidigh, J.W., Abad, J.L., Jones, R.A., and Peterson, L.A. (2006) Detection of DNA adducts derived from the reactive metabolite of furan, *cis*-2-butene-1,4-dial. *Chemical Research in Toxicology,* **19** (3), 414–420.

65 Kellert, M., Wagner, S., Lutz, U., and Lutz, W.K. (2008) Biomarkers of furan exposure by metabolic profiling of rat urine with liquid-chromatography tandem mass spectrometry and principal component analysis. *Chemical Research in Toxicology,* **21** (3), 761–768.

66 Spirtas, R. and Kaminski, R. (1978) Angiosarcoma of the liver in vinyl chloride/polyvinyl chloride workers. 1977 update of the NIOSH register. *Journal of Occupational Medicine,* **20** (6), 427–429.

67 Guengerich, F.P., Persmark, M., and Humphreys, W.G. (1993) Formation of 1, N2- and N2,3-ethenoguanine from 2-halooxiranes: isotopic labeling studies and isolation of a hemiaminal derivative of N2-(2-oxoethyl)guanine. *Chemical Research in Toxicology,* **6** (5), 635–648.

68 Guengerich, F.P., Mason, P.S., Scott, W.T., Fox, T.R., and Watanabe, P.G. (1981) Roles of 2-haloethylene oxides and 2-haloacetaldehydes derived from vinyl bromide and vinyl chloride in irreversible binding to protein and DNA. *Cancer Research,* **41** (11 Pt 1), 4391–4398.

69 Dahl, G.A., Miller, E.C., and Miller, J.A. (1980) Comparative carcinogenicities and mutagenicities of vinyl carbamate, ethyl carbamate, and ethyl N-hydroxycarbamate. *Cancer Research,* **40** (4), 1194–1203.

70 Dahl, G.A., Miller, J.A., and Miller, E.C. (1978) Vinyl carbamate as a promutagen and a more carcinogenic analog of ethyl carbamate. *Cancer Research,* **38** (11 Pt 1), 3793–3804.

71 Leithauser, M.T., Liem, A., Stewart, B.C., Miller, E.C., and Miller, J.A. (1990) 1,N6-Ethenoadenosine formation, mutagenicity and murine tumor induction as indicators of the generation of an electrophilic epoxide metabolite of the closely related carcinogens ethyl carbamate (urethane) and vinyl carbamate. *Carcinogenesis,* **11** (3), 463–473.

72 Guengerich, F.P. and Kim, D.H. (1991) Enzymatic oxidation of ethyl carbamate to vinyl carbamate and its role as an intermediate in the formation of 1,N6-ethenoadenosine. *Chemical Research in Toxicology,* **4** (4), 413–421.

73 Forkert, P.G. (2010) Mechanisms of lung tumorigenesis by ethyl carbamate and vinyl carbamate. *Drug Metabolism Reviews,* **42** (2), 355–378.

74 Rannug, U., Sundvall, A., and Ramel, C. (1978) The mutagenic effect of 1,2-dichloroethane on *Salmonella typhimurium*. I. Activation through conjugation with glutathione in vitro.

Chemico-Biological Interactions, **20** (1), 1–16.

75 Rannug, U. (1980) Genotoxic effects of 1,2-dibromoethane and 1,2-dichloroethane. *Mutation Research*, **76** (3), 269–295.

76 van Bladeren, P.J., Breimer, D.D., Rotteveel-Smijs, G.M.T., de Knijff, P., Mohn, G.R., van Meeteren-Walchli, B., and van der Gen, A. (1981) The relation between the structure of vicinal dihalogen compounds and their mutagenic activation via conjugation to glutathione. *Carcinogenesis*, **2** (6), 499–505.

77 Ozawa, N. and Guengerich, F.P. (1983) Evidence for formation of an *S*-[2-(*N*7-guanyl)ethyl]glutathione adduct in glutathione-mediated binding of 1,2-dibromoethane to DNA. *Proceedings of the National Academy of Sciences of the United States of America*, **80** (17), 5266–5270.

78 Koga, N., Inskeep, P.B., Harris, T.M., and Guengerich, F.P. (1986) *S*-[2-(*N*7-Guanyl) ethyl]glutathione, the major DNA adduct formed from 1,2-dibromoethane. *Biochemistry*, **25** (8), 2192–2198.

79 Peterson, L.A., Harris, T.M., and Guengerich, F.P. (1988) Evidence for an episulfonium ion intermediate in the formation of *S*-[2-(*N*7-guanyl)ethyl] glutathione in DNA. *Journal of the American Chemical Society*, **110**, 3284–3291.

80 Humphreys, W.G., Kim, D.H., Cmarik, J. L., Shimada, T., and Guengerich, F.P. (1990) Comparison of the DNA alkylating properties and mutagenic responses caused by a series of *S*-(2-haloethyl)-substituted cysteine and glutathione derivatives. *Biochemistry*, **29** (45), 10342–10350.

81 Webb, W.W., Elfarra, A.A., Webster, K.D., Thom, R.E., and Anders, M.W. (1987) Role for an episulfonium ion in *S*-(2-chloroethyl)-DL-cysteine-induced cytotoxicity and its reaction with glutathione. *Biochemistry*, **26** (11), 3017–3023.

82 Their, R., Pemble, S.E., Taylor, J.B., Humphreys, W.G., Persmark, M., Ketterer, B., and Guengerich, F.P. (1993) Expression of mammalian glutathione *S*-transferase 5-5 in *Salmonella typhimurium* TA1535 leads to base-pair mutations upon exposure to dihalomethanes. *Proceedings of the National Academy of Sciences of the United States of America*, **90** (18), 8576–8580.

83 Ames, B.N., McCann, J., and Yamasaki, E. (1975) Methods for detecting carcinogens and mutagens with the *Salmonella/*mammalian-microsomes mutagenicity test. *Mutation Research*, **31** (6), 347–364.

84 McCann, J., Choi, E., Yamasaki, E., and Ames, B.N. (1975) Detection of carcinogens as mutagens in the *Salmonella*/microsome test: assay of 300 chemicals. *Proceedings of the National Academy of Sciences of the United States of America*, **72** (12), 5135–5139.

85 Maron, D.M. and Ames, B.N. (1983) Revised method for the *Salmonella* mutagenicity test. *Mutation Research*, **113** (3–4), 173–215.

86 Kim, B.S. and Margolin, B.H. (1999) Prediction of rodent carcinogenicity utilizing a battery of in vitro and in vivo genotoxicity tests. *Environmental and Molecular Mutagenicity*, **34** (4), 297–304.

87 Zeiger, E. (1998) Identification of rodent carcinogens and noncarcinogens using genetic toxicity tests: premises, promises, and performance. *Regulatory Toxicology and Pharmacology*, **28** (2), 85–95.

88 Evans, H.J. (1997) Historical perspectives on the development of the in vitro micronucleus test: a personal view. *Mutation Research*, **392**, 5–10.

89 Schmid, W. (1975) The micronucleus test. *Mutation Research*, **31**, 9–15.

90 Kalgutkar, A.S., Dalvie, D.K., Aubrecht, J., Smith, E.B., Coffing, S.L., Cheung, J.R., Vage, C., Lame, M.E., Chiang, P., McClure, K.F., Maurer, T.S., Coelho, R.V. Jr., Soliman, V.F., and Schildknegt, K. (2007) Genotoxity of 2-(3-chlorobenzyloxy)-6-(piperazinyl)pyrazine, a novel 5-hydroxytryptamine2c receptor agonist for the treatment of obesity: role of metabolic activation. *Drug Metabolism and Disposition*, **35** (6), 848–858.

91 Kalgutkar, A.S., Bauman, J.N., McClure, K.F., Aubrecht, J., Cortina, S.R., and Paralkar, J. (2009) Biochemical basis for differences in metabolism-dependent genotoxicity by two diazinylpiperazine-

based 5-HT2C receptor agonists. *Bioorganic Medicinal Chemistry Letters*, **19** (6), 1559–1563.

92 Chen, H., Murray, J., Kornberg, B., Dethloff, L., Rock, D., Nikam, S., and Mutlib, A.E. (2006) Metabolism-dependent mutagenicity of a compound containing a piperazinyl indazole motif: role of a novel P450-mediated metabolic reaction involving a putative oxaziridine intermediate. *Chemical Research in Toxicology*, **19** (10), 1341–1350.

93 Lim, H.-K., Chen, J., Sensenhauser, C., Cook, K., Preston, R., Thomas, T., Shook, B., Jackson, P.F., Rassnick, S., Rhodes, K., Gopaul, V., Salter, R., Silva, J., and Evans, D.C. (2011) Overcoming the genotoxicity of a pyrrolidine substituted arylindenopyrimidine as a potent dual adenosine A_{2A}/A_1 antagonist by minimizing bioactivation to an iminium ion reactive intermediate. *Chemical Research in Toxicology*, **24** (7), 1012–1030.

94 Ku, W.W., Bigger, A., Brambilla, G., Glatt, H., Gocke, E., Guzzie, P.J., Hakura, A., Honma, M., Martus, H.-J., Obach, R.S., and Roberts, S. (2007) Strategy for genotoxicity testing – metabolic considerations. *Mutation Research*, **627**, 59–77.

95 Kalgutkar, A.S., Griffith, D.A., Ryder, T., Sun, H., Miao, Z., Bauman, J.N., Didiuk, M.T., Frederick, K.S., Zhao, S.X., Prakash, C., Soglia, J.R., Bagley, S.W., Bechle, B.M., Kelley, R.M., Dirico, K., Zawistoski, M., Li, J., Oliver, R., Guzman-Perez, A., Liu, K.K.C., Walker, D.P., Benbow, J.W., and Morris, J. (2010) Discovery tactics to mitigate toxicity risks due to reactive metabolite formation with 2-(2-hydroxyaryl)-5-(trifluoromethyl)pyrido [4,3-*d*]pyrimidin-4(3*H*)-one derivatives, potent calcium-sensing receptor antagonists and clinical candidate(s) for the treatment of osteoporosis. *Chemical Research in Toxicology*, **23** (6), 1115–1126.

96 Dobo, K.L., Obach, R.S., Luffer-Atlas, D., and Bercu, J.P. (2009) A strategy for the risk assessment of human genotoxic metabolites. *Chemical Research in Toxicology*, **22** (2), 348–356.

3
Bioactivation and Inactivation of Cytochrome P450 and Other Drug-Metabolizing Enzymes

Abbreviations

1-ABT	1-Aminobenzotriazole
AUC	Area under the plasma concentration versus time curve
CL	Clearance
CL_{int}	Intrinsic clearance
DDI	Drug–drug interaction
[I]	Inhibitor/inactivator concentration
k_{inact}	Maximum inactivation rate constant
K_I	Inactivator concentration required to achieve half k_{inact}
MAO	Monoamine oxidase
MDMA	Methylenedioxymethamphetamine
MI	Metabolite-intermediate
MPTP	N-Methyl-1,2,3,6-tetrahydropyridine
V_{max}	Maximum reaction velocity

3.1
Introduction

In Chapter 1, the biological ramifications of the generation of reactive metabolites of drugs and xenobiotics were described. These effects arise via the reaction of these metabolites with biological macromolecules, such as nucleic acids and proteins. An important subset of proteins affected by reactive metabolites includes the very enzymes that generate them: cytochrome P450 enzymes in the majority of examples. This can result in the inactivation of these enzymes, the end result being the potential for reduction of clearance (CL) of the drug and other drugs metabolized by the affected enzyme and a concomitant increase in exposure *in vivo*. This process has been referred to as time-dependent inhibition, mechanism-based inactivation, catalysis-dependent inhibition, and suicide inactivation (the inactivators referred to as suicide substrates).

Reactive Drug Metabolites, First Edition. Amit S. Kalgutkar, Deepak Dalvie, R. Scott Obach, and Dennis A. Smith.
© 2012 Wiley-VCH Verlag GmbH & Co. KGaA. Published 2012 by Wiley-VCH Verlag GmbH & Co. KGaA.

3.2
Pharmacokinetic and Enzyme Kinetic Principles Underlying Mechanism-Based Inactivation and Drug–Drug Interactions

3.2.1
Enzyme Kinetic Principles of Mechanism-Based Inactivation

A mechanism-based inactivator is necessarily a substrate of the enzyme that it inactivates. Thus, unlike simple reversible enzyme inhibitors that block the activity of an enzyme through reversible binding to the enzyme, a mechanism-based inactivator must be acted upon by the enzyme to generate a product or intermediate that will chemically react with the enzyme and irreversibly damage it such that it can no longer catalyze reactions. The kinetic description of a mechanism-based inactivator more closely resembles that of a substrate of the enzyme than an inhibitor of the enzyme (Scheme 3.1).

In the Michaelis–Menten equation, the reversible inhibitor will lower the rate of catalysis (v) by influencing the Michaelis constant (K_M) term in the Michaelis–Menten equation:

$$v = \frac{V_{max} \cdot [S]}{K_M + [S]} \rightarrow v = \frac{V_{max} \cdot [S]}{K_M \cdot [(1 + [I])/K_i] + [S]} \tag{3.1}$$

where V_{max} is the maximum reaction velocity at a theoretical infinite substrate concentration [S], K_i is the reversible binding constant between enzyme and inhibitor, and [I] is the concentration of inhibitor. In contrast, a mechanism-based inactivator decreases the rate of catalytic reaction by reducing the amount of active enzyme, thereby decreasing the maximum velocity (V_{max}) term in the Michaelis–Menten equation as a function of time:

$$v = \frac{V_{max} \cdot [S]}{K_M + [S]} \rightarrow v = \frac{V_{max} \cdot e^{(-t \cdot [I] \cdot k_{inact})/(K_I + [I])} \cdot [S]}{K_M + [S]} \tag{3.2}$$

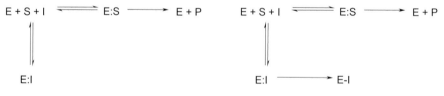

| reversible inhibition | mechanism-based inhibition |

E = free enzyme
S = substrate
I = inhibitor or inactivator
P = product
E:S = enzyme-substrate complex
E:I = enzyme-inhibitor or inactivator complex
E-I = irreversibly bound enzyme-inactivator adduct

Scheme 3.1 Kinetic description of a mechanism-based inhibitor.

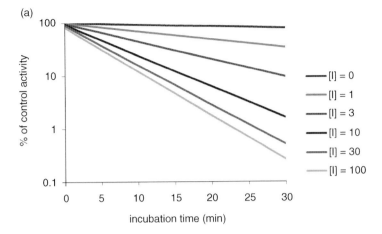

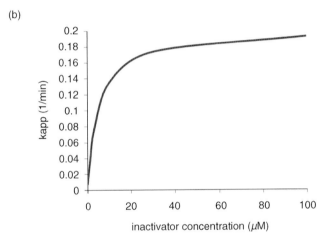

Figure 3.1 Plots of enzyme inactivation over time (a) and relationship between inactivation constants and inactivator concentrations (b).

Since the generation of the inactivated enzyme proceeds via a catalytic process (and not merely via reversible binding), its kinetics can also be described. By definition, mechanism-based inactivation is dependent on time so that an inactivator will cause a greater decrease in enzyme activity with increasing time. This is via a first-order process (Figure 3.1). The first-order rate constant describing this process (k) will be dependent on the inactivator concentration in a hyperbolic relationship wherein there is a maximum inactivation rate constant (k_{inact}) that would be observed at a theoretical infinite concentration of inactivator [I]:

$$k = \frac{k_{inact} \cdot [I]}{K_I + [I]} \qquad (3.3)$$

It is important to note that for inactivators, the term K_I is not a binding constant (like K_i is for reversible inhibitors), but rather it is a constant describing the relationship between the first-order inactivation rate constant and inactivator concentration. The k_{inact} and K_I terms are important in determining the extent of enzyme inactivation, and thereby magnitude of drug–drug interactions (DDIs) that will occur in the presence of concentrations of inactivator *in vivo* (see below).

3.2.2
Pharmacokinetic Principles Underlying DDIs Caused by Mechanism-Based Inactivation

In order to understand the basis of pharmacokinetic DDIs arising via mechanism-based inactivation of drug-metabolizing enzymes, we must first visit some basic clearance concepts. The systemic exposure to a drug, as defined by the area under the plasma concentration versus time curve (AUC) projected to $t = \infty$, that is, $AUC_{(0 \to \infty)}$, will be dependent on the dose that is administered and the rate at which the drug is cleared:

$$AUC_{(0 \to \infty)} = \frac{dose}{CL} \tag{3.4}$$

The CL of a drug is performed by various organs in the body, most notably the liver. The CL is defined by three parameters: the rate at which the drug is presented to the organ (as defined by the flow of blood to the clearing organ, Q), the fraction of the drug in blood that is not bound to macromolecules and thereby can penetrate into the clearing organ (free fraction, f_u), and the intrinsic capability of the organ to clear the drug (intrinsic clearance, CL_{int}). The CL is defined by these three parameters in the following relationship [1]:

$$CL = \frac{Q \cdot f_u \cdot CL_{int}}{Q + f_u \cdot CL_{int}} \tag{3.5}$$

For an enzyme-catalyzed metabolic process, the CL_{int} term is defined by its underlying enzyme kinetic terms:

$$CL_{int} = \frac{V_{max}}{K_M + [S]} \tag{3.6}$$

The V_{max} term is dependent on the amount of active enzyme. If that amount is decreased because of exposure to a mechanism-based inactivator, then V_{max} will decrease proportionally, thus giving rise to a decrease in CL_{int} that will in turn cause a decrease in CL and an increase in exposure (AUC). This is the underpinning for a pharmacokinetic-based DDI caused by a mechanism-based inactivator of a drug-metabolizing enzyme.

In vivo under normal conditions, the amount of active enzyme in a clearing organ will be at steady state, such that the rate of biosynthesis and the rate of degradation of the enzyme will be equal. When an inactivator is present, the rate of active enzyme degradation will be increased because now there is a second process contributing to degradation (i.e., mechanism-based inactivation).

This decreases the amount of active enzyme at steady state, thereby decreasing the maximum velocity:

$$V_{max} \propto [E] \propto \frac{k_{syn}}{k_{deg}} \rightarrow V_{max} \propto [E] \propto \frac{k_{syn}}{k_{deg} + [([I] \cdot k_{inact})/([I] + K_I)]} \tag{3.7}$$

Since CL_{int} is directly proportional to V_{max}, it will decrease by the same factor as V_{max} decreases in the presence of an inactivator:

$$\frac{CL_{int,inactivated}}{CL_{int}} = \frac{V_{max,inactivated}}{V_{max}} = \frac{k_{syn}/\{k_{deg} + [([I] \cdot k_{inact})/([I] + K_I)]\}}{k_{syn}/k_{deg}}$$

$$= \frac{k_{deg}}{k_{deg} + [([I] \cdot k_{inact})/([I] + K_I)]} \tag{3.8}$$

Thus, CL will decrease:

$$CL = \frac{Q \cdot f_u \cdot CL_{int}}{Q + f_u \cdot CL_{int}} \rightarrow CL = \frac{Q \cdot f_u \cdot CL_{int} \cdot \{k_{deg}/[k_{deg} + [([I] \cdot k_{inact})/([I] + K_I)]]\}}{Q + f_u \cdot CL_{int} \cdot \{k_{deg}/[k_{deg} + [([I] \cdot k_{inact})/([I] + K_I)]]\}} \tag{3.9}$$

And hence the exposure (i.e., AUC from Eq. (3.4)) will increase. This is a simplified version that disregards when there are other pathways that can contribute to CL of the impacted drug and thereby diminish the effect of the inactivator[2–4]. The exposure to the inactivator (i.e., value for [I]) will also be important and will be driven by the total dose of inactivator, its distribution to the site of action (most likely the liver and intestine), and the rate at which it is removed from the body. Furthermore, whether the increase in exposure will actually lead to a DDI that is clinically meaningful (i.e., cause side effects or toxicity) depends on the margin of safety of the affected drug.

3.3
Mechanisms of Inactivation of Cytochrome P450 Enzymes

There are three mechanisms described for mechanism-based inactivation of cytochrome P450 enzymes: quasi-irreversible metabolite-intermediate (MI) complex formation, heme adduction, and protein adduction [5]:

3.3.1
Quasi-Irreversible Inactivation

In quasi-irreversible inactivation, a substrate is bioactivated to an intermediate that can form a tight, noncovalent interaction with the ferrous heme intermediate form in the cytochrome P450 reaction cycle. These are uncovered through UV/Vis spectral experiments, as they typically result in an altered P450 spectrum with an absorbance peak in the 455–460 nm region. *In vivo*, the formation of this complex is irreversible; the term quasi-irreversible refers to the fact that in *in vitro* experiments with amines, enzyme activity can be restored by the addition of ferricyanide

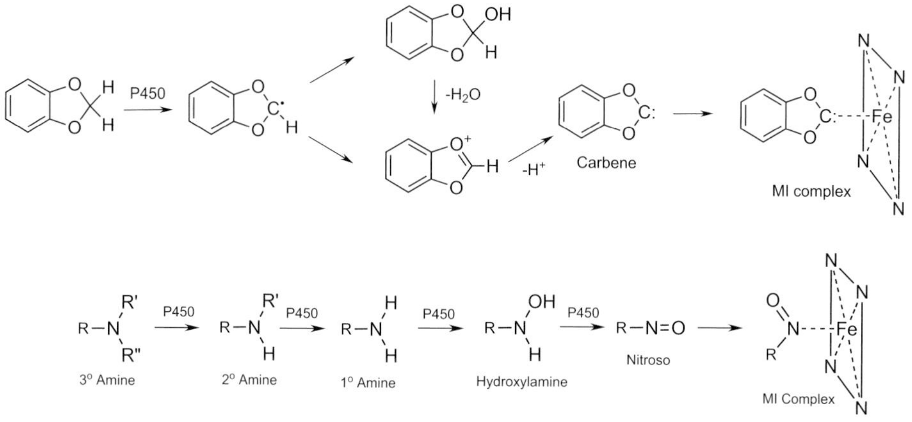

Figure 3.2 Bioactivation of methylenedioxyphenyl derivatives and amines to quasi-irreversible MI complex formation with cytochrome P450s.

that will dissipate the MI complex [6]. The two most commonly studied mechanisms of quasi-irreversible P450 inactivation are for primary amines and methylenedioxyphenyl compounds. Primary amines are oxidized to nitroso intermediates, and these can complex to the ferrous heme intermediate. Secondary and tertiary amines can also participate in MI complex formation provided they are first *N*-dealkylated to the primary amine metabolite. Methylenedioxyphenyl compounds are hydroxylated at the methylene carbon and spontaneous dehydration yields a carbene that will form a ligand complex to the heme iron (Figure 3.2) [7].

3.3.2
Heme Adducts

Cytochrome P450 bioactivation to a reactive intermediate can also result in the reactive species escaping the active site of the enzyme and undergoing reaction elsewhere (e.g., phase 2 conjugation reaction, quenching with water or other small molecule nucleophiles, or adduction to other proteins) or reacting with a nucleophile on the P450 enzyme that generates it. Among the latter category, reaction can occur at a position on the protein itself (see Section 3.3.3) or with the porphyrin. Reaction with the porphyrin renders the enzyme inactive. Porphyrin is not a very nucleophilic entity, and it is the pyrrole nitrogens that have the greatest nucleophilicity on the molecule, albeit the nucleophilicity of pyrrole nitrogens is considerably lower than most biological nucleophiles. However, the porphyrin will be proximal to any formed electrophile, so that reactions may occur by virtue of this proximity and the reactivity of the intermediate metabolite. Also, reaction of porphyrin with reactive radical intermediates is a common mechanism for adduct formation. Experimentally, demonstration of heme adduct formation is most readily accomplished by their detection using HPLC–UV or HPLC–MS after extraction of the porphyrin from an *in vitro* incubation treated with inactivator, a source of NADPH, and a source of P450 enzyme. The UV spectrum will likely be altered by adduction, and the retention time on HPLC will differ between unreacted porphyrin and adducted porphyrin [8]. Porphyrin adducts have been demonstrated for terminal alkenes, alkynes (both terminal and internal), dihydropyridines, hydrazines, cyclopropylamines, and triazenes [9–14].

3.3.3
Protein Adducts

The P450 apoprotein contains amino acids that have nucleophilic side chains, such as cysteine and lysine. Thus, if a reactive electrophile is generated during oxidation, that reactive metabolite can react with these nucleophilic groups and this can result in either complete inactivation of the enzyme or alteration of its activity [15]. Protein adduct formation can also occur if a radical intermediate is formed. Determination that an adduct has formed with the P450 protein itself is usually done by incubating a radiolabeled analogue of the inactivator with P450 and NADPH and analyzing the radioactivity that is bound to the enzyme. More recently, advances in mass spectrometry have permitted the determination of covalent adducts to P450 without requiring radiolabeled inactivator [16–19]. In addition to enzyme inactivation, P450 adducts have been shown to be immunogenic [20, 21].

3.4
Examples of Drugs and Other Compounds that are Mechanism-Based Inactivators of Cytochrome P450 Enzymes

In this section, an example of each of the various bioactivation mechanisms that result in inactivation of a cytochrome P450 enzyme and that result in a DDI will be illustrated. A list of drugs known to be time-dependent inhibitors that have been shown to cause DDI is included in Table 3.1.

3.4.1
Amines

Several drugs cause mechanism-based inactivation by oxidation of an amino group to a nitroso intermediate that will form an MI complex with the heme iron. These include several antibiotics (e.g., troleandomycin, erythromycin, clarithromycin) and other drugs such as verapamil and diltiazem. Such compounds are all substituted amines and must first undergo *N*-dealkylation to yield the primary amines that can undergo further oxidation to hydroxylamine and nitroso compounds. *In vitro* incubations of P450 with amines such as troleandomycin result in enzyme inactivation and the formation of the complex that has unique spectral properties with a Soret maximum at 455 nm. This complex can be broken with the addition of ferricyanide to yield active enzyme, consistent with its quasi-irreversible nature. The stability of the inactivated complex has been shown through treatment of rats with

Table 3.1 Drugs known as cytochrome P450 time-dependent inhibitors that have been shown to cause DDIs in humans.

Drug/Chemical	Enzymes
Amiodarone	P4502C9 and 3A
Amlodipine	P4503A
Azithromycin	P4503A
Cimetidine	P4502D6
Clarithromycin	P4503A
Cyclosporin	P4503A
Diethyldithiocarbamate (disulfiram metabolite)	P4502E1
6,7-Dihydroxybergamottin (grapefruit juice component)	P4503A
Diltiazem	P4503A
Erlotinib	P4503A
Erythromycin	P4503A
Ethinylestradiol	P4503A
Furafylline	P4501A2
Gemfibrozil glucuronide (gemfibrozil metabolite)	P4502C8
Isoniazid	Several P450s
Itraconazole	P4503A
Methoxsalen	P4502A6
Methylenedioxymethamphetamine	P4502D6
Mibefradil	P4503A
Nefazodone	P4503A
Nelfinavir	P4503A
Oltipraz	P4501A2
Omeprazole	P4503A
Paroxetine	P4501A2
Propoxyphene	P4503A
Ritonavir	P4502D6
Rofecoxib	P4501A2
Saquinavir	P4503A
Thiabendazole	P4501A2
Ticlopidine	P4502C19
Tienilic acid	P4502C9
Troleandomycin	P4503A
Verapamil	P4503A
Zileuton	P4501A2

troleandomycin, isolation of the liver microsomes, and demonstration that the P450 spectral properties mimicked those that are observed with *in vitro* incubation [22]. The proposal that the amines must be sequentially oxidized to the nitroso metabolite to generate inactivation is supported by the observation that *N*-hydroxylamphetamine also yields the MI complex [23]. Amine-containing drugs can show marked DDIs with P4503A-cleared compounds such as midazolam, alfentanil, and many others [24]. A list of interactions with midazolam (the most frequently employed P4503A probe substrate for clinical DDI studies) is given in Table 3.2.

Table 3.2 Amine-containing drugs that cause drug interactions with midazolam in humans presumed to occur via MI complex formation.

Drug	Dose (mg)	DDI (fold increase)
Troleandomycin	500 (single)	14.8
Clarithromycin	500 (BID)	8.4
Diltiazem	120 (BID)	4.0
Erythromycin	500 (TID)	3.8
Verapamil	80 (TID)	2.9
Roxithromycin	300 (QD)	1.5
Azithromycin	500 (QD)	1.3

3.4.2
Methylenedioxyphenyl Compounds

Both paroxetine and methylenedioxymethamphetamine (MDMA) contain methylenedioxy phenyl substituents and have been demonstrated to cause DDIs via inactivation of P4502D6 (Figure 3.3) [25, 26]. Metabolism of the methylene group

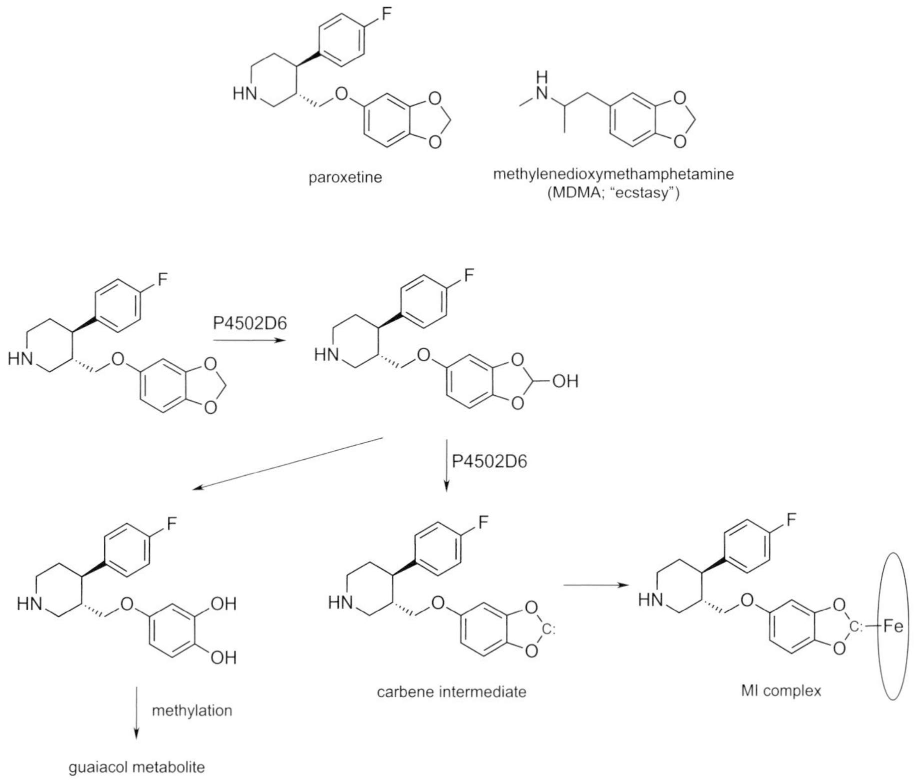

Figure 3.3 Structures of paroxetine and MDMA and mechanism of P4502D6 inactivation by paroxetine.

to the carbene results in the formation of an MI complex with the carbene coordinating with the heme iron. Demethylenation yields a catechol intermediate that can be subsequently methylated to the corresponding guaiacol metabolite by catechol-*O*-methyl transferase. Paroxetine has been shown to cause marked increases in the exposure to P4502D6-cleared drugs and, interestingly, it also inactivates its own metabolism that results in increases in systemic exposure following multiple doses that would not be predicted from single-dose pharmacokinetic data [27, 28]. MDMA also has been shown to cause an inactivation of P4502D6 *in vivo*, presumably by the same mechanism [29].

3.4.3
Quinones, Quinone Imines, and Quinone Methides

Nefazodone has been shown to inactivate P4503A and it has been shown to cause fivefold increase in exposure to P4503A-cleared drugs such as midazolam [30, 31]. The proposed mechanism for the inactivation is via generation of a reactive quinone imine metabolic intermediate(s) (Figure 3.4). Raloxifene has been shown to be a catalysis-dependent inhibitor of human P4503A4; however, since raloxifene is subject to very high extraction in the gut by glucuronidation, it is unlikely that this drug causes pharmacokinetic interactions *in vivo*. Nevertheless, the bioactivation mechanism has been well characterized and is instructive as an example of reactive quinones causing P450 inactivation [19, 32, 33]. Raloxifene possesses a conjugated bis-phenol that is electronically equivalent to a hydroquinone. Oxidation yields an extended quinone structure and this reacts with a specific cysteine thiol

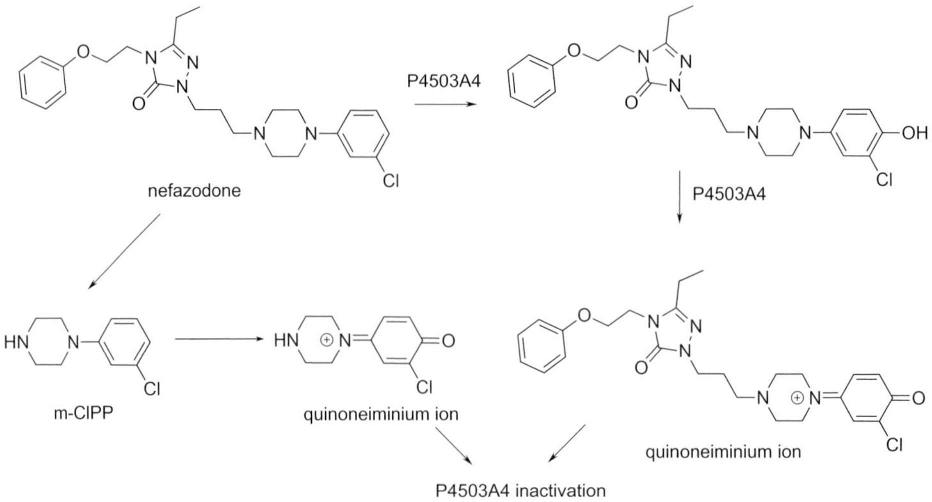

Figure 3.4 Proposed bioactivation pathway of nefazodone leading to P4503A4 inactivation.

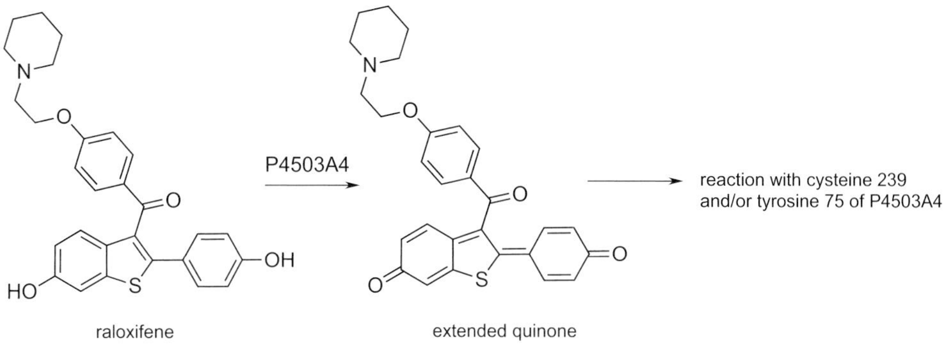

Figure 3.5 Bioactivation of raloxifene to an inactivator of P4503A4.

nucleophile in P4503A4 to cause the inactivation; a separate analysis suggested a tyrosine phenol nucleophile reacts with raloxifene (Figure 3.5).

Two examples of drugs that generate quinone methides are tamoxifen and phencyclidine, but there is controversy in each case regarding the role of this type of reactive intermediate in P450 inactivation. In the case of tamoxifen, metabolism to the quinone methide via initial generation of 4-hydroxytamoxifen is a well-characterized bioactivation pathway for which glutathione adducts have been observed (see Chapter 2). Tamoxifen has been shown to be a substrate and inactivator of P4502B6 [34]. However, 4-hydroxytamoxifen does not cause inactivation, and since tamoxifen also undergoes *N*-demethylation reactions, it is possible that P450 inactivation arises by MI complex formation via the primary amine (Figure 3.6) [35]. Phencyclidine has been shown to be an inactivator of P4502B6. Initially, a radical pathway was proposed to explain this observation, while later on the generation of a quinone methide was proposed (Figure 3.6) [36, 37]. In neither case (tamoxifen or phencyclidine) has an *in vivo* DDI been shown that could be attributed to this *in vitro* inactivation.

3.4.4
Thiophenes

Tienilic acid, suprofen, and zileuton contain thiophene rings and all three cause inactivation of cytochrome P450 enzymes, the first two on P4502C9 and the last on P4501A2 (Figure 3.7) [21, 38–41]. Tienilic acid, a diuretic agent, was only briefly used *in vivo* before being withdrawn from clinical use due to hepatotoxicity (see Chapter 4), but there was a report of a threefold increase in the exposure to warfarin, a drug cleared in large part by P4502C9, when coadministered with tienilic acid [42]. Zileuton has been shown to cause a 1.9-fold increase in theophylline exposure [43]. The proposed mechanism of the inactivation of P450 enzymes by thiophenes involves covalent bonding to the protein. Initial oxidation occurs to generate either an *S*-oxide or an epoxide; there is evidence to suggest the existence of both of these

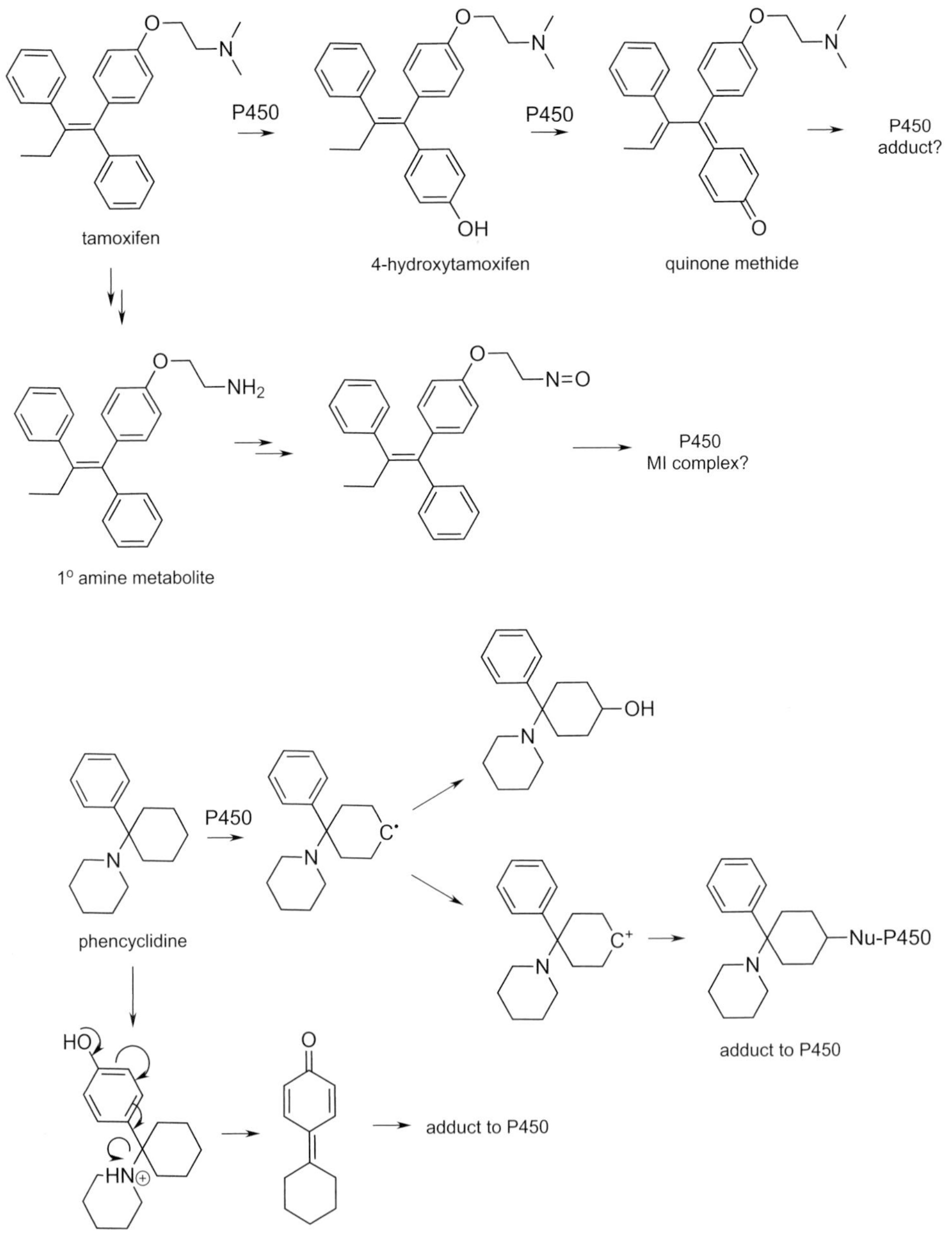

Figure 3.6 Proposed bioactivation pathways of tamoxifen yielding quinone methides that could inactivate cytochrome P450.

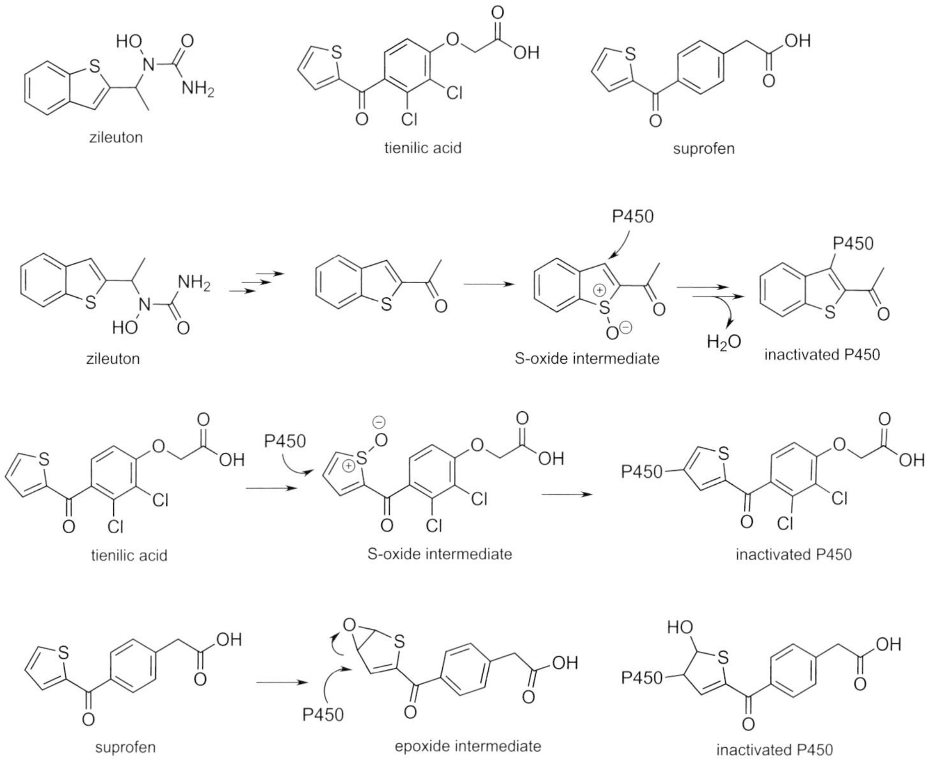

Figure 3.7 Proposed bioactivation of thiophene-containing drugs resulting in inactivation of P450 enzymes.

pathways, depending on the drug being examined. These electrophilic intermediates can react with thiol nucleophiles on the protein. For tienilic acid, covalent bonding has been supported by the observation of radiolabeled P4502C9 when incubated with radiolabeled tienilic acid and analyzed by electrophoresis. Furthermore, antibodies to P4502C9 were shown to be generated in patients treated with tienilic acid [44]. The *S*-oxide of tienilic acid is proposed as the reactive intermediate [21]. For zileuton bioactivation is also via an *S*-oxide metabolite that reacts with nucleophiles; an *N*-acetylcysteine adduct to the 3-position of the thiophene has been identified [45]. Whether this is the mechanism of inactivation of P4501A2 remains uncharacterized.

3.4.5
Furans

Methoxsalen (8-methoxypsoralen; Figure 3.8) is a furan-containing drug used as a topical agent for the treatment of psoriasis, and it is also a very effective inactivator of human P4502A6 (with k_{inact} values greater than 1/min). The

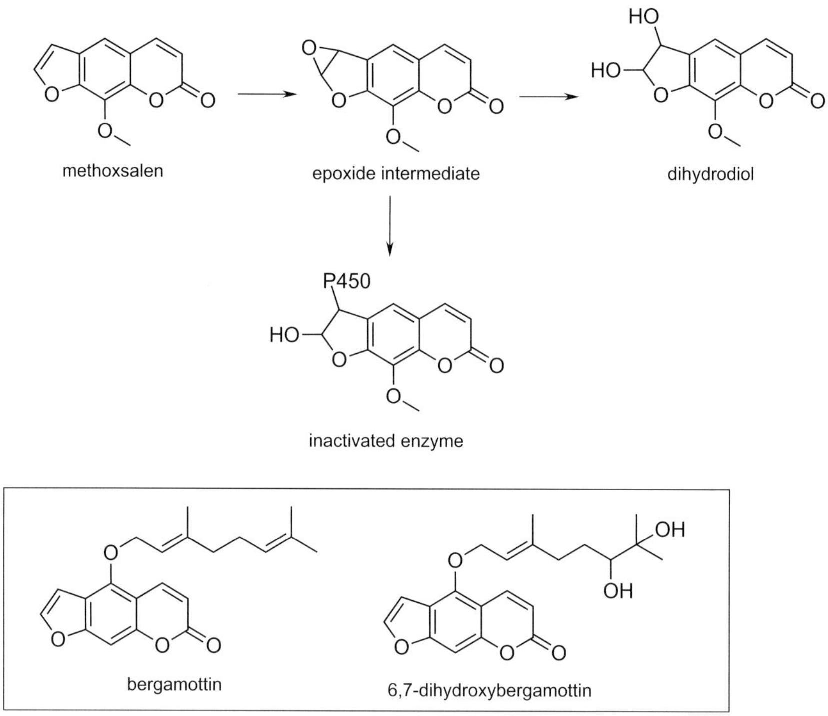

Figure 3.8 Proposed bioactivation pathways of furan-containing drugs that result in cytochrome P450 inactivation.

proposed mechanism is via epoxidation of the furan ring followed by adduct formation [46], which could arise via epoxide ring opening or via addition to a γ-ketoenal form. Considerable evidence obtained using human and rat systems has shown that the mechanism of inactivation is not via alterations in the heme, but that the P450 spectrum is altered, and mass spectral data on the protein show an adduct [46–48]. The furanocoumarins in grapefruit juice, bergamottin, and its 6,7-dihydrodiol metabolite have been shown to be mechanism-based inactivators of P4503A, and protein adducts were shown to be generated after incubation [49].

3.4.6
Alkynes

Alkyne functionalities are not frequent in drugs; however, there are some examples of these and there have been instances of DDIs arising due to bioactivation of a drug containing one of these substituents. Alkynes have been frequently used as tool compounds to probe the biochemical function of P450 enzymes. Examples of drugs containing alkynes that result in the inactivation of P450 enzymes include ethinylestradiol, mifepristone, and efavirenz. The mechanism of bioactivation of

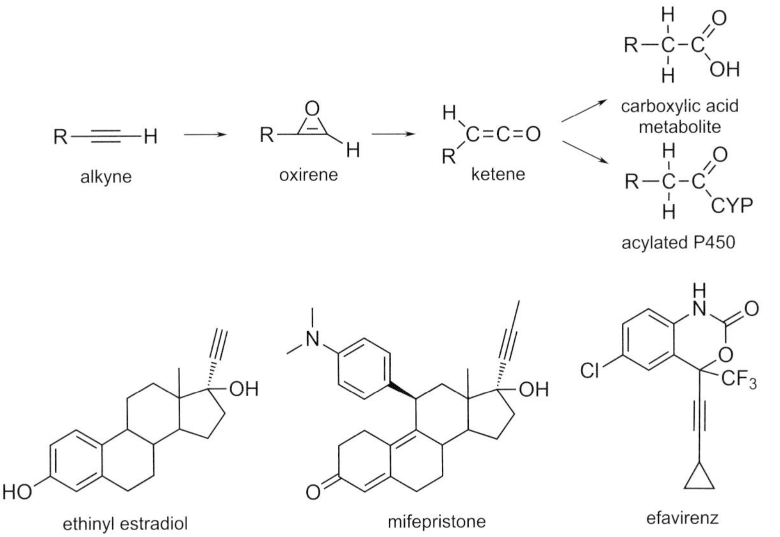

Figure 3.9 Bioactivation of alkynes to inactivate cytochrome P450 and structures of alkenes that can inactivate P450 enzymes.

alkynes that can result in inactivation of P450 enzymes is shown in Figure 3.9. Initial oxidation across the triple bond yields an unstable oxirene ring that rearranges to a highly electrophilic ketene intermediate. This can either undergo reaction with water to yield stable acetic acid metabolites or react with the P450 enzyme to yield adducts. Adduction has frequently been shown to occur to the heme prosthetic group, and various alkynes have been used to probe the architecture of P450 enzymes by determination of the structures of heme adducts [13]. Ethinylestradiol itself is dosed at a very low level when used in contraception (typically <0.05 mg/day), so DDIs caused by this agent are small, despite its capability as a mechanism-based inactivator of P4503A. Mifepristone, an agent used as a single dose of 200 mg to induce abortion, has not been well studied as a perpetrator of DDIs *in vivo*, but it is a reasonable expectation that it would cause substantial increases in exposures of drugs metabolized by P4503A.

3.4.7
2-Alkylimidazoles

Furafylline is commonly used as an *in vitro* tool to determine whether a compound is a substrate for CYP1A2 since it is a selective inactivator of that enzyme [50]. It is not used as a drug, so information about the possibility of *in vivo* DDI is restricted to one report wherein it was shown to cause an increase in exposure to the P4501A2-cleared drug theophylline [51]. It possesses a furan ring; nevertheless, its mechanism of inactivation does not involve metabolism on this portion. Rather, activation arises via hydroxylation of the 8-methyl group, which after elimination

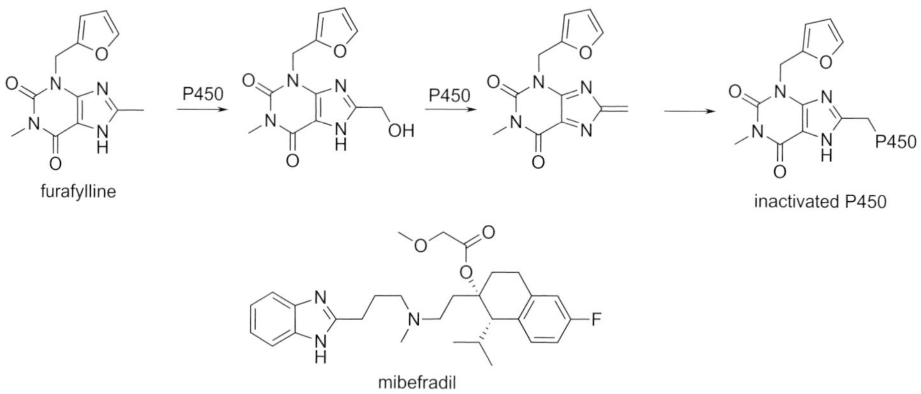

furafylline

inactivated P450

mibefradil

Figure 3.10 Proposed bioactivation pathway of furafylline resulting in enzyme inactivation and structure of mibefradil.

of water yields an imine-methide that reacts with a nucleophile on P4501A2 (Figure 3.10) [52]. Mibefradil also has an 8-alkylimidazole group and is a very effective time-dependent inhibitor of P4503A, to the extent that it was withdrawn from clinical use partially due to this property. It has been shown to cause increases in exposure to P4503A-cleared drugs such as midazolam [53]. Its mechanism is not truly understood; however, data obtained suggest that after activation it causes destruction of the heme [54].

3.4.8
Other Noteworthy Cytochrome P450 Inactivators

1-Aminobenzotriazole (ABT) has been used for years as a tool compound that can inactivate multiple cytochrome P450 enzymes of humans and laboratory animals and has been applied both *in vitro* and *in vivo* [55–57]. The mechanism of bioactivation of ABT has been described based on data gathered regarding the heme adducts that are formed wherein there is a bridging benzene ring (Figure 3.11) [58]. Gemfibrozil was shown to cause marked DDIs with P4502C8-cleared drugs such as cerivastatin and repaglinide [59, 60]. Gemfibrozil itself was shown to be only a weak inhibitor of P4502C8; however, the major glucuronide metabolite of gemfibrozil was demonstrated to be a mechanism-based inactivator [61]. While gemfibrozil glucuronide is an acyl glucuronide and these types of metabolites have been associated with reactivity and protein adduct formation, it is actually a simple benzylic tradical generated in the normal course of a P450 hydroxylation reaction that has been attributed to cause the inactivation via formation of an adduct to the porphyrin (Figure 3.12) [62]. Thus, it must be appreciated that during the normal reaction mechanism of P450 hydroxylation, reactive radicals are formed that would typically undergo a rebound reaction with the iron-oxo intermediate to form the stable hydroxyl product, but that these reactive species could still react with the P450 enzyme itself if properly oriented.

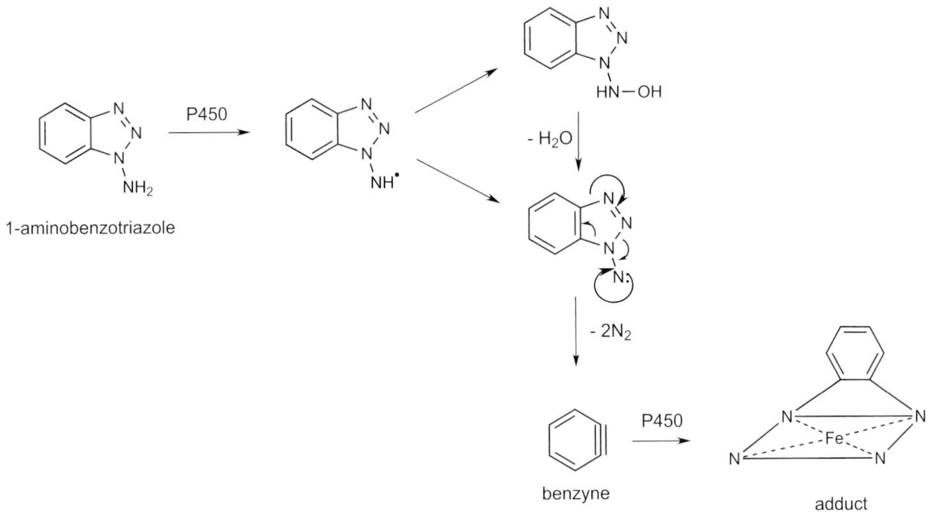

Figure 3.11 Proposed bioactivation pathway of 1-aminobenzotriazole (ABT) to inactivate cytochrome P450 enzymes.

Isoniazid has been shown to inactivate several human P450 enzymes [63, 64] and causes DDIs with drugs cleared by P4502E1 and P4503A4 [65, 66]. It contains an acyl hydrazine moiety and it is metabolism at this substituent that is responsible for inactivation. A spectral change is observed yielding a peak at 449 nm and this can be dissipated with addition of ferricyanide, showing that isoniazid forms an MI complex with the reduced iron center on P450 [67]. Inactivation caused by hydrazines is proposed to occur via a nitrene radical (Figure 3.13).

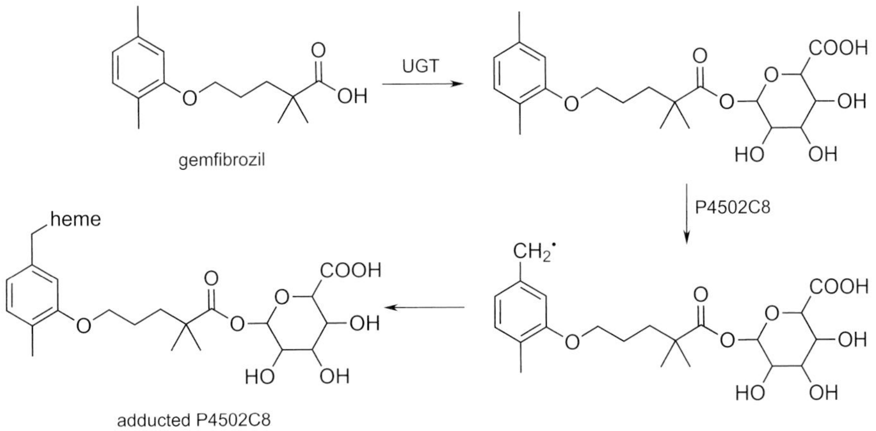

Figure 3.12 Proposed bioactivation mechanism for gemfibrozil.

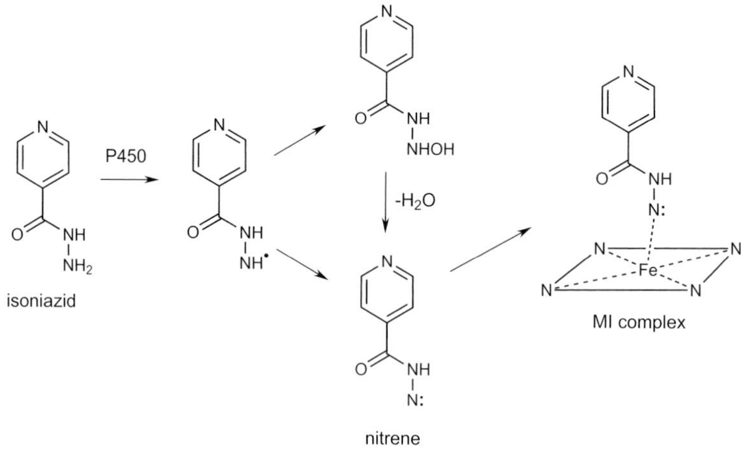

Figure 3.13   Proposed bioactivation of isoniazid resulting in cytochrome P450 inactivation.

3.5
Mechanism-Based Inactivation of Other Drug-Metabolizing Enzymes

3.5.1
Aldehyde Oxidase

The molybdenum cofactor containing enzyme aldehyde oxidase, which oxidizes aldehydes, heterocyclic aza-aromatic compounds, and iminium ions, and reduces compounds containing N—O bonds, has been shown to be a target for mechanism-based inactivation; however, the mechanisms of these have not been delineated. Hydralazine (Figure 3.14) has been shown to be an inactivator of aldehyde oxidase activity in guinea pigs, rabbits, and baboons [68], and after administration to guinea pigs it can cause a DDI with aldehyde oxidase–cleared drugs [69]. The mechanism of hydralazine inactivation of aldehyde oxidase is not known; however, it has been shown to generate phthalazine as a product, which means that reactivity could be a consequence of metabolism of the hydrazine moiety. Quinazoline has also been described as causing mechanism-based inactivation of rabbit aldehyde oxidase, as shown with a decrease in activity within a few minutes that was not due to the 4-hydroxyquinazoline product [70]. Nitroso-imidacloprid (Figure 3.14) has been shown to undergo

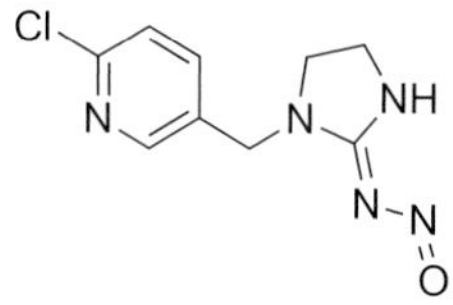

Figure 3.14   Structure of nitroso-imidacloprid, an irreversible inactivator of rabbit aldehyde oxidase.

rabbit aldehyde oxidase–catalyzed reduction to the corresponding amine, and it has also been shown to inactivate the enzyme while generating a covalent adduct [71]. Again, the exact mechanism of this inactivation is unknown. But it does depend on reduction, since the inactivation requires addition of *N*-methyl-nicotinamide, an electron donor substrate. The relevance of all three of these inactivators to human aldehyde oxidase is not known.

3.5.2
Monoamine Oxidases

Monoamine oxidase (MAO) dysfunction is thought to be responsible for a number of neurological disorders (e.g., depression, schizophrenia, substance abuse, attention deficit disorder, etc.), given their pivotal role in neurotransmitter metabolism. MAO inhibitors are one of the major classes of drug prescribed for the treatment of depression, although they are often the last line of treatment due to risks of the DDIs with dietary components or other drugs. MAO-A inhibitors act as antidepressant and antianxiety agents, whereas MAO-B inhibitors are used alone or in combination to treat Alzheimer's and Parkinson's diseases [72].

The antituberculosis drug iproniazid (a hydrazine derivative) was the first MAO inhibitor to be described in the literature. Its discovery was the result of a profound antidepressant "side effect" observed in tuberculosis patients [73]. After ~5 years of clinical observations in tuberculosis patients, iproniazid was introduced into the market as the first antidepressant drug. Compounds belonging to the first generation of MAO inhibitors were mechanism-based inactivators, which acted via formation of reactive metabolites that covalently modified the enzyme [74]. As such, most of the MAO inhibitors also inactivated hepatic P450 enzymes in a manner consistent with mechanism-based inactivation. Because of the propensity to form reactive intermediates in the liver, most irreversible MAO inhibitors have been associated with hepatotoxicity [75]. A second, more serious side effect with irreversible MAO inhibitors is the occurrence of the so-called cheese effect, a phenomenon that leads to severe hypertensive crisis induced by elevated tyramine levels resulting from MAO inactivation [76]. The hepatotoxic and hypertensive liabilities led to a sharp decline in the popularities of MAO inhibitors as antidepressant agents and led toward efforts directed toward the identification of reversible isozyme-selective MAO inhibitors [77]. The propargylic amine *R*-deprenyl (selegiline, Figure 3.15) is the only irreversible MAO inhibitor used clinically. Deprenyl is used on its own or in combination with L-DOPA for the treatment of early stage Parkinson's disease. At normal clinical doses, the drug selectively inactivates MAO-B; however, in larger doses, deprenyl loses its specificity and also inhibits MAO-A.

A general strategy that has allowed the facile design of selective, irreversible MAO inhibitors involves the placement of functional groups on the nitrogen atom of isozyme-selective substrates, which undergo MAO-catalyzed conversion to reactive metabolites that alkylate the flavin and/or a complementary amino acid residue in the active site of the enzyme. *N*-Substituents that are capable of imparting irreversible inhibition properties to MAO substrates include amino

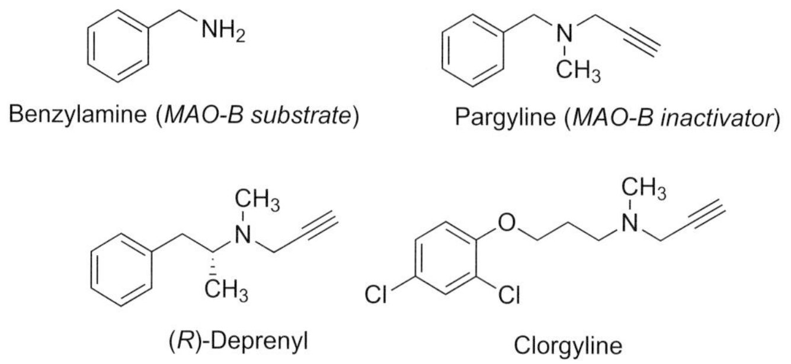

Benzylamine (*MAO-B substrate*)

Pargyline (*MAO-B inactivator*)

(*R*)-Deprenyl

Clorgyline

Figure 3.15 Inactivators of monoamine oxidases.

(hydrazines), allyl, propargyl, cyclopropyl, and oxazolidinonyl groups. For example, the MAO-B-selective substrate benzylamine is converted to the MAO-B-selective and irreversible inhibitor pargyline by incorporating a propargyl group on the nitrogen atom that is susceptible to enzyme-mediated oxidation [78]. Extending the distance between this electron-rich center and the aromatic ring or incorporating a bulky group on the aromatic ring of irreversible MAO-B-selective inhibitors affords irreversible MAO-A-selective inhibitors. This is apparent from structural differences between (*R*)-deprenyl (MAO-B selective) and clorgyline (MAO-A selective) (Figure 3.15).

The mechanism of MAO inactivation by hydrazine derivatives such as iproniazid and phenyl hydrazine (Figure 3.16) is thought to involve an initial MAO-catalyzed dehydrogenation to a corresponding phenyldiazine intermediate that in turn loses a H atom and N_2 to afford an electrophilic phenyl radical. On the basis of results obtained from model studies, covalent attachment of the phenyl radical has been proposed to occur at the 4a-position on the flavin group in MAO-B [79]. Allylamines and propargylamines undergo MAO-catalyzed oxidation to the corresponding electrophilic dieniminium and eyniminium species, respectively (Figure 3.16). These highly electrophilic Michael acceptors then inactivate the enzyme by bonding covalently to an active site residue or the flavin group [80, 81]. Unlike hydrazines, covalent bond formation with allylamines or propargylamines does not occur on the 4a-position on the flavin moiety. Comparison of the spectral properties of the inactivated enzyme to those observed in model studies on the photoreduction of synthetic flavins with propargylamines suggests the N5 position on the flavin as the site of covalent modification [80–82]. The pathway(s) responsible for the mechanism-based inhibition by cyclopropylamines is thought to involve an initial single-electron transfer from the amine to the flavin cofactor to generate the aminium radical cation followed by spontaneous ring opening of the cyclopropyl group to afford the primary carbon-centered radical that alkylates an active site residue leading to covalent inactivation (Figure 3.16) [83, 84]. Peptide mapping studies followed by mass spectral analysis for *N*-cyclopropyl-α-methylbenzylamine revealed the attachment of the carbon-centered radical to a cysteine residue in bovine liver MAO-B [85]. Mechanism-based inactivation by oxazolidinones (e.g., MD

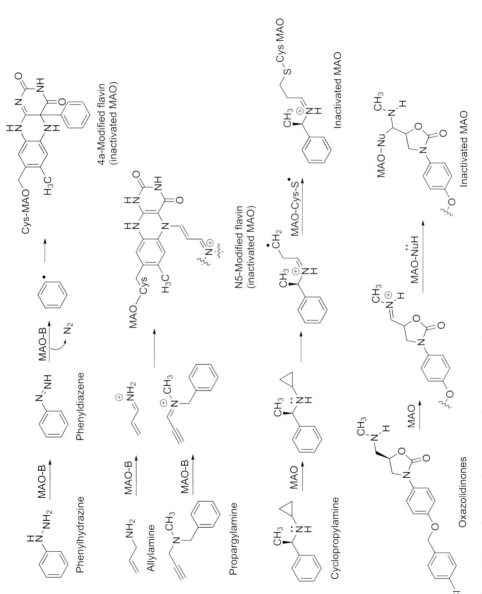

Figure 3.16 Mechanisms of inactivation of monoamine oxidase.

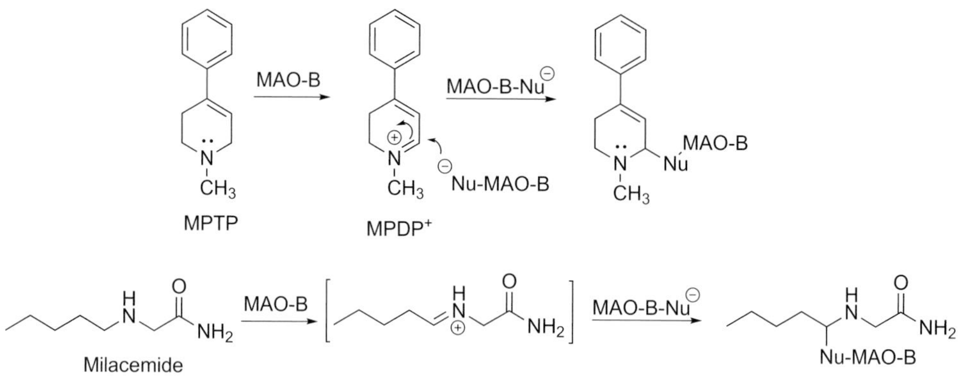

Figure 3.17 Irreversible MAO inactivation by the nigrostriatal neurotoxin MPTP and the anticonvulsant agent milacemide.

780236, Figure 3.16) is dependent on the presence of the aminomethyl group, since replacement of nitrogen with other heteroatoms alters the mode of inhibition from irreversible to reversible. The proposed mechanism of inhibition involves initial α-carbon oxidation of the aminomethyl group to give an iminium species that covalently modifies MAO by reacting with an active site residue [86, 87].

Additional examples of irreversible MAO inactivators that demonstrate such behavior include the nigrostriatal neurotoxin *N*-methyl-1,2,3,6-tetrahydropyridine (MPTP) and the anticonvulsant drug milacemide (Figure 3.17). Oxidation of MPTP, particularly by MAO-A, is accompanied by irreversible inactivation [88]. The most likely pathway involves the alkylation of an active site residue by *N*-methyl-3-phenyl-2,3-dihydropyridinium species, which is the two-electron oxidation product of MPTP. A second example is provided with the anticonvulsant drug milacemide, which undergoes selective MAO-B-catalyzed oxidation to the iminium species that is thought to alkylate the protein [89].

3.6
Concluding Remarks

When studying drugs and other chemicals that can generate chemically reactive metabolites, consideration of the potential for these reactive entities to react with the very enzyme molecules that generated them and irreversibly inactivate them is an important phenomenon. In a drug design setting, observation of time-dependent inhibition of cytochrome P450 enzymes for a newly synthesized compound should send a warning sign that a chemically reactive intermediate may be generated. This should warrant follow-up experiments to better understand the chemical mechanism responsible for the time-dependent inhibition. Finally, DDI must be added to the list of deleterious outcomes potentially caused by chemically reactive metabolites that are described in this book.

References

1 Pang, K.S. and Rowland, M. (1977) Hepatic clearance of drugs. I. Theoretical considerations of a "well-stirred" model and a "parallel tube" model. Influence of hepatic blood flow, plasma and blood cell binding, and the hepatocellular enzymatic activity on hepatic drug clearance. *Journal of Pharmacokinetics and Biopharmaceutics*, **5** (6), 625–653.

2 Mayhew, B.S., Jones, D.R., and Hall, S.D. (2000) An in vitro model for predicting in vivo inhibition of cytochrome P450 3A4 by metabolic intermediate complex formation. *Drug Metabolism and Disposition*, **28** (9), 1031–1037.

3 Venkatakrishnan, K. and Obach, R.S. (2005) In vitro–in vivo extrapolation of CYP2D6 inactivation by paroxetine: prediction of nonstationary pharmacokinetics and drug interaction magnitude. *Drug Metabolism and Disposition*, **33** (6), 845–852.

4 Obach, R.S., Walsky, R.L., and Venkatakrishnan, K. (2007) Mechanism-based inactivation of human cytochrome p450 enzymes and the prediction of drug–drug interactions. *Drug Metabolism and Disposition*, **35** (2), 246–255.

5 Hollenberg, P.F., Kent, U.M., and Bumpus, N.N. (2008) Mechanism-based inactivation of human cytochromes p450s: experimental characterization, reactive intermediates, and clinical implications. *Chemical Research in Toxicology*, **21** (1), 189–205.

6 Pessayre, D., Larrey, D., Vitaux, J., Breil, P., Belghiti, J., and Benhamou, J.P. (1982) Formation of an inactive cytochrome P-450 Fe(II)-metabolite complex after administration of troleandomycin in humans. *Biochemical Pharmacology*, **31** (9), 1699–1704.

7 Franklin, M.R. (1971) Enzymic formation of a methylenedioxyphenyl derivative exhibiting an isocyanide-like spectrum with reduced cytochrome P-450 in hepatic microsomes. *Xenobiotica*, **1** (6), 581–591.

8 Ortiz de Montellano, P.R., Mico, B.A., and Yost, G.S. (1978) Suicidal inactivation of cytochrome P 450. Formation of a heme-substrate covalent adduct. *Biochemical and Biophysical Research Communications*, **83** (1), 132–137.

9 Grab, L.A., Swanson, B.A., and Ortiz de Montellano, P.R. (1988) Cytochrome P-450 inactivation by 3-alkylsydnones. Mechanistic implications of *n*-alkyl and *n*-alkenyl heme adduct formation. *Biochemistry*, **27** (13), 4805–4814.

10 Muakkassah, S.F. and Yang, W.C. (1981) Mechanism of the inhibitory action of phenelzine on microsomal drug metabolism. *Journal of Pharmacology and Experimental Therapeutics*, **219** (1), 147–155.

11 de Matteis, F., Hollands, C., Gibbs, A.H., de Sa, N., and Rizzardini, M. (1982) Inactivation of cytochrome P-450 and production of *N*-alkylated porphyrins caused in isolated hepatocytes by substituted dihydropyridines. Structural requirements for loss of heme and alkylation of the pyrrole nitrogen atom. *FEBS Letters*, **145** (1), 87–92.

12 Ortiz de Montellano, P.R., Mico, B.A., Mathews, J.M., Kunze, K.L., Miwa, G.T., and Lu, A.Y.H. (1981) Selective inactivation of cytochrome P-450 isozymes by suicide substrates. *Archives of Biochemistry and Biophysics*, **210** (2), 717–728.

13 Kunze, K.L., Mangold, B.L., Wheeler, C., Beilan, H.S., and Ortiz de Montellano, P.R. (1983) The cytochrome P-450 active site. Regiospecificity of prosthetic heme alkylation by olefins and acetylenes. *Journal of Biological Chemistry*, **258** (7), 4202–4207.

14 Hanzlik, R.P. and Tullman, R.H. (1982) Suicidal inactivation of cytochrome P-450 by cyclopropylamines. Evidence for cation-radical intermediates. *Journal of the American Chemical Society*, **104** (7), 2048–2050.

15 Kang, P., Liao, M., Wester, M.R., Leeder, J.S., Pearce, R.E., and Correia, M.A. (2008) CYP3A4-mediated carbamazepine (CBZ) metabolism: formation of a covalent CBZ–CYP3A4 adduct and alteration of the enzyme kinetic profile. *Drug Metabolism and Disposition*, **36** (3), 490–499.

16 Lightning, L.K. and Trager, W.F. (2002) Characterization of covalent adducts to intact cytochrome P450s by mass spectrometry. *Methods in Enzymology*, **357**, 296–300.

17 Koenigs, L.L., Peter, R.M., Hunter, A.P., Haining, R.L., Rettie, A.E., Friedberg, T., Pritchard, M.P., Shou, M., Rushmore, T.H., and Trager, W.F. (1999) Electrospray ionization mass spectrometric analysis of intact cytochrome P450: identification of tienilic acid adducts to P450 2C9. *Biochemistry*, **38** (8), 2312–2319.

18 Regal, K.A., Schrag, M.L., Kent, U.M., Wienkers, L.C., and Hollenberg, P.F. (2000) Mechanism-based inactivation of cytochrome P450 2B1 by 7-ethynylcoumarin. Verification of apo-P450 adduction by electrospray ion trap mass spectrometry. *Chemical Research in Toxicology*, **13** (4), 262–270.

19 Baer, B.R., Wienkers, L.C., and Rock, D.A. (2007) Time-dependent inactivation of P450 3A4 by raloxifene: identification of Cys239 as the site of apoprotein alkylation. *Chemical Research in Toxicology*, **20** (6), 954–964.

20 Leeder, J.S., Riley, R.J., Cook, V.A., and Spielberg, S.P. (1992) Human anti-cytochrome P450 antibodies in aromatic anticonvulsant-induced hypersensitivity reactions. *Journal of Pharmacology and Experimental Therapeutics*, **263** (1), 360–367.

21 Lopez Garcia, M.P., Dansette, P.M., Valadon, P., Amar, C., Beaune, P.H., Guengerich, F.P., and Mansuy, D. (1993) Human liver cytochromes P-450 expressed in yeast as tools for reactive-metabolite formation studies. Oxidative activation of tienilic acid by cytochromes P-450 2C9 and 2C10. *European Journal of Biochemistry*, **213** (1), 223–232.

22 Pessayre, D., Konstantinova-Mitcheva, M., Descatoire, V., Cobert, B., Wandscheer, J.C., Level, R., Feldmann, G., Mansuy, D., and Benhamou, J.P. (1981) Hypoactivity of cytochrome P-450 after triacetyloleandomycin administration. *Biochemical Pharmacology*, **30** (6), 559–564.

23 Franklin, M.R. (1974) Formation of a 455 nm complex during cytochrome P 450-dependent N-hydroxyamphetamine metabolism. *Molecular Pharmacology*, **10** (6), 975–985.

24 Zhou, S., Chan, E., Lee, Y.L., Boelsterli, U.A., Li, S.C., Wang, J., Zhang, Q., Huang, M., and Xu, A. (2004) Therapeutic drugs that behave as mechanism-based inhibitors of cytochrome P450 3A4. *Current Drug Metabolism*, **5** (5), 415–442.

25 Bertelsen, K.M., Venkatakrishnan, K., Von Moltke, L.L., Obach, R.S., and Greenblatt, D.J. (2003) Apparent mechanism-based inhibition of human CYP2D6 in vitro by paroxetine: comparison with fluoxetine and quinidine. *Drug Metabolism and Disposition*, **31** (3), 289–293.

26 Heydari, A., Yeo, K.R., Lennard, M.S., Ellis, S.W., Tucker, G.T., and Rostami-Hodjegan, A. (2004) Mechanism-based inactivation of CYP2D6 by methylenedioxymethamphetamine. *Drug Metabolism and Disposition*, **32** (11), 1213–1217.

27 Brosen, K., Hansen, J.G., Nielsen, K.K., Sindrup, S.H., and Gram, L.F. (1993) Inhibition by paroxetine of desipramine metabolism in extensive but not in poor metabolizers of sparteine. *European Journal of Clinical Pharmacology*, **44** (4), 349–355.

28 Sindrup, S.H., Brosen, K., and Gram, L.F. (1992) Pharmacokinetics of the selective serotonin reuptake inhibitor paroxetine: nonlinearity and relation to the sparteine oxidation polymorphism. *Clinical Pharmacology and Therapeutics*, **51** (3), 288–295.

29 O'Mathuna, B., Farre, M., Rostami-Hodjegan, A., Yang, J., Cuyas, E., Torrens, M., Pardo, R., Abanades, S., Maluf, S., Tucker, G.T., and de la Torre, R. (2008) The consequences of 3,4-methylenedioxymethamphetamine induced CYP2D6 inhibition in humans. *Journal of Clinical Psychopharmacology*, **28** (5), 525–531.

30 Kalgutkar, A.S., Vaz, A.D.N., Lame, M.E., Henne, K.R., Soglia, J., Zhao, S.X., Abramov, Y.A., Lombardo, F., Collin, C., Hendsch, Z.S., and Hop Cornelis, E.C.A. (2005) Bioactivation of the nontricyclic antidepressant nefazodone to a reactive quinone-imine species in human liver microsomes and recombinant cytochrome

P450 3A4. *Drug Metabolism and Disposition*, **33** (2), 243–253.

31 Lam, Y.W., Alfaro, C.L., Ereshefsky, L., and Miller, M. (2003) Pharmacokinetic and pharmacodynamic interactions of oral midazolam with ketoconazole, fluoxetine, fluvoxamine, and nefazodone. *Journal of Clinical Pharmacology*, **43** (11), 1274–1282.

32 Chen, Q., Ngui, J.S., Doss, G.A., Wang, R. W., Cai, X., DiNinno, F.P., Blizzard, T.A., Hammond, M.L., Stearns, R.A., Evans, D.C., Baillie, T.A., and Tang, W. (2002) Cytochrome P450 3A4-mediated bioactivation of raloxifene: irreversible enzyme inhibition and thiol adduct formation. *Chemical Research in Toxicology*, **15** (7), 907–914.

33 Yukinaga, H., Takami, T., Shioyama, S.-H., Tozuka, Z., Masumoto, H., Okazaki, O., and Sudo, K. (2007) Identification of cytochrome P450 3A4 modification site with reactive metabolite using linear ion trap-Fourier transform mass spectrometry. *Chemical Research in Toxicology*, **20** (10), 1373–1378.

34 Sridar, C.K., Ute, M., Notley, L.M., Gillam, E.M.J., and Hollenberg, P.F. (2002) Effect of tamoxifen on the enzymatic activity of human cytochrome CYP2B6. *Journal of Pharmacology and Experimental Therapeutics*, **301** (3), 945–952.

35 Zhao, X.-J., Jones, D.R., Wang, Y.-H., Grimm, S.W., and Hall, S.D. (2002) Reversible and irreversible inhibition of CYP3A enzymes by tamoxifen and metabolites. *Xenobiotica*, **32** (10), 863–878.

36 Driscoll, J.P., Kornecki, K., Wolkowski, J.P., Chupak, L., Kalgutkar, A.S., and O'Donnell, J.P. (2007) Bioactivation of phencyclidine in rat and human liver microsomes and recombinant P450 2B enzymes: evidence for the formation of a novel quinone methide intermediate. *Chemical Research in Toxicology*, **20** (10), 1488–1497.

37 Jushchyshyn, M.I., Wahlstrom, J.L., Hollenberg, P.F., and Wienkers, L.C. (2006) Mechanism of inactivation of human cytochrome P450 2B6 by phencyclidine. *Drug Metabolism and Disposition*, **34** (9), 1523–1529.

38 Ha-Duong, N.-T., Dijols, S., Macherey, A.-C., Goldstein, J.A., Dansette, P.M., and Mansuy, D. (2001) Ticlopidine as a selective mechanism-based inhibitor of human cytochrome P450 2C19. *Biochemistry*, **40** (40), 12112–12122.

39 Lu, P., Schrag, M.L., Slaughter, D.E., Raab, C.E., Shou, M., and Rodrigues, A.D. (2003) Mechanism-based inhibition of human liver microsomal cytochrome P450 1A2 by zileuton, a 5-lipoxygenase inhibitor. *Drug Metabolism and Disposition*, **31** (11), 1352–1360.

40 O'Donnell, J.P., Dalvie, D.K., Kalgutkar, A.S., and Obach, R.S. (2003) Mechanism-based inactivation of human recombinant P450 2C9 by the nonsteroidal anti-inflammatory drug suprofen. *Drug Metabolism and Disposition*, **31** (11), 1369–1377.

41 Hutzler, J.M., Balogh, L.M., Zientek, M., Kumar, V., and Tracy, T.S. (2009) Mechanism-based inactivation of cytochrome P450 2C9 by tienilic acid and suprofen: a comparison of kinetics and probe substrate selection. *Drug Metabolism and Disposition*, **37** (1), 59–65.

42 O'Reilly, R.A. (1982) Ticrynafen-racemic warfarin interaction: hepatotoxic or stereoselective? *Clinical Pharmacology and Therapeutics*, **32** (3), 356–361.

43 Granneman, G.R., Braeckman, R.A., Locke, C.S., Cavanaugh, J.H., Dube, L.M., and Awni, W.M. (1995) Effect of zileuton on theophylline pharmacokinetics. *Clinical Pharmacokinetics*, **29** (Suppl. 2), 77–83.

44 Beaune, P.H., Lecoeur, S., Bourdi, M., Gauffre, A., Belloc, C., Dansette, P., and Mansuy, D. (1996) Anti-cytochrome P450 autoantibodies in drug-induced disease. *European Journal of Haematology Supplement*, **60**, 89–92.

45 Joshi, E.M., Heasley, B.H., Chordia, M.D., and Macdonald, T.L. (2004) In vitro metabolism of 2-acetylbenzothiophene: relevance to zileuton hepatotoxicity. *Chemical Research in Toxicology*, **17** (2), 137–143.

46 Koenigs, L.L. and Trager, W.F. (1998) Mechanism-based inactivation of P450 2A6 by furanocoumarins. *Biochemistry*, **37** (28), 10047–10061.

47 Letteron, P., Descatoire, V., Larrey, D., Tinel, M., Geneve, J., and Pessayre, D.

(1986) Inactivation and induction of cytochrome P-450 by various psoralen derivatives in rats. *Journal of Pharmacology and Experimental Therapeutics*, **238** (2), 685–692.

48 Labbe, G., Descatoire, V., Beaune, P., Letteron, P., Larrey, D., and Pessayre, D. (1989) Suicide inactivation of cytochrome P-450 by methoxsalen. Evidence for the covalent binding of a reactive intermediate to the protein moiety. *Journal of Pharmacology and Experimental Therapeutics*, **250** (3), 1034–1042.

49 Lin, H.-L., Kent, U.M., and Hollenberg, P.F. (2005) The grapefruit juice effect is not limited to cytochrome P450 (P450) 3A4: evidence for bergamottin-dependent inactivation, heme destruction, and covalent binding to protein in P450s 2B6 and 3A5. *Journal of Pharmacology and Experimental Therapeutics*, **313** (1), 154–164.

50 Kunze, K.L. and Trager, W.F. (1993) Isoform-selective mechanism-based inhibition of human cytochrome P450 1A2 by furafylline. *Chemical Research in Toxicology*, **6** (5), 649–656.

51 Tarrus, E., Cami, J., Roberts, D.J., Spickett, R.G., Celdran, E., and Segura, J. (1987) Accumulation of caffeine in healthy volunteers treated with furafylline. *British Journal of Clinical Pharmacology*, **23** (1), 9–18.

52 Racha, J.K., Rettie, A.E., and Kunze, K.L. (1998) Mechanism-based inactivation of human cytochrome P450 1A2 by furafylline: detection of a 1:1 adduct to protein and evidence for the formation of a novel imidazomethide intermediate. *Biochemistry*, **37** (20), 7407–7419.

53 Veronese, M.L., Gillen, L.P., Dorval, E.P., Hauck, W.W., Waldman, S.A., and Greenberg, H.E. (2003) Effect of mibefradil on CYP3A4 in vivo. *Journal of Clinical Pharmacology*, **43** (10), 1091–1100.

54 Foti, R.S., Rock, D.A., Pearson, J.T., Wahlstrom, J.L., and Wienkers, L.C. (2011) Mechanism-based inactivation of cytochrome P450 3A4 by mibefradil through heme destruction. *Drug Metabolism and Disposition*, **39** (7), 1188–1195.

55 Linder, C.D., Renaud, N.A., and Hutzler, J.M. (2009) Is 1-aminobenzotriazole an appropriate in vitro tool as a nonspecific cytochrome P450 inactivator? *Drug Metabolism and Disposition*, **37** (1), 10–13.

56 Emoto, C., Murase, S., Sawada, Y., Jones, B.C., and Iwasaki, K. (2003) In vitro inhibitory effect of 1-aminobenzotriazole on drug oxidations catalyzed by human cytochrome P450 enzymes: a comparison with SKF-525A and ketoconazole. *Drug Metabolism and Pharmacokinetics*, **18** (5), 287–295.

57 Balani, S.K., Zhu, T., Yang, T.J., Liu, Z., He, B., and Lee, F.W. (2002) Effective dosing regimen of 1-aminobenzotriazole for inhibition of antipyrine clearance in rats, dogs, and monkeys. *Drug Metabolism and Disposition*, **30** (10), 1059–1062.

58 Ortiz de Montellano, P.R., Mathews, J.M., and Langry, K.C. (1984) Autocatalytic inactivation of cytochrome P-450 and chloroperoxidase by 1-aminobenzotriazole and other aryne precursors. *Tetrahedron*, **40** (3), 511–519.

59 Backman, J.T., Kyrklund, C., Neuvonen, M., and Neuvonen, P.J. (2002) Gemfibrozil greatly increases plasma concentrations of cerivastatin. *Clinical Pharmacology and Therapeutics*, **72** (6), 685–691.

60 Kalliokoski, A., Backman, J.T., Kurkinen, K.J., Neuvonen, P.J., and Niemi, M. (2008) Effects of gemfibrozil and atorvastatin on the pharmacokinetics of repaglinide in relation to SLCO1B1 polymorphism. *Clinical Pharmacology and Therapeutics*, **84** (4), 488–496.

61 Ogilvie, B.W., Zhang, D., Li, W., Rodrigues, A.D., Gipson, A.E., Holsapple, J., Toren, P., and Parkinson, A. (2006) Glucuronidation converts gemfibrozil to a potent, metabolism-dependent inhibitor of CYP2C8: implications for drug–drug interactions. *Drug Metabolism and Disposition*, **34** (1), 191–197.

62 Baer, B.R., DeLisle, R.K., and Allen, A. (2009) Benzylic oxidation of gemfibrozil-1-*O*-beta-glucuronide by P450 2C8 leads to heme alkylation and irreversible inhibition. *Chemical Research in Toxicology*, **22** (7), 1298–1309.

63 Polasek, T.M., Elliot, D.J., Somogyi, A.A., Gillam, E.M.J., Lewis, B.C., and Miners, J.O. (2006) An evaluation of potential

mechanism-based inactivation of human drug metabolizing cytochromes P450 by monoamine oxidase inhibitors, including isoniazid. *British Journal of Clinical Pharmacology*, **61** (5), 570–584.

64 Wen, X., Wang, J.-S., Neuvonen, P.J., and Backman, J.T. (2002) Isoniazid is a mechanism-based inhibitor of cytochrome P450 1A2, 2A6, 2C19 and 3A4 isoforms in human liver microsomes. *European Journal of Clinical Pharmacology*, **57** (11), 799–804.

65 Yew, W.W. (2002) Clinically significant interactions with drugs used in the treatment of tuberculosis. *Drug Safety*, **25** (2), 111–133.

66 Ochs, H.R., Greenblatt, D.J., and Knuchel, M. (1983) Differential effect of isoniazid on triazolam oxidation and oxazepam conjugation. *British Journal of Clinical Pharmacology*, **16** (6), 743–746.

67 Muakkassah, S.F., Bidlack, W.R., and Yang, W.C. (1982) Reversal of the effects of isoniazid on hepatic cytochrome P-450 by potassium ferricyanide. *Biochemical Pharmacology*, **31** (2), 249–251.

68 Johnson, C., Stubley-Beedham, C., Stell, J., and Godfrey, P. (1985) Hydralazine: a potent inhibitor of aldehyde oxidase activity in vitro and in vivo. *Biochemical Pharmacology*, **34** (24), 4251–4256.

69 Critchley, D.J.P., Rance, D.J., and Beedham, C. (1994) Biotransformation of carbazeran in guinea pig: effect of hydralazine pretreatment. *Xenobiotica*, **24** (1), 37–47.

70 McCormack, J.J., Allen, B.A., and Hodnett, C.N. (1978) Oxidation of quinazoline and quinoxaline by xanthine oxidase and aldehyde oxidase. *Journal of Heterocyclic Chemistry*, **15** (8), 1249–1254.

71 Dick, R.A., Kanne, D.B., and Casida, J.E. (2007) Nitroso-imidacloprid irreversibly inhibits rabbit aldehyde oxidase. *Chemical Research in Toxicology*, **20** (12), 1942–1946.

72 Wimbiscus, M., Kostenko, O., and Malone, D. (2010) MAO inhibitors: risks, benefits, and lore. *Cleveland Clinical Journal of Medicine*, **77** (12), 859–882.

73 Fowler, C.J. and Ross, R.B. (1984) Selective inhibitors of monoamine oxidase

A and B: biochemical, pharmacological, and clinical properties. *Medicinal Research Reviews*, **4** (3), 323–358.

74 Dostert, P. and Strolin-Benedetti, M. (1986) New monoamine oxidase inhibitors. *Actual Chimica Therapeutics*, **13**, 269–287.

75 Amrein, R., Allen, S.R., Guentert, T.W., Hartmann, D., Lorscheid, T., Schoerlin, M.P., and Vranesic, D. (1989) The pharmacology of reversible monoamine oxidase inhibitors. *British Journal of Psychiatry Supplement*, **6**, 66–71.

76 Davies, B., Bannister, R., and Sever, P. (1978) Pressor amines and monoamine-oxidase inhibitors for treatment of postural hypotension in autonomic failure. Limitations and hazards. *Lancet*, **1** (8057), 172–175.

77 Kalgutkar, A.S., Dalvie, D.K., Castagnoli, N. Jr., and Taylor, T.J. (2001) Interactions of nitrogen-containing xenobiotics with monoamine oxidase (MAO) isozymes A and B: SAR studies on MAO substrates and inhibitors. *Chemical Research in Toxicology*, **14** (9), 1139–1162.

78 Knoll, J., Escery, Z., Magyar, K., and Satory, E. (1978) Novel (−)-deprenyl-derived selective inhibitors of B-type monoamine oxidase. The relation of structure to their action. *Biochemical Pharmacology*, **27** (13), 1739–1747.

79 Patek, D. and Hellerman, L. (1974) Mitochondiral monoamine oxidase. Mechanism of inhibition of phenyl hydrazine and by aralkylhydrazines. Role of enzymic oxidations. *Journal of Biological Chemistry*, **249** (8), 2373–2380.

80 Silverman, R.B., Hiebert, C.K., and Vazquez, M.L. (1985) Inactivation of monoamine oxidase by allylamine does not result in flavin attachment. *Journal of Biological Chemistry*, **260** (27), 14648–14652.

81 Maycock, A.L., Abeles, R.H., Salach, J.I., and Singer, T.P. (1976) The structure of the covalent adduct formed by the interaction of 3-dimethyalmino-1-propyne and the flavine of mitochondrial amine oxidase. *Biochemistry*, **15** (1), 114–125.

82 Maycock, A.L. (1980) Flavin suicide inhibitor adducts. *Methods in Enzymology*, **66**, 294–302.

83 Silverman, R.B. and Hoffman, S.J. (1980) Mechanism of inactivation of mitochondrial monoamine oxidase by N-cyclopropyl-N-arylalkylamines. *Journal of the American Chemical Society*, **102**, 884–886.

84 Silverman, R.B. and Yamasaki, R.B. (1984) Mechanism-based inactivation of mitochondrial monoamine oxidase by N-(1-methylcyclopropyl)benzylamine. *Biochemistry*, **23** (6), 1322–1332.

85 Vazquez, M.L. and Silverman, R.B. (1985) Revised mechanism for inactivation of mitochondrial monoamine oxidase by N-cyclopropylbenzylamine. *Biochemistry*, **24** (23), 6538–6543.

86 Gates, K.S. and Silverman, R.B. (1989) Model studies for the mechanism of inactivation of monoamine oxidase by 5-(aminomethyl)-3-aryl-2-oxazolidinones.

Journal of the American Chemical Society, **111**, 8891–8895.

87 Gates, K.S. and Silverman, R.B. (1990) 5-(Aminomethyl)-3-aryl-2-oxazolidinones. A novel class of mechanism-based inactivators of monoamine oxidase B. *Journal of the American Chemical Society*, **112**, 9364–9372.

88 Krueger, M.J., McKeown, K., Ramsay, R.R., Youngster, S.K., and Singer, T.P. (1990) Mechanism-based inactivation of monoamine oxidases A and B by tetrahydropyridines and dihydropyridines. *Biochemical Journal*, **268** (1), 219–224.

89 Silverman, R.B., Nishimura, K., and Lu, X. (1993) Mechanism of inactivation of monoamine oxidase-B by the anticonvulsant agent milacemide (2-(n-pentylamino)acetamide). *Journal of the American Chemical Society*, **115**, 4949–4954.

4

Role of Reactive Metabolites in Drug-Induced Toxicity – The Tale of Acetaminophen, Halothane, Hydralazine, and Tienilic Acid

Abbreviations

DMPO	5,5-Dimethyl-1-pyrroline-*N*-oxide
GSH	Glutathione
HOCl	Hypochlorous acid
NAPQI	*N*-Acetyl-*para*-benzoquinone imine
NAT	*N*-Acetyltransferase
CYP	Cytochrome P450
TA	Tienilic acid
TFA	Trifluoroacetic acid
UGT	Uridine glucuronosyl transferase

4.1
Introduction

The concept of reactive metabolite formation as a causative factor in drug-induced hepatic and immunological toxicity is explored in detail with acetaminophen, halothane, hydralazine, and tienilic acid (TA) [1–6].

4.2
Acetaminophen

First synthesized in 1888 as an intermediate for the synthesis of phenacetin, acetaminophen (Figure 4.1) is one of the world's most widely used analgesic and antipyretic agent. At therapeutic doses, it has been shown to be a remarkably safe drug. Consumption of high doses can lead to fulminant hepatic necrosis and even death in humans and preclinical species [4, 7–11].

Reactive Drug Metabolites, First Edition. Amit S. Kalgutkar, Deepak Dalvie, R. Scott Obach, and Dennis A. Smith.
© 2012 Wiley-VCH Verlag GmbH & Co. KGaA. Published 2012 by Wiley-VCH Verlag GmbH & Co. KGaA.

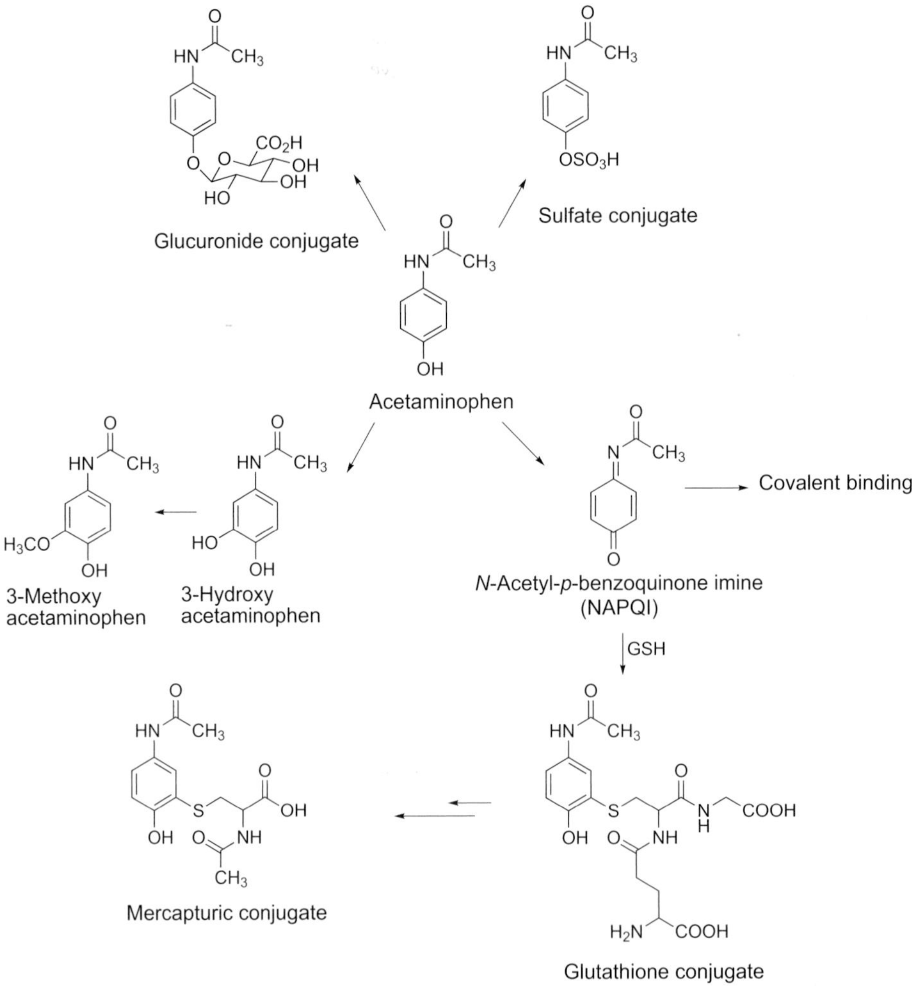

Figure 4.1 Metabolism of acetaminophen.

4.2.1
Metabolism of Acetaminophen

Acetaminophen is primarily metabolized via conjugative reactions [12–16]. Its phenolic group is susceptible to glucuronidation and sulfation, which are essentially detoxification pathways of the compound. At therapeutic doses, about one-half and one-third of the excreted urinary metabolites are in the forms of acetaminophen O-glucuronide and acetaminophen O-sulfate, respectively (Figure 4.1) [17, 18]. Acetaminophen glucuronidation is catalyzed by uridine glucuronosyl transferase (UGT) 1A family (UGT1A1, 1A6, and 1A9) as well as UGT2B15 [19]. The sulfation pathway of acetaminophen metabolism can be saturated at high acetaminophen doses, because of either limited supply of 3′-phosphoadenosine 5′-phosphosulfate substrate or limited sulfotransferase enzyme capacity [20]. Studies with the UGT-deficient Gunn rat and other animal models have demonstrated that impairment of glucuronidation results in enhanced acetaminophen toxicity [21, 22]. This increased sensitivity is also discerned in humans with Gilbert's syndrome, in which glucuronidation activity is impaired [23]. Acetaminophen is also metabolized via a third pathway that involves a cytochrome P450 (CYP)–catalyzed oxidation of the compound to the electrophilic N-acetyl-*para*-benzoquinone imine (NAPQI) metabolite (Figure 4.1) [24]. Glutathione (GSH) conjugates (1,4-Michael adduct) of NAPQI and the corresponding cysteine conjugate and mercapturic acid breakdown products have been found *in vivo* in human urine after ingestion of acetaminophen as well as *in vitro* liver microsomal incubations [17, 25, 26]. Although a minor oxidation reaction, hydroxylation of acetaminophen to 3-hydroxyacetaminophen (Figure 4.1) probably also occurs in humans as methylated 3-hydroxyacetaminophen has been found in urine of patients who had taken an overdose of acetaminophen [26]. Quantitatively, only a small percentage of administered dose undergoes oxidative metabolism. However, there is compelling evidence to indicate that acetaminophen bioactivation is mediated via the oxidative bioactivation pathway.

4.2.2
Metabolic Activation of Acetaminophen

There is general consensus that hepatotoxicity of acetaminophen is the result of its oxidative metabolism to NAPQI in the liver by P450 [9, 11, 27–29] or other oxidative enzymes such as prostaglandin H synthetase [30, 31], myeloperoxidase, chloroperoxidase, and lactoperoxidase [32]. The second oxidative metabolite of acetaminophen, 3-hydroxyacetaminophen, does not exhibit hepatotoxicity [33]. Several human CYP enzymes can oxidize acetaminophen to NAPQI, including 3A4, 1A2, 2A6, 2D6, and 2E1 [34–36]. The formation of NAPQI was initially thought to result from dehydration of the N-hydroxyacetaminophen (Figure 4.2, pathway A) or the 3,4-epoxyacetaminophen (Figure 4.2, pathway B) metabolites [37]. Subsequent reports indicated a direct two-electron oxidation to NAPQI (Figure 4.2, pathway C) [38, 39]. Alternatively, one-electron oxidation of acetaminophen to a semiquinone radical (NAPSQI) followed by a subsequent one-electron oxidation of the semiquinone radical also yielded NAPQI (Figure 4.2, pathway D) [37, 40].

The hepatotoxicity of acetaminophen is a result of covalent binding of NAPQI to proteins in the liver. NAPQI generally binds to low-molecular-weight nucleophiles such as the antioxidant GSH *in vivo*, and is detoxified via this pathway [41, 42]. However, GSH stores can also be depleted during NAPQI detoxification, which can lead to covalent adduction of NAPQI with proteins. Covalent binding to protein has been shown to correlate with the centrilobular hepatic necrosis commonly seen after acetaminophen overdose [7, 43–45]. The covalent binding of acetaminophen to hepatic proteins was initially demonstrated using [3]H- or ^{14}C-acetaminophen in seminal studies by Gillette and coworkers [27, 28, 41, 46]. The major nucleophilic targets in proteins are the thiol groups of cysteine residues [47, 48]. Binding was

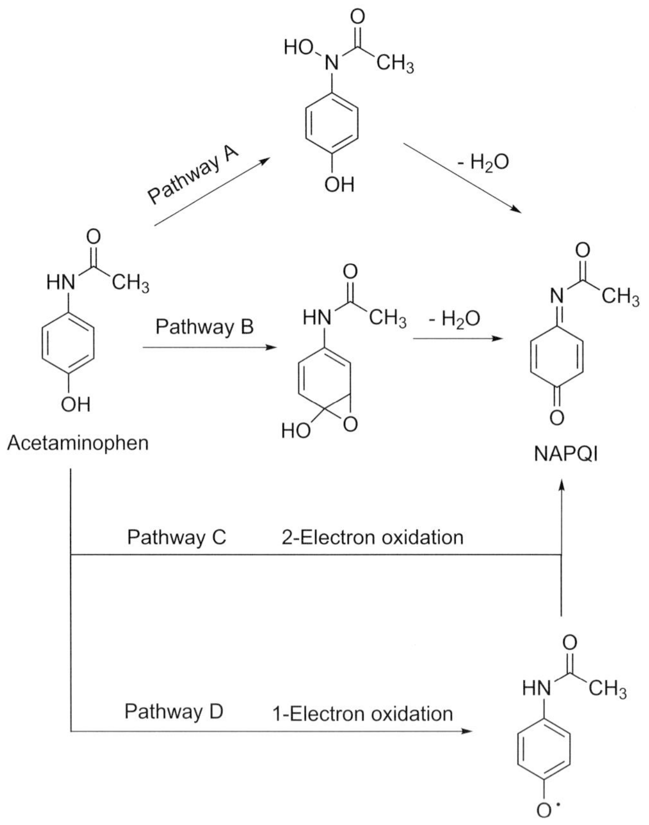

Figure 4.2 Proposed CYP-catalyzed metabolic activation pathways of acetaminophen [37].

observed in all subcellular compartments examined: nuclear, mitochondrial, endoplasmic reticulum, and cytosol. This binding was far greater in liver than in nontarget tissues (e.g., muscle). Pretreatment of mice with CYP inhibitors decreased both the covalent binding and the hepatotoxicity, whereas pretreatment with CYP inducers increased both parameters. Later studies used immunohistochemistry with antibodies against acetaminophen–protein adducts to show that the histological pattern of covalent adduction matches that of the toxicity, with damage to the centrilobular rather than the periportal regions [49, 50]. Gillette and coworkers also demonstrated the protective role of GSH. Understanding the significance of GSH for acetaminophen detoxification led directly to improved clinical therapy for acetaminophen poisoning. Administration of *N*-acetyl-ʟ-cysteine, which replenishes GSH stores [51], remains the treatment of choice in human overdose cases [52].

Radiolabeling, immunological, and proteomic methods, including mass spectrometry, have been used to identify proteins adducted/inactivated by acetaminophen [53]. No single protein or set of proteins, and no specific subcellular compartment, has been found to be a uniquely sensitive target of acetaminophen

Table 4.1 Some hepatic proteins adducted by acetaminophen mouse liver [4, 10].

Enzyme/Protein	Compartment
Aldehyde dehydrogenase	Cytosol, mitochondria
ATP synthase α-subunit	Mitochondria
Glutamine synthase	Endoplasmic reticulum
Glutathione peroxidase	Cytosol, mitochondria
Glutathione transferase	Cytosol, mitochondria
Glycine N-methyltransferase	Cytosol
3-Hydroxyanthranilate 3,4-dioxygenase	Cytosol
Tropomyosin 5	Cytoskeleton
Urate oxidase	Peroxisomes
Carbamyl phosphate synthetase I	Mitochondrial
N10-Formyltetrahydrofolate dehydrogenase	Cytosol
Selenium-binding protein	Cytosol
Lamin A	Nuclear
Aldehyde dehydrogenase	Mitochondrial

adduction. The plasma membrane fraction contains the highest level of binding on a per milligram protein basis, followed by the mitochondrial fraction, and the highest overall level of binding was in the cytosol. Two mitochondrial targets of acetaminophen have been identified. A 50 kDa acetaminophen–protein adduct was purified by chromatography followed by preparative electrophoresis and was identified as glutamate dehydrogenase [54], which catalyzes the reversible oxidative deamination of glutamate to yield 2-ketoglutarate and ammonia. The activity of glutamate dehydrogenase is significantly decreased in a dose-dependent manner following treatment with acetaminophen. Another 54 kDa mitochondrial adduct has recently been identified as aldehyde dehydrogenase [55]. Other adducts detected by staining were the microsomal 44 kDa protein and plasma membrane adducts of 72 and 82 kDa [3, 4]. A sample of acetaminophen target proteins that have been identified is shown in Table 4.1 [3, 10]. It is speculated that the mitochondrial adducts may play a critical role in the toxicity [4, 56–58].

Several other hypotheses have also been presented as the mechanism for acetaminophen toxicity. These include oxidative stress, disruption of calcium homeostasis [8], DNA fragmentation leading to apoptosis [59, 60], and Kuppfer cell activation [61]. How these mechanisms will ultimately lead to hepatotoxicity is less clear.

4.3
Halothane

Halothane (2-bromo-2-chloro-1,1,1-trifluoroethane, Figure 4.3) is a general inhalation anesthetic that was first synthesized by C.W. Suckling of Imperial

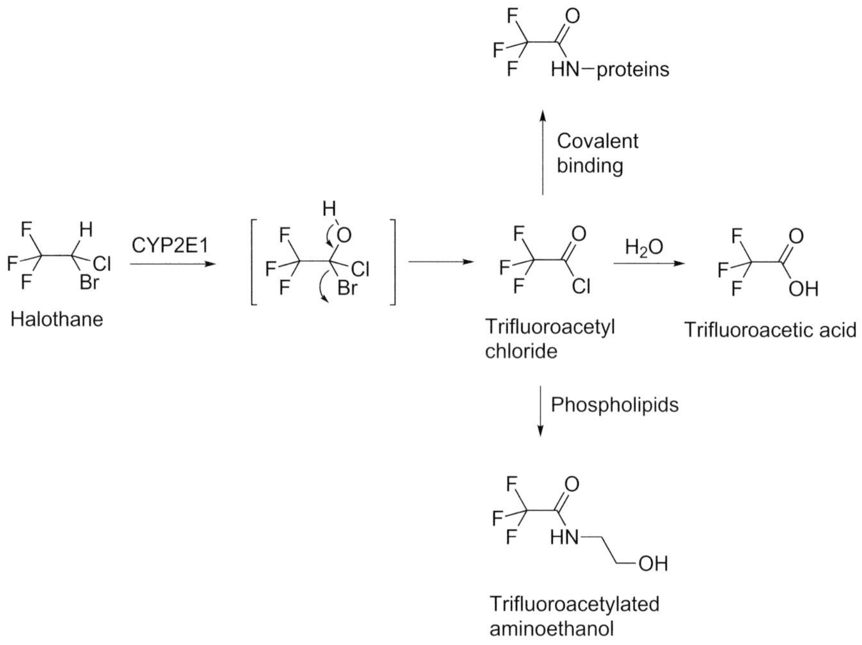

Figure 4.3 Oxidative metabolism of halothane.

Chemical Industries (ICI) in 1951 and used clinically by M. Johnstone in Manchester in 1956. It became popular as a nonflammable general anesthetic replacing other volatile anesthetics such as diethyl ether and cyclopropane and was given to millions of adult and pediatric patients worldwide since its introduction in 1956 to the 1980s. Its lack of airway irritation made it a common inhalation induction agent in pediatric anesthesia. Use of the anesthetic was phased out during the 1980s and 1990s as newer anesthetic agents became popular. Halothane still retains some use in veterinary surgery and in the Third World because of its lower cost.

4.3.1
Metabolism of Halothane

Biotransformation appears to be a prerequisite for the development of halothane-associated hepatotoxicity. About 20% of absorbed halothane is metabolized in the body [62–64]. The metabolism takes place via oxidative and reductive pathways, although the primary route of metabolism is oxidative in nature and is mediated by CYP enzymes [65–68]. Using reconstituted CYP enzymes, antibodies directed against discrete CYP isozymes, and CYP-inducing agents, CYP2El has been identified as the major halothane-metabolizing isozyme [69, 70]. Oxidative metabolism by CYP2E1 is also believed to be a primary pathway in halothane bioactivation that results in idiosyncratic hepatotoxicity. The mechanism of oxidation involves initial conversion of halothane to a geminal bromohydrin intermediate, which spontaneously degenerates to afford trifluoroacetyl chloride (Figure 4.3). Hydrolysis of the acyl chloride yields trifluoroacetic acid (TFA). Analysis of human urine samples following administration of ^{14}C halothane (radiolabel on the fluorinated carbon) revealed only one metabolite that was identified as TFA [63, 65, 71]. TFA is also a major urinary metabolite of halothane metabolism in dogs [72] and rats [73]. Alternatively, the trifluoroacetyl chloride intermediate may react with any nucleophile available at the site of its generation [65, 74–76]. The primary targets are probably lysine residues in proteins resulting in formation of trifluoroacetamide derivatives (Figure 4.3) and ethanolamine moiety of the phosphatidylethanolamines [65, 73, 74, 77]. Mass spectrometric analysis of urinary samples reveals that N-trifluoroacetyl-2-aminoethanol (Figure 4.3) is one of the urinary metabolites, most likely arising through the oxidative biotransformation of halothane in humans [65]. GSH or cysteine is also capable of scavenging the reactive trifluoroacetyl chloride in incubations of halothane with rat liver microsomes in the presence of NADPH *in vitro*; the presence of GSH or cysteine dramatically reduces the extent of trifluoroacetyl–protein adduct formation when monitored with a monospecific anti-TFA antibody on immunoblots [78–80].

Reductive metabolism of halothane generally occurs under low levels of oxygen [81, 82]. Anaerobic incubations of halothane with rat liver microsomes that are fortified with NADPH yield 2-chloro-1,1,1-trifluoroethane as a primary metabolite (Figure 4.4). The reaction proceeds via donation of one electron from CYP to the substrate followed by the loss of a bromine ion to give the carbon-centered 2-chloro-1,1,1-trifluoroethyl radical. Subsequent abstraction of hydrogen atom from a suitable donor may lead to formation of the corresponding 2-chloro-1,1,1-

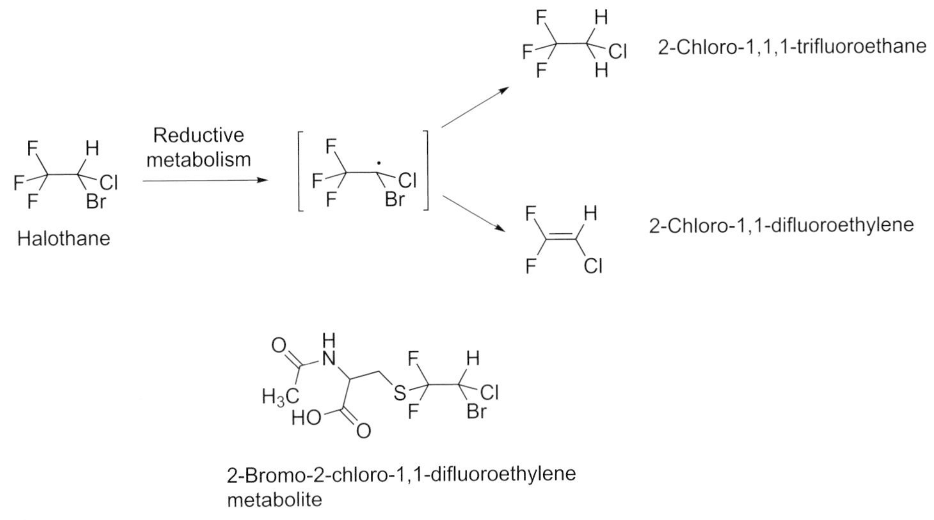

Figure 4.4 Reductive metabolism of halothane.

trifluoroethane [83, 84]. Alternatively, donation of a second electron results in the formation of the carbanion [84], which under rearrangement and loss of fluoride ion gives rise to 2-chloro-1,1-difluoroethylene [83]. The metabolism is blocked by oxygen and carbon monoxide [85, 86]. Two reductive dehalogenated metabolites of halothane, namely, 2-chloro-1,1,1-trifluoroethane and 2-chloro-1,1-difluoroethylene (Figure 4.4), have been identified in the expired gas of halothane-anesthetized rabbits and humans [87, 88]. The radical formed during the formation of the hydrocarbon metabolites has the potential to adduct with microsomal endoplasmic proteins and microsomal phospholipids [75, 89–91]. The isolation of *S*-(2-bromo-2-chloro-1,1-difluoroethyl)-*N*-acetyl-L-cysteine (Figure 4.4) as a urinary metabolite of halothane is suggestive of yet another reductive pathway in humans [65, 92]. The formation of the cysteinyl adduct is a result of CYP-mediated proton abstraction followed by a loss of fluoride ion to yield the 2-bromo-2-chloro-1,1-difluoroethylene metabolite. This possibly forms the glutathione transferase–catalyzed adduct with cellular GSH, which can enter the mercapturic acid pathway, and, after processing, may be excreted in the urine as the observed L-cysteine conjugate [93].

4.3.2
Hepatotoxicity following Halothane Administration

Halothane is well known to cause severe liver dysfunction. Two major forms of hepatotoxic events are observed in patients following halothane administration [78]. The two forms appear to be unrelated and are termed type I (mild) and type II (fulminant) [94–96]. Type I hepatotoxicity is benign, self-limiting, and relatively common (up to 25–30% of patients who receive halothane). This type is marked by mild transient increases in serum transaminase and glutathione transferase concentrations and by altered postoperative drug metabolism [97–99]. The mild hepatocellular damage is due to a direct effect of halothane or its metabolites on the liver [4]. The effect could be attributed to binding of halothane-related material to the cellular constituents either reversibly or irreversibly.

Fulminant or type II hepatotoxicity (also referred to as halothane hepatitis) is unpredictable and is associated with massive centrilobular liver necrosis that leads to liver failure and can sometimes be fatal. The incidence is 1 in 10 000 to 1 in 35 000 following a single exposure to the anesthetic and increases to about 1 in 3000 following multiple exposures. Type II hepatotoxicity has a mortality rate of 30–70%. Fulminant necrosis is now believed to be an immune phenomenon occurring in genetically susceptible individuals and is a result of repeated exposure to halothane [4, 78]. The sera of patients with halothane hepatitis contain antibodies that are reactive against a number of heterologous trifluoroacetylated liver microsomal proteins (so-called TFA–protein adducts) [100–104]. These antibodies and lymphocytes are also reactive against liver tissue from halothane-treated rabbits [105–107]. As outlined above, TFA–protein adducts are trifluoroacetylated predominantly at the lysine moieties [73]. Trifluoroacetylation renders the proteins antigenic and this process stimulates the formation of antibodies to this metabolite–protein complex. Reexposure to halothane, thus, initiates an immune-mediated

Table 4.2 Identification of TFA–protein adducts [4, 78].

Molecular Mass (kDa)	Identified proteins
27	Glutathione S-transferase
50	CYP2E1
54	CYP450
57	Protein disulfide isomerase
58	Isomerase
59	Carboxyesterase
63	Calreticulin
80	Erp72
82	BiP/GRP78
100	Erp99
170	UDP-glucose:glycoprotein glucosyltransferase

necrosis. Studies by Kenna, Pohl, and others have demonstrated that the antisera of halothane hepatitis patients seem to react with specific trifluoroacetylated proteins of apparent molecular masses of 170, 100, 82, 80, 76, 63, 59, 57, 58, 54, 50, and 27 (Table 4.2) [4, 78].

Autoantibodies to human hepatic proteins were detected in sera of most patients susceptible to hepatitis following halothane administration [108]. These proteins included three of the major luminal endoplasmic reticulum proteins, carboxyesterases, as well as the primary enzyme that metabolizes halothane to the reactive intermediate, CYP2E1 [109–113]. It has been shown that patients with halothane hepatitis not only develop an immune response that is directed against the TFA-adducted protein but also have antibodies that are directed against the native protein [109].

4.4
Hydralazine

Hydralazine is a potent vasodilator, which has been used for many years in the treatment of essential hypertension and is associated with an autoimmune, lupus-like syndrome [114, 115]. Although antinuclear antibodies occur in up to 50% of patients exposed to hydralazine, the drug-induced immune reaction is observed in very few patients [115, 116]. Hydralazine undergoes metabolism by two pathways: oxidation and acetylation. N-Acetylation, which is catalyzed by the polymorphic N-acetyltransferase-2 (NAT-2), is the primary route of hydralazine metabolism yielding an inactive, nontoxic metabolite (Figure 4.5) [117–121]. Given the polymorphic nature of NAT-2, the rate of acetylation of hydralazine is genetically controlled and the population can generally be divided into slow and fast acetylators, depending on the rate of metabolism [122, 123]. Interestingly, slow acetylators appear to be more susceptible to hydralazine-induced lupus [114, 124–126].

It has been shown that this population metabolizes less of the drug by acetylation, but compensates by oxidizing a greater proportion of the drug. The lupus syndrome

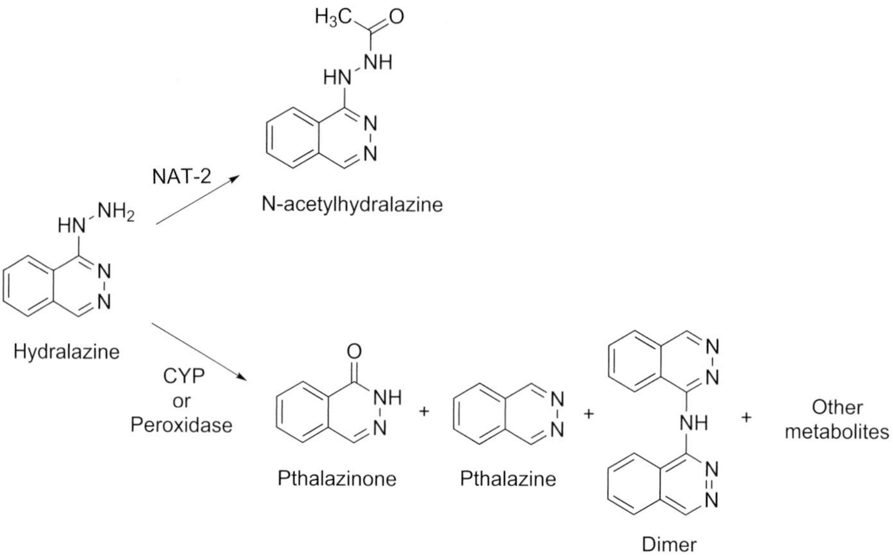

Figure 4.5 Metabolism of hydralazine.

therefore is ascribed to the oxidative metabolism of hydralazine in these patients [126]. Oxidatively, hydralazine is primarily metabolized to phthalazinone, phthalazine, and the corresponding dimer in liver microsomes in the presence of NADPH (Figure 4.5) [123, 127, 128]. In slow acetylators, the urinary excretion of phthalazinone is three times greater than it is in fast acetylators. The metabolism of hydralazine by rat liver microsomes leads to covalent binding, presumably of a reactive species, and the formation of phthalazinone [123, 127, 128]. Hydralazine is also oxidized by activated leukocytes to phthalazinone, phthalazine, and a product that is capable of covalently binding to protein [129, 130]. The covalent binding is a result of the reactive metabolite formed by P450 as well as myeloperoxidase. Studies by LaCagnin *et al.* as well as Streeter and Timbrell have shown that microsomal incubations fortified with GSH result in reduction of covalent binding to microsomal proteins and the formation of oxidative metabolites [127, 128]. The results of the electron spin resonance experiments indicate that the reactive microsomal metabolite of hydralazine involved in the covalent binding may be a nitrogen-centered radical. Addition of a spin trapping agent such as 5,5-dimethyl-1-pyrroline-*N*-oxide (DMPO) in the incubation mixture results in a DMPO adduct in a NADPH-dependent fashion. A nitrogen-centered DMPO adduct, similar to that produced by hepatic microsomes, was also detected during hydralazine incubation with horseradish peroxidase suggesting that a similar free radical oxidation pathway is involved in both systems [128, 131, 132]. Although the intermediate that forms a DMPO adduct is unknown, the metabolic activation of hydralazine is thought to involve a two-electron oxidation of hydralazine, which proceeds through several intermediates, including the nitrogen-centered phthalazinylhydrazyl (RNNH•) and diazene (RN=NH) radicals. The diazene radical decomposes to molecular nitrogen (N_2) and a carbon-

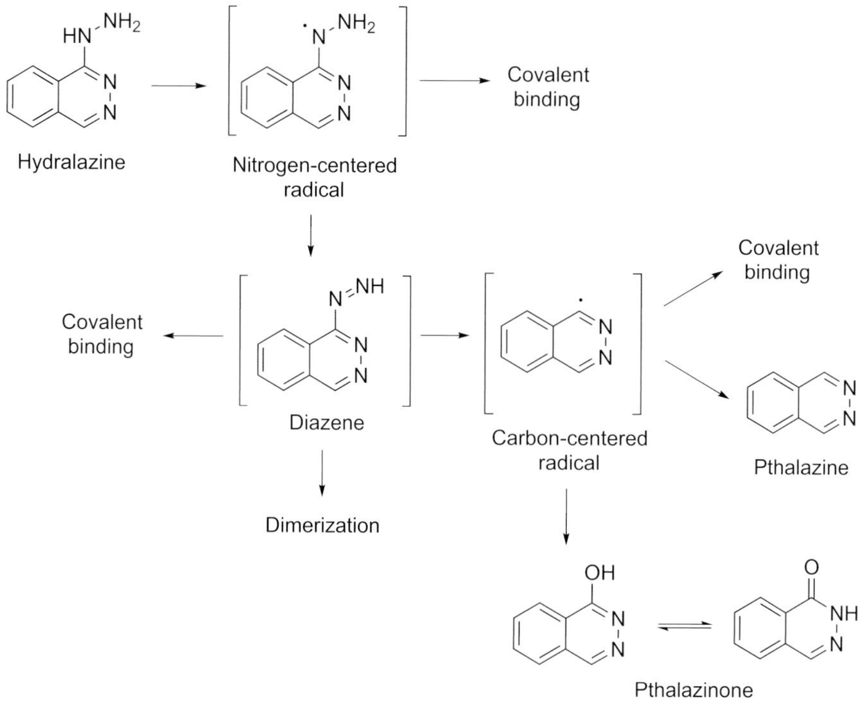

Figure 4.6 Metabolic activation of hydralazine [128].

centered phthalazinyl (R•) radical (Figure 4.6). This pathway includes two different nitrogen-centered radicals and provides a mechanism for the formation of phthalazine, phthalazinone, and the dimer via free radical intermediates [128].

Further, studies by LaCagnin *et al.* also demonstrate that there is a strong correlation between the formation of the oxidative metabolites, nitrogen radicals, and covalent binding [128]. Therefore, the oxidative metabolism of hydralazine may represent a bioactivation pathway for the drug. Since drug-induced lupus is a systemic disease, the metabolic activation of hydralazine may also be catalyzed by enzymes similar to horseradish peroxidase, such as prostaglandin synthetase, which is found in almost all mammalian cell types. The formation of a diazene intermediate has also been proposed by Hofstra and Uetrecht (Figure 4.7) [129]. In addition, this group also proposed the formation of a diazonium salt as an intermediate in the metabolic activation by myeloperoxidase. This was rationalized by the results of incubation of hydralazine by hypochlorous acid (HOCl) generated by activated leukocytes that lead to a reactive intermediate that was trapped with *N*-acetylcysteine. The adduct was identified as 1-phthalazylmercapturic acid (Figure 4.7).

The protein adducts formed by either mechanism could induce the formation of antihydralazine antibodies that cross-react with nuclear material and thus lead to the generation of antinuclear antibodies [1]. Induction of antibodies that recognized nuclear antigens was obtained by immunization of rabbits with hydralazine human

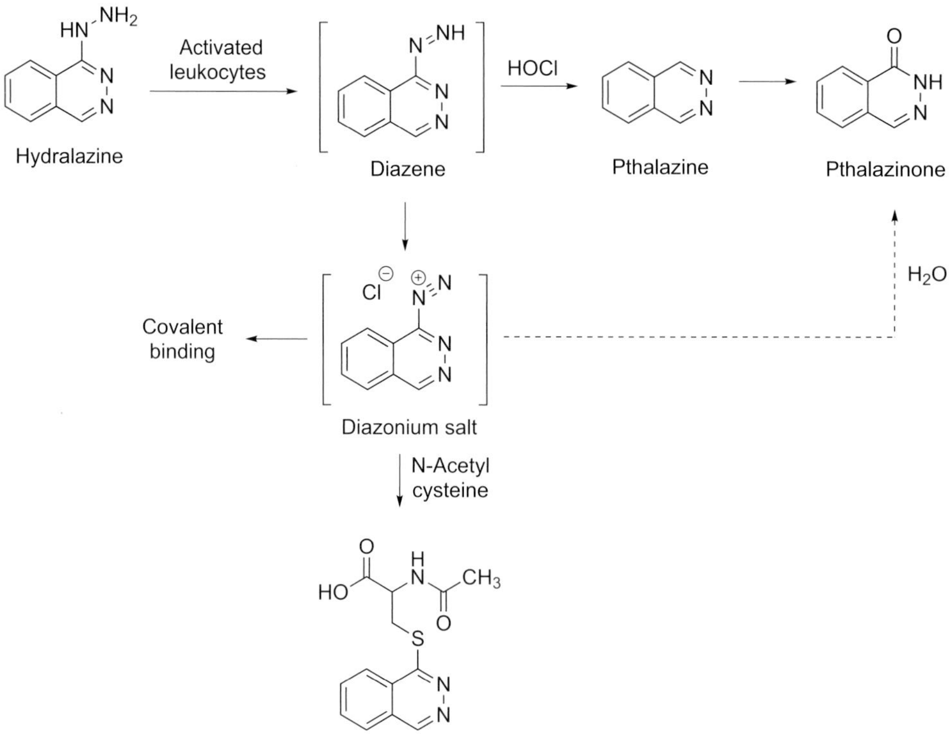

Figure 4.7 Proposed reaction pathway for oxidation of hydralazine by activated leukocytes or HOCl [129].

serum albumin conjugates [133]. Studies in humans demonstrated that hydralazine also induced antibodies to single- and double-stranded RNA and DNA [134, 135].

4.5
Tienilic Acid

TA is a thiophene ring-containing drug that causes immunoallergic hepatitis in susceptible individuals. This uricosuric diuretic was withdrawn from clinical use in the United States after more than 500 cases of hepatic injury and 25 fatalities were reported to the manufacturer [136]. Patients with TA hepatitis exhibit type 2 anti-liver kidney microsome autoantibodies that recognize unalkylated CYP2C9 in humans and also react with CYP2C11 in rats (a major isoform in adult male liver that exhibits 85% sequence identity with CYP2C9) [113, 137–141]. Immunoblotting of serum from persons with TA-induced hepatitis demonstrated that the antibodies recognized CYP2C9, but not 2C8 or 2C19 [138].

TA is metabolized by CYP2C9 in the presence of NADPH to 5-hydroxytienilic acid, which is derived from the hydroxylation of the thiophene ring (Figure 4.8). Besides this hydroxylation, the thiophene ring also undergoes a CYP2C9-catalyzed

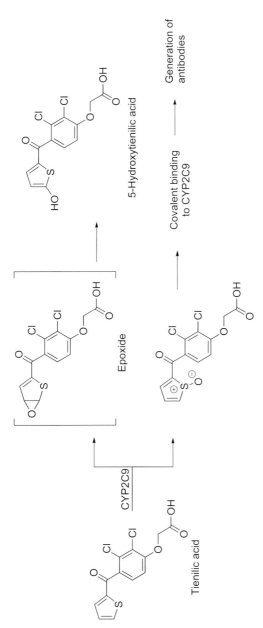

Figure 4.8 Metabolism of tienilic acid by P4502C9.

oxidation to yield a reactive thiophene-*S*-oxide metabolite that can bind covalently with the enzyme and inactivate it [142–146]. It is hypothesized that covalent adduction of CYP with this reactive intermediate is responsible for the immune-mediated hepatitis. TA is very specific in binding to protein targets, unlike acute hepatotoxins such as acetaminophen that bind to a large number of cellular proteins. These specific protein targets (e.g., CYP2C9) may then interact with the immune system, and somehow result in an autoimmune response and the appearance of anti-liver kidney microsome antibodies.

References

1 Park, B.K. and Kitteringham, N.R. (1990) Drug–protein conjugation and its immunological consequences. *Drug Metabolism Reviews*, **22** (1), 87–144.

2 Park, B.K., Kitteringham, N.R., Maggs, J.L., Pirmohamed, M., and Williams, D. P. (2005) The role of metabolic activation in drug-induced hepatotoxicity. *Annual Reviews in Pharmacology and Toxicology*, **45**, 177–202.

3 Pumford, N.R., Halmes, N.C., and Hinson, J.A. (1997) Covalent binding of xenobiotics to specific proteins in the liver. *Drug Metabolism Reviews*, **29** (1–2), 39–57.

4 Pumford, N.R. and Halmes, N.C. (1997) Protein targets of xenobiotic reactive intermediates. *Annual Reviews in Pharmacology and Toxicology*, **37**, 91–117.

5 Mitchell, J.R., Snodgrass, W.R., and Gillette, J.R. (1976) The role of biotransformation in chemical-induced liver injury. *Environmental Health Perspectives*, **15**, 27–38.

6 Mitchell, J.R., Nelson, S.D., Thorgeirsson, S.S., McMurtry, R.J., and Dybing, E. (1976) Metabolic activation: biochemical basis for many drug-induced liver injuries. *Progress in Liver Disease*, **5**, 259–279.

7 Bessems, J.G. and Vermeulen, N.P. (2001) Paracetamol (acetaminophen)-induced toxicity: molecular and biochemical mechanisms, analogues and protective approaches. *Critical Reviews in Toxicology*, **31** (1), 55–138.

8 Vermeulen, N.P., Bessems, J.G., and Van de Straat, R. (1992) Molecular aspects of paracetamol-induced hepatotoxicity and its mechanism-based prevention. *Drug Metabolism Reviews*, **24** (3), 367–407.

9 Nelson, S.D. (1990) Molecular mechanisms of the hepatotoxicity caused by acetaminophen. *Seminars in Liver Disease*, **10** (4), 267–278.

10 David, J.P. (2005) The molecular toxicology of acetaminophen. *Drug Metabolism Reviews*, **37** (4), 581–594.

11 Hinson, J.A. (1980) Biochemical toxicology of acetaminophen. *Reviews in Biochemical Toxicology*, **12**, 103–130.

12 Bock, K.W., Forster, A., Gschaidmeier, H., Bruck, M., Munzel, P., Schareck, W., Fournel-Gigleux, S., and Burchell, B. (1993) Paracetamol glucuronidation by recombinant rat and human phenol UDP-glucuronosyltransferases. *Biochemical Pharmacology*, **45** (9), 1809–1814.

13 Clements, J.A., Critchley, J.A., and Prescott, L.F. (1984) The role of sulphate conjugation in the metabolism and disposition of oral and intravenous paracetamol in man. *British Journal of Clinical Pharmacology*, **18** (4), 481–485.

14 Court, M.H. (2001) Acetaminophen UDP-glucuronosyltransferase in ferrets: species and gender differences, and sequence analysis of ferret UGT1A6. *Journal of Veterinary Pharmacology and Therapeutics*, **24** (6), 415–422.

15 Court, M.H., Duan, S.X., von Moltke, L.L., Greenblatt, D.J., Patten, C.J., Miners, J.O., and Mackenzie, P.I. (2001) Interindividual variability in acetaminophen glucuronidation by human liver microsomes: identification of relevant acetaminophen UDP-

glucuronosyltransferase isoforms. *Journal of Pharmacology and Experimental Therapeutics*, **299** (3), 998–1006.

16 Thomas, S.H. (1993) Paracetamol (acetaminophen) poisoning. *Pharmacology and Therapeutics*, **60** (1), 91–120.

17 Howie, D., Adriaenssens, P.I., and Prescott, L.F. (1977) Paracetamol metabolism following overdosage: application of high performance liquid chromatography. *Journal of Pharmacy and Pharmacology*, **29** (4), 235–237.

18 Tone, Y., Kawamata, K., Murakami, T., Higashi, Y., and Yata, N. (1990) Dose-dependent pharmacokinetics and first-pass metabolism of acetaminophen in rats. *Journal of Pharmacobio-Dynamics*, **13** (6), 327–335.

19 Mutlib, A.E., Goosen, T.C., Bauman, J.N., Williams, J.A., Kulkarni, S., and Kostrubsky, S. (2006) Kinetics of acetaminophen glucuronidation by UDP-glucuronosyltransferases 1A1, 1A6, 1A9 and 2B15. Potential implications in acetaminophen-induced hepatotoxicity. *Chemical Research in Toxicology*, **19** (5), 701–709.

20 Liu, L. and Klaassen, C.D. (1996) Different mechanism of saturation of acetaminophen sulfate conjugation in mice and rats. *Toxicology and Applied Pharmacology*, **139** (1), 128–134.

21 de Morais, S.M. and Wells, P.G. (1989) Enhanced acetaminophen toxicity in rats with bilirubin glucuronyl transferase deficiency. *Hepatology*, **10** (2), 163–167.

22 de Morais, S.M., Chow, S.Y., and Wells, P.G. (1992) Biotransformation and toxicity of acetaminophen in congenic RHA rats with or without a hereditary deficiency in bilirubin UDP-glucuronosyltransferase. *Toxicology and Applied Pharmacology*, **117** (1), 81–87.

23 de Morais, S.M., Uetrecht, J.P., and Wells, P.G. (1992) Decreased glucuronidation and increased bioactivation of acetaminophen in Gilbert's syndrome. *Gastroenterology*, **102** (2), 577–586.

24 Dahlin, D.C., Miwa, G.T., Lu, A.Y., and Nelson, S.D. (1984) *N*-Acetyl-*p*-benzoquinone imine: a cytochrome P-450-mediated oxidation product of acetaminophen. *Proceedings of the National Academy of Sciences of the United States of America*, **81** (5), 1327–1331.

25 Rosen, G.M., Rauckman, E.J., Ellington, S.P., Dahlin, D.C., Christie, J.L., and Nelson, S.D. (1984) Reduction and glutathione conjugation reactions of *N*-acetyl-*p*-benzoquinone imine and two dimethylated analogues. *Molecular Pharmacology*, **25** (1), 151–157.

26 Knox, J.H. and Jurand, J. (1977) Determination of paracetamol and its metabolites in urine by high-performance liquid chromatography using reversed-phase bonded supports. *Journal of Chromatography*, **142**, 651–670.

27 Mitchell, J.R., Jollow, D.J., Potter, W.Z., Davis, D.C., Gillette, J.R., and Brodie, B.B. (1973) Acetaminophen-induced hepatic necrosis. I. Role of drug metabolism. *Journal of Pharmacology and Experimental Therapeutics*, **187** (1), 185–194.

28 Potter, W.Z., Davis, D.C., Mitchell, J.R., Jollow, D.J., Gillette, J.R., and Brodie, B.B. (1973) Acetaminophen-induced hepatic necrosis. 3. Cytochrome P-450-mediated covalent binding in vitro. *Journal of Pharmacology and Experimental Therapeutics*, **187** (1), 203–210.

29 Cohen, S.D. and Khairallah, E.A. (1997) Selective protein arylation and acetaminophen-induced hepatotoxicity. *Drug Metabolism Reviews*, **29** (1–2), 59–77.

30 Potter, D.W. and Hinson, J.A. (1987) Mechanisms of acetaminophen oxidation to *N*-acetyl-*P*-benzoquinone imine by horseradish peroxidase and cytochrome P-450. *Journal of Biological Chemistry*, **262** (3), 966–973.

31 Potter, D.W. and Hinson, J.A. (1987) The 1- and 2-electron oxidation of acetaminophen catalyzed by prostaglandin H synthase. *Journal of Biological Chemistry*, **262** (3), 974–980.

32 Potter, D.W. and Hinson, J.A. (1989) Acetaminophen peroxidation reactions. *Drug Metabolism Reviews*, **20** (2–4), 341–358.

33 Forte, A.J., Wilson, J.M., Slattery, J.T., and Nelson, S.D. (1984) The formation and toxicity of catechol metabolites of

acetaminophen in mice. *Drug Metabolism and Disposition*, **12** (4), 484–491.

34 Dong, H., Haining, R.L., Thummel, K.E., Rettie, A.E., and Nelson, S.D. (2000) Involvement of human cytochrome P450 2D6 in the bioactivation of acetaminophen. *Drug Metabolism and Disposition*, **28** (12), 1397–1400.

35 Chen, W., Koenigs, L.L., Thompson, S.J., Peter, R.M., Rettie, A.E., Trager, W.F., and Nelson, S.D. (1998) Oxidation of acetaminophen to its toxic quinone imine and nontoxic catechol metabolites by baculovirus-expressed and purified human cytochromes P450 2E1 and 2A6. *Chemical Research in Toxicology*, **11** (4), 295–301.

36 Thummel, K.E., Lee, C.A., Kunze, K.L., Nelson, S.D., and Slattery, J.T. (1993) Oxidation of acetaminophen to *N*-acetyl-*p*-aminobenzoquinone imine by human CYP3A4. *Biochemical Pharmacology*, **45** (8), 1563–1569.

37 van de Straat, R., Vromans, R.M., Bosman, P., de Vries, J., and Vermeulen, N.P. (1988) Cytochrome P-450-mediated oxidation of substrates by electron-transfer; role of oxygen radicals and of 1- and 2-electron oxidation of paracetamol. *Chemico-Biological Interactions*, **64** (3), 267–280.

38 van de Straat, R., de Vries, J., and Vermeulen, N.P. (1987) Role of hepatic microsomal and purified cytochrome P-450 in one-electron reduction of two quinone imines and concomitant reduction of molecular oxygen. *Biochemical Pharmacology*, **36** (5), 613–619.

39 Loew, G.H. and Goldblum, A. (1985) Metabolic activation and toxicity of acetaminophen and related analogs. A theoretical study. *Molecular Pharmacology*, **27** (3), 375–386.

40 de Vries, J. (1981) Hepatotoxic metabolic activation of paracetamol and its derivatives phenacetin and benorilate: oxygenation or electron transfer? *Biochemical Pharmacology*, **30** (5), 399–402.

41 Jollow, D.J., Mitchell, J.R., Potter, W.Z., Davis, D.C., Gillette, J.R., and Brodie, B.B. (1973) Acetaminophen-induced

hepatic necrosis. II. Role of covalent binding in vivo. *Journal of Pharmacology and Experimental Therapeutics*, **187** (1), 195–202.

42 Hinson, J.A., Monks, T.J., Hong, M., Highet, R.J., and Pohl, L.R. (1982) 3-(Glutathion-*S*-yl)acetaminophen: a biliary metabolite of acetaminophen. *Drug Metabolism and Disposition*, **10** (1), 47–50.

43 Bartolone, J.B., Sparks, K., Cohen, S.D., and Khairallah, E.A. (1987) Immunochemical detection of acetaminophen-bound liver proteins. *Biochemical Pharmacology*, **36** (8), 1193–1196.

44 Pumford, N.R., Hinson, J.A., Benson, R.W., and Roberts, D.W. (1990) Immunoblot analysis of protein containing 3-(cystein-*S*-yl) acetaminophen adducts in serum and subcellular liver fractions from acetaminophen-treated mice. *Toxicology and Applied Pharmacology*, **104** (3), 521–532.

45 Pumford, N.R., Roberts, D.W., Benson, R.W., and Hinson, J.A. (1990) Immunochemical quantitation of 3-(cystein-*S*-yl)acetaminophen protein adducts in subcellular liver fractions following a hepatotoxic dose of acetaminophen. *Biochemical Pharmacology*, **40** (3), 573–579.

46 Mitchell, J.R., Jollow, D.J., Potter, W.Z., Gillette, J.R., and Brodie, B.B. (1973) Acetaminophen-induced hepatic necrosis. IV. Protective role of glutathione. *Journal of Pharmacology and Experimental Therapeutics*, **187** (1), 211–217.

47 Hoffmann, K.J., Streeter, A.J., Axworthy, D.B., and Baillie, T.A. (1985) Identification of the major covalent adduct formed in vitro and in vivo between acetaminophen and mouse liver proteins. *Molecular Pharmacology*, **27** (5), 566–573.

48 Hoffmann, K.J., Streeter, A.J., Axworthy, D.B., and Baillie, T.A. (1985) Structural characterization of the major covalent adduct formed in vitro between acetaminophen and bovine serum albumin. *Chemico-Biological Interactions*, **53** (1–2), 155–172.

49 Hinson, J.A., Pike, S.L., Pumford, N.R., and Mayeux, P.R. (1998) Nitrotyrosine–protein adducts in hepatic centrilobular areas following toxic doses of acetaminophen in mice. *Chemical Research in Toxicology*, **11** (6), 604–607.

50 Salminen, W.F. Jr., Roberts, S.M., Pumford, N.R., and Hinson, J.A. (1998) Immunochemical comparison of 3′-hydroxyacetanilide and acetaminophen binding in mouse liver. *Drug Metabolism and Disposition*, **26** (3), 267–271.

51 Hazelton, G.A., Hjelle, J.J., and Klaassen, C.D. (1986) Effects of cysteine pro-drugs on acetaminophen-induced hepatotoxicity. *Journal of Pharmacology and Experimental Therapeutics*, **237** (1), 341–349.

52 Smilkstein, M.J., Bronstein, A.C., Linden, C., Augenstein, W.L., Kulig, K.W., and Rumack, B.H. (1991) Acetaminophen overdose: a 48-hour intravenous N-acetylcysteine treatment protocol. *Annals of Emergency Medicine*, **20** (10), 1058–1063.

53 Ruepp, S.U., Tonge, R.P., Shaw, J., Wallis, N., and Pognan, F. (2002) Genomics and proteomics analysis of acetaminophen toxicity in mouse liver. *Toxicological Sciences*, **65** (1), 135–150.

54 Halmes, N.C., Hinson, J.A., Martin, B. M., and Pumford, N.R. (1996) Glutamate dehydrogenase covalently binds to a reactive metabolite of acetaminophen. *Chemical Research in Toxicology*, **9** (2), 541–546.

55 Landin, J.S., Cohen, S.D., and Khairallah, E.A. (1996) Identification of a 54-kDa mitochondrial acetaminophen-binding protein as aldehyde dehydrogenase. *Toxicology and Applied Pharmacology*, **141** (1), 299–307.

56 Coen, M., Lenz, E.M., Nicholson, J.K., Wilson, I.D., Pognan, F., and Lindon, J.C. (2003) An integrated metabonomic investigation of acetaminophen toxicity in the mouse using NMR spectroscopy. *Chemical Research in Toxicology*, **16** (3), 295–303.

57 Reid, A.B., Kurten, R.C., McCullough, S.S., Brock, R.W., and Hinson, J.A. (2005) Mechanisms of acetaminophen-induced hepatotoxicity: role of oxidative stress and mitochondrial permeability transition in freshly isolated mouse hepatocytes. *Journal of Pharmacology and Experimental Therapeutics*, **312** (2), 509–516.

58 Hinson, J.A., Reid, A.B., McCullough, S.S., and James, L.P. (2004) Acetaminophen-induced hepatotoxicity: role of metabolic activation, reactive oxygen/nitrogen species, and mitochondrial permeability transition. *Drug Metabolism Reviews*, **36** (3–4), 805–822.

59 Shen, W., Kamendulis, L.M., Ray, S.D., and Corcoran, G.B. (1992) Acetaminophen-induced cytotoxicity in cultured mouse hepatocytes: effects of Ca (2+)-endonuclease, DNA repair, and glutathione depletion inhibitors on DNA fragmentation and cell death. *Toxicology and Applied Pharmacology*, **112** (1), 32–40.

60 Ray, S.D., Sorge, C.L., Raucy, J.L., and Corcoran, G.B. (1990) Early loss of large genomic DNA in vivo with accumulation of Ca2+ in the nucleus during acetaminophen-induced liver injury. *Toxicology and Applied Pharmacology*, **106** (2), 346–351.

61 Laskin, D.L. and Pendino, K.J. (1995) Macrophages and inflammatory mediators in tissue injury. *Annual Reviews in Pharmacology and Toxicology*, **35**, 655–677.

62 Rehder, K., Forbes, J., Alter, H., Hessler, O., and Stier, A. (1967) Halothane biotransformation in man: a quantitative study. *Anesthesiology*, **28** (4), 711–715.

63 Casorbi, H.F., Vesell, E.S., Blake, D.A., and Helrich, M. (1971) Halothane biotransformation in man. *Annals of the New York Academy of Sciences*, **179**, 244–248.

64 Casorbi, H.F., Blake, D.A., and Heerich, M. (1970) Differences in biotransformation of halothane in man. *Anesthesiology*, **32** (2), 119–123.

65 Cohen, E.N., Trudell, J.R., Edmunds, H.N., and Watson, E. (1975) Urinary metabolites of halothane in man. *Anesthesiology*, **43** (4), 392–401.

66 Karashima, D., Hirokata, Y., Shigematsu, A., and Furukawa, T. (1977) The in vitro metabolism of halothane (2-bromo-2-chloro-1,1,1-trifluoroethane) by hepatic microsomal cytochrome P-450. *Journal of Pharmacology and Experimental Therapeutics*, **203** (2), 409–416.

67 Gandolfi, A.J., White, R.D., Sipes, I.G., and Pohl, L.R. (1980) Bioactivation and covalent binding of halothane in vitro: studies with [3H]- and [14C]halothane. *Journal of Pharmacology and Experimental Therapeutics*, **214** (3), 721–725.

68 Sipes, I.G., Gandolfi, A.J., Pohl, L.R., Krishna, G., and Brown, B.R. Jr. (1980) Comparison of the biotransformation and hepatotoxicity of halothane and deuterated halothane. *Journal of Pharmacology and Experimental Therapeutics*, **214** (3), 716–720.

69 Gruenke, L.D. and Waskell, L.A. (1988) A gas chromatographic mass spectrometric method for the analysis of trifluoroacetic acid: application to the metabolism of halothane by in vitro preparations. *Biomedical and Environmental Mass Spectrometry*, **17** (6), 471–475.

70 Gruenke, L.D., Konopka, K., Koop, D.R., and Waskell, L.A. (1988) Characterization of halothane oxidation by hepatic microsomes and purified cytochromes P-450 using a gas chromatographic mass spectrometric assay. *Journal of Pharmacology and Experimental Therapeutics*, **246** (2), 454–459.

71 Stier, A. (1964) Trifluoroacetic acid as metabolite of halothane. *Biochemical Pharmacology*, **13**, 1544.

72 Sakai, T., Yoshida, H., Fukui, A., and Takaori, M. (1991) Urinary and biliary excretion of metabolites of halothane in dogs. *Drug Metabolism and Disposition*, **19** (2), 419–422.

73 Harris, J.W., Pohl, L.R., Martin, J.L., and Anders, M.W. (1991) Tissue acylation by the chlorofluorocarbon substitute 2,2-dichloro-1,1,1-trifluoroethane. *Proceedings of the National Academy of Sciences of the United States of America*, **88** (4), 1407–1410.

74 Muller, R. and Stier, A. (1982) Modification of liver microsomal lipids by halothane metabolites; a multi nuclear NMR spectroscopic study. *Naunyn Schmiedeberg's Archives of Pharmacology*, **321** (3), 234–237.

75 Van Dyke, R.A. and Gandolf, A.J. (1974) Studies on irreversible binding of radioactivity from (14C)halothane to rat hepatic microsomal lipids and protein. *Drug Metabolism and Disposition*, **2** (5), 469–476.

76 Edmunds, H.N., Trudell, J.R., and Cohen, E.N. (1981) Low-level binding of halothane metabolites to rat liver histones in vivo. *Anesthesiology*, **54** (4), 298–304.

77 Harris, J.W. and Anders, M.W. (1991) The use of 19F NMR in the study of protein alkylation by fluorinated reactive intermediates. *Advances in Experimental Medicine and Biology*, **283**, 735–738.

78 Gut, J., Christen, U., and Huwyler, J. (1993) Mechanisms of halothane toxicity: novel insights. *Pharmacology and Therapeutics*, **58** (2), 133–155.

79 Huwyler, J., Aeschlimann, D., Christen, U., and Gut, J. (1992) The kidney as a novel target tissue for protein adduct formation associated with metabolism of halothane and the candidate chlorofluorocarbon replacement 2,2-dichloro-1,1,1-trifluoroethane. *European Journal of Biochemistry*, **207** (1), 229–238.

80 Huwyler, J. and Gut, J. (1992) Exposure to the chlorofluorocarbon substitute 2,2-dichloro-1,1,1-trifluoroethane and the anesthetic agent halothane is associated with transient protein adduct formation in the heart. *Biochemistry Biophysics Research Communications*, **184** (3), 1344–1349.

81 Nastainczyk, W. and Ullrich, V. (1978) Effect of oxygen concentration on the reaction of halothane with cytochrome P450 in liver microsomes and isolated perfused rat liver. *Biochemical Pharmacology*, **27** (4), 387–392.

82 Nastainczyk, W., Ahr, H.J., and Ullrich, V. (1982) The reductive metabolism of halogenated alkanes by liver microsomal cytochrome P450. *Biochemical Pharmacology*, **31** (3), 391–396.

83 Ahr, H.J., King, L.J., Nastainczyk, W., and Ullrich, V. (1982) The mechanism of reductive dehalogenation of halothane by liver cytochrome P450. *Biochemical Pharmacology*, **31** (3), 383–390.

84 Ruf, H.H., Schuhn, D., and Nastainczyk, W. (1984) EPR titration of ovine prostaglandin H synthase with hemin. *FEBS Letters*, **165** (2), 293–296.

85 Fujii, K., Miki, N., Sugiyama, T., Morio, M., Yamano, T., and Miyake, Y. (1981) Anaerobic dehalogenation of halothane by reconstituted liver microsomal cytochrome P-450 enzyme system. *Biochemistry Biophysics Research Communications*, **102** (1), 507–512.

86 Fujii, K., Morio, M., and Kikuchi, H. (1981) A possible role of cytochrome P450 in anaerobic dehalogenation of halothane. *Biochemistry Biophysics Research Communications*, **101** (4), 1158–1163.

87 Mukai, S., Morio, M., and Fuji, K. (1975) Volatile metabolites of halothane in the rabbit. *Anesthesiology*, **47** (3), 392–401.

88 Sharp, J.H., Trudell, J.R., and Cohen, E.N. (1979) Volatile metabolites and decomposition products of halothane in man. *Anesthesiology*, **50** (1), 2–8.

89 Uehleke, H., Hellmer, K.H., and Tabarelli-Poplawski, S. (1973) Metabolic activation of halothane and its covalent binding to liver endoplasmic proteins in vitro. *Naunyn-Schmiedeberg's Archives of Pharmacology*, **279** (1), 39–52.

90 Van Dyke, R.A. (1975) Metabolism of halothane. *Anesthesiology*, **43** (4), 386–387.

91 Van Dyke, R.A. and Wood, C.L. (1975) In vitro studies on irreversible binding of halothane metabolite to microsomes. *Drug Metabolism and Disposition*, **3** (1), 51–57.

92 Wark, H., Earl, J., Chau, D.D., Overton, J., and Cheung, H.T. (1990) A urinary cysteine–halothane metabolite: validation and measurement in children. *British Journal of Anesthesia*, **64** (4), 469–473.

93 Ullrich, V. and Schnabel, K.H. (1973) Formation and binding of carbanions by cytochrome P-450 of liver microsomes. *Drug Metabolism and Disposition*, **1** (1), 176–183.

94 Pohl, L.R. and Gillette, J.R. (1982) A perspective on halothane-induced hepatotoxicity. *Anesthesia and Analgesia*, **61** (10), 809–811.

95 Allan, L.G., Hussey, A.J., Howie, J., Beckett, G.J., Smith, A.F., Hayes, J.D., and Drummond, G.B. (1987) Hepatic glutathione S-transferase release after halothane anaesthesia: open randomised comparison with isoflurane. *Lancet*, **1** (8536), 771–774.

96 Neuberger, J. (ed.) (1989) *Halothane Hepatitis – An Example of Possibly Immune-Mediated Heptotoxicity*, Elsevier, Amsterdam.

97 Wright, R., Crampton-Smith, A., Hawksley, M., Lloyd, B., Moles, T.M., Trowell, J., Chisholm, M., Eade, O.C., and Edwards, J.C. (1975) Proceedings: a controlled prospective trial of the effect of multiple exposures to halothane on liver function. *Gut*, **16** (5), 403.

98 Trowell, J., Peto, R., and Smith, A.C. (1975) Controlled trial of repeated halothane anaesthetics in patients with carcinoma of the uterine cervix treated with radium. *Lancet*, **1** (7911), 821–824.

99 Stock, J.G. and Strunin, L. (1985) Unexplained hepatitis following halothane. *Anesthesiology*, **63** (4), 424–439.

100 Kenna, J.G., Satoh, H., Christ, D.D., and Pohl, L.R. (1988) Metabolic basis for a drug hypersensitivity: antibodies in sera from patients with halothane hepatitis recognize liver neoantigens that contain the trifluoroacetyl group derived from halothane. *Journal of Pharmacology and Experimental Therapeutics*, **245** (3), 1103–1109.

101 Kenna, J.G., Neuberger, J., and Williams, R. (1987) Specific antibodies to halothane-induced liver antigens in halothane-associated hepatitis. *British Journal of Anaesthesia*, **59** (10), 1286–1290.

102 Kenna, J.G., Neuberger, J., and Williams, R. (1987) Identification by immunoblotting of three halothane-induced liver microsomal polypeptide antigens recognized by antibodies in sera from patients with halothane-associated hepatitis. *Journal of Pharmacology and Experimental Therapeutics*, **242** (2), 733–740.

103 Kenna, J.G., Neuberger, J., and Williams, R. (1988) Evidence for expression in

human liver of halothane-induced neoantigens recognized by antibodies in sera from patients with halothane hepatitis. *Hepatology*, **8** (6), 1635–1641.

104 Kenna, J.G. (1991) The molecular basis of halothane-induced hepatitis. *Biochemical Society Transactions*, **19** (1), 191–195.

105 Vergani, D., Tsantoulas, D., Eddleston, A.L., Davis, M., and Williams, R. (1978) Sensitisation to halothane-altered liver components in severe hepatic necrosis after halothane anaesthesia. *Lancet*, **2** (8094), 801–803.

106 Vergani, D., Mieli-Vergani, G., Alberti, A., Neuberger, J., Eddleston, A.L., Davis, M., and Williams, R. (1980) Antibodies to the surface of halothane-altered rabbit hepatocytes in patients with severe halothane-associated hepatitis. *New England Journal of Medicine*, **303** (2), 66–71.

107 Davis, M., Eddleston, A.L., Neuberger, J.M., Vergani, D., Mieli-Vergani, G., and Williams, R. (1980) Halothane hepatitis. *New England Journal of Medicine*, **303** (19), 1123–1124.

108 Kitteringham, N.R., Kenna, J.G., and Park, B.K. (1995) Detection of autoantibodies directed against human hepatic endoplasmic reticulum in sera from patients with halothane-associated hepatitis. *British Journal of Clinical Pharmacology*, **40** (4), 379–386.

109 Pohl, L.R., Pumford, N.R., and Martin, J.L. (1996) Mechanisms, chemical structures and drug metabolism. *European Journal of Haemotology Supplement*, **60**, 98–104.

110 Smith, G.C., Kenna, J.G., Harrison, D.J., Tew, D., and Wolf, C.R. (1993) Autoantibodies to hepatic microsomal carboxylesterase in halothane hepatitis. *Lancet*, **342** (8877), 963–964.

111 Eliasson, E. and Kenna, J.G. (1996) Cytochrome P450 2E1 is a cell surface autoantigen in halothane hepatitis. *Molecular Pharmacology*, **50** (3), 573–582.

112 Bourdi, M., Chen, W., Peter, R.M., Martin, J.L., Buters, J.T., Nelson, S.D., and Pohl, L.R. (1996) Human cytochrome P450 2E1 is a major autoantigen associated with halothane

hepatitis. *Chemical Research in Toxicology*, **9** (7), 1159–1166.

113 Beaune, P.H., Lecoeur, S., Bourdi, M., Gauffre, A., Belloc, C., Dansette, P., and Mansuy, D. (1996) Anti-cytochrome P450 autoantibodies in drug-induced disease. *European Journal of Haemotology Supplement*, **60**, 89–92.

114 Hahn, B.H., Sharp, G.C., Irvin, W.S., Kantor, O.S., Gardner, C.A., Bagby, M.K., Perry, H.M. Jr., and Osterland, C.K. (1972) Immune responses to hydralazine and nuclear antigens in hydralazine-induced lupus erythematosus. *Annals of Internal Medicine*, **76** (3), 365–374.

115 Perry, H.M. Jr. (1973) Late toxicity to hydralazine resembling systemic lupus erythematosus or rheumatoid arthritis. *American Journal of Medicine*, **54** (1), 58–72.

116 Alarcon-Segovia, D., Wakim, K.G., Worthington, J.W., and Ward, L.E. (1967) Clinical and experimental studies on the hydralazine syndrome and its relationship to systemic lupus erythematosus. *Medicine (Baltimore)*, **46** (1), 1–33.

117 Ludden, T.M., McNay, J.L. Jr., Shepherd, A.M., and Lin, M.S. (1982) Clinical pharmacokinetics of hydralazine. *Clinical Pharmacokinetics*, **7** (3), 185–205.

118 Reidenberg, M.M., Drayer, D., DeMarco, A.L., and Bello, C.T. (1973) Hydralazine elimination in man. *Clinical Pharmacology and Therapeutics*, **14** (6), 970–977.

119 Facchini, V., Streeter, A.J., and Timbrell, J.A. (1980) Determination of hydralazine and its acetylated metabolites in urine by gas chromatography and high-pressure liquid chromatography. *Journal of Chromatography*, **187** (1), 218–223.

120 Timbrell, J.A., Harland, S.J., and Facchini, V. (1980) Polymorphic acetylation of hydralazine. *Clinical Pharmacology and Therapeutics*, **28** (3), 350–355.

121 Lesser, J.M., Israili, Z.H., Davis, D.C., and Dayton, P.G. (1974) Metabolism and disposition of hydralazine-14C in man and dog. *Drug Metabolism and Disposition*, **2** (4), 351–360.

122 Evans, D.A.P. and White, T.A. (1964) Human acetylation polymorphism. *Journal of Laboratory and Clinical Medicine*, **63**, 394–403.

123 LaCagnin, L.B., Colby, H.D., and O'Donnell, J.P. (1986) The oxidative metabolism of hydralazine by rat liver microsomes. *Drug Metabolism and Disposition*, **14** (5), 549–554.

124 Ramsay, L.E. and Cameron, H.A. (1984) The lupus syndrome induced by hydralazine. *British Medical Journal (Clinical Research Edition)*, **289** (6454), 1310–1311.

125 Cameron, H.A. and Ramsay, L.E. (1984) The lupus syndrome induced by hydralazine: a common complication with low dose treatment. *British Medical Journal (Clinical Research Edition)*, **289** (6442), 410–412.

126 Timbrell, J.A., Facchini, V., Harland, S.J., and Mansilla-Tinoco, R. (1984) Hydralazine-induced lupus: is there a toxic metabolic pathway? *European Journal of Clinical Pharmacology*, **27** (5), 555–559.

127 Streeter, A.J. and Timbrell, J.A. (1985) The in vitro metabolism of hydralazine. *Drug Metabolism and Disposition*, **13** (2), 255–259.

128 LaCagnin, L.B., Colby, H.D., Dalal, N.S., and O'Donnell, J.P. (1987) Metabolic activation of hydralazine by rat liver microsomes. *Biochemical Pharmacology*, **36** (16), 2667–2672.

129 Hofstra, A.H. and Uetrecht, J.P. (1993) Reactive intermediates in the oxidation of hydralazine by HOCl: the major oxidant generated by neutrophils. *Chemico-Biological Interactions*, **89** (2–3), 183–196.

130 Hofstra, A.H., Matassa, L.C., and Uetrecht, J.P. (1991) Metabolism of hydralazine by activated leukocytes: implications for hydralazine induced lupus. *Journal of Rheumatology*, **18** (11), 1673–1680.

131 Sinha, B.K. and Patterson, M.A. (1983) Free radical metabolism of hydralazine. Binding and degradation of nucleic acids. *Biochemical Pharmacology*, **32** (22), 3279–3284.

132 Sinha, B.K. (1983) Enzymatic activation of hydrazine derivatives. A spin-trapping study. *Journal of Biological Chemistry*, **258** (2), 796–801.

133 Yamauchi, Y., Litwin, A., Adams, L., Zimmer, H., and Hess, E.V. (1975) Induction of antibodies to nuclear antigens in rabbits by immunization with hydralazine-human serum albumin conjugates. *Journal of Clinical Investigation*, **56** (4), 958–969.

134 Litwin, A., Adams, L.E., Zimmer, H., and Hess, E.V. (1981) Immunologic effects of hydralazine in hypertensive patients. *Arthritis and Rheumatism*, **24** (8), 1074–1078.

135 Litwin, A., Adams, L.E., Zimmer, H., Foad, B., Loggie, J.H., and Hess, E.V. (1981) Prospective study of immunologic effects of hydralazine in hypertensive patients. *Clinical Pharmacology and Therapeutics*, **29** (4), 447–456.

136 Zimmerman, H.J., Lewis, J.H., Ishak, K.G., and Maddrey, W.C. (1984) Ticrynafen-associated hepatic injury: analysis of 340 cases. *Hepatology*, **4** (2), 315–323.

137 Homberg, J.C., Andre, C., and Abuaf, N. (1984) A new anti-liver-kidney microsome antibody (anti-LKM2) in tienilic acid-induced hepatitis. *Clinical and Experimental Immunology*, **55** (3), 561–570.

138 Lecoeur, S., Bonierbale, E., Challine, D., Gautier, J.C., Valadon, P., Dansette, P.M., Catinot, R., Ballet, F., Mansuy, D., and Beaune, P.H. (1994) Specificity of in vitro covalent binding of tienilic acid metabolites to human liver microsomes in relationship to the type of hepatotoxicity: comparison with two directly hepatotoxic drugs. *Chemical Research in Toxicology*, **7** (3), 434–442.

139 Pons, C., Dansette, P.M., Amar, C., Jaouen, M., Wolf, C.R., Gregeois, J., Homberg, J.C., and Mansuy, D. (1991) Detection of human hepatitis anti-liver kidney microsomes (LKM2) autoantibodies on rat liver sections is predominantly due to reactivity with rat liver P-450 IIC11. *Journal of Pharmacology and Experimental Therapeutics*, **259** (3), 1328–1334.

140 Beaune, P., Dansette, P.M., Mansuy, D., Kiffel, L., Finck, M., Amar, C., Leroux, J. P., and Homberg, J.C. (1987) Human anti-endoplasmic reticulum autoantibodies appearing in a drug-induced hepatitis are directed against a human liver cytochrome P-450 that hydroxylates the drug. *Proceedings of the National Academy of Sciences of the United States of America*, **84** (2), 551–555.

141 Lecoeur, S., Andre, C., and Beaune, P.H. (1996) Tienilic acid-induced autoimmune hepatitis: anti-liver and -kidney microsomal type 2 autoantibodies recognize a three-site conformational epitope on cytochrome P4502C9. *Molecular Pharmacology*, **50** (2), 326–333.

142 Dansette, P.M., Amar, C., Smith, C., Pons, C., and Mansuy, D. (1990) Oxidative activation of the thiophene ring by hepatic enzymes. Hydroxylation and formation of electrophilic metabolites during metabolism of tienilic acid and its isomer by rat liver microsomes. *Biochemical Pharmacology*, **39** (5), 911–918.

143 Lopez-Garcia, M.P., Dansette, P.M., and Mansuy, D. (1994) Thiophene derivatives as new mechanism-based inhibitors of cytochromes P-450: inactivation of yeast-expressed human liver cytochrome P-450

2C9 by tienilic acid. *Biochemistry*, **33** (1), 166–175.

144 Lopez Garcia, M.P., Dansette, P.M., Valadon, P., Amar, C., Beaune, P.H., Guengerich, F.P., and Mansuy, D. (1993) Human-liver cytochromes P-450 expressed in yeast as tools for reactive-metabolite formation studies. Oxidative activation of tienilic acid by cytochromes P-450 2C9 and 2C10. *European Journal of Biochemistry*, **213** (1), 223–232.

145 Dansette, P.M., Amar, C., Valadon, P., Pons, C., Beaune, P.H., and Mansuy, D. (1991) Hydroxylation and formation of electrophilic metabolites of tienilic acid and its isomer by human liver microsomes. Catalysis by a cytochrome P450 IIC different from that responsible for mephenytoin hydroxylation. *Biochemical Pharmacology*, **41** (4), 553–560.

146 Koenigs, L.L., Peter, R.M., Hunter, A.P., Haining, R.L., Rettie, A.E., Friedberg, T., Pritchard, M.P., Shou, M., Rushmore, T. H., and Trager, W.F. (1999) Electrospray ionization mass spectrometric analysis of intact cytochrome P450: identification of tienilic acid adducts to P450 2C9. *Biochemistry*, **38** (8), 2312–2319.

5

Pathways of Reactive Metabolite Formation with Toxicophores/-Structural Alerts

Abbreviations

AIA	2-Allylisopropylacetamide
GSH	Glutathione
MI complex	Metabolic-intermediate complex
P450	Cytochrome P450

5.1
Introduction

Toxic properties of xenobiotics are intimately connected to functional groups present within the chemical structures. Organ-directed toxicity can arise from a direct reaction/interaction of proteins and/or DNA with a functional group(s) present in the xenobiotic. Alternatively, the functionality can undergo metabolic activation (also referred to as bioactivation) to a chemically reactive metabolite that can form a covalent adduct with the enzyme that catalyzes its formation or with amino acid residues on proteins and nucleoside bases on DNA. Functionalities capable of reacting directly (intrinsic electrophiles) or via reactive metabolite formation are referred to as toxicophores or structural alerts. This chapter discusses some of the well-known toxicophores that have been associated with bioactivation leading to reactive metabolite formation.

5.2
Intrinsically Reactive Toxicophores

Functional groups that belong to this category can be characterized as those that are intrinsically electrophilic and are associated with direct covalent interactions with DNA and/or proteins via alkylation (so-called "frank" electrophiles). Substituents capable of complexation with metal ion(s) present in enzyme active sites also belong to this category (referred to as metal chelators). Metal chelators can elicit their adverse effects by interacting with or inhibiting important drug-metabolizing

Reactive Drug Metabolites, First Edition. Amit S. Kalgutkar, Deepak Dalvie, R. Scott Obach, and Dennis A. Smith.
© 2012 Wiley-VCH Verlag GmbH & Co. KGaA. Published 2012 by Wiley-VCH Verlag GmbH & Co. KGaA.

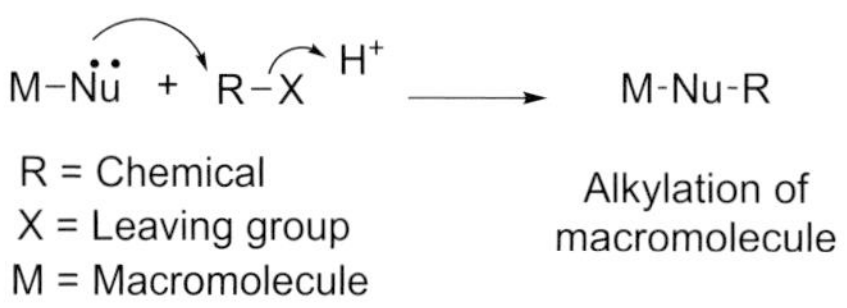

M−N̈u + R−X H⁺ ⟶ M-Nu-R

R = Chemical
X = Leaving group
M = Macromolecule

Alkylation of
macromolecule

Figure 5.1 Schematic representation of reaction of electrophiles with nucleophilic centers on protein macromolecules.

enzymes such as cytochrome P450 (P450) through metal chelation with the heme prosthetic group and causing significant drug–drug interactions via alteration of exposures of concomitantly administered drugs. Alternatively, these toxicophores can indirectly manifest their toxicity by inhibiting critical cellular pathophysiological functions, such as signal transduction and transport and storage of important cellular constituents.

5.2.1
Electrophilic Functional Groups

In the case of electrophiles, which elicit their toxic effects by formation of covalent bonds with nucleophiles (e.g., nucleoside bases on DNA and amino acid residues on proteins), the process often involves transfer of an alkyl/acyl group from the electrophile to a nucleophile (Figure 5.1).

Typical reactions that toxicophores can undergo include alkylation, arylation, and/or acylation. Tables 5.1 and 5.2 highlight the important toxicophores and the corresponding reactions associated with these functional groups. Chemical reactivity is obviously a key parameter with toxicophores that alkylate or acylate proteins or DNA. Highly electrophilic functional groups are often very toxic because they can react nonspecifically with various cellular nucleophiles resulting in cytotoxicity. DNA is the most common target for most alkylating agents. As a consequence of DNA modification, mutations are also triggered, explaining the higher incidence of cancer following their exposure.

Given their ability to alkylate DNA, some electrophilic functional groups have also been exploited as anticancer drugs in the form of alkylating antineoplastic agents. Most of these compounds are dialkylating agents that react with two different guanosine residues present in opposing double-helical DNA strands leading to cross-links. Alkylated DNA does not either coil or uncoil properly, or cannot be processed by information-decoding enzymes leading to tumor suppression. However, in some cases, the electrophile reacts with two guanine groups on the same strand of DNA, resulting in a limpet attachment of the drug molecule to the DNA. Such a covalent attachment does not prevent separation of the two DNA strands and is the main cause of mutations. A classic example of electrophilic chemotherapeutic agents includes nitrogen mustards (Figure 5.2). DNA alkylation by a representative nitrogen mustard scaffold is shown in Figure 5.3.

Table 5.1 Toxicophores that do not require metabolic activation.

Class	[0,2–3]Group	
Alkyl Halides	R-X	$R = sp^3$ carbon; $X = Cl, Br, I, SO_2CH_3$
Michael acceptors	R⌒EWG	R = any functionality; EWG = electron-withdrawing group; COX (X = H, CH_3, OCH_3, NH_2); SO_2CH_3; NO_2
Epoxides	R_1, R, O, R_3, R_2	R, R_1, R_2, R_3 = any alkyl or aryl groups
Thiols and disulfides	R-SH; R-S-S-R	R = alkyl or aryl groups
Activated heterocycles	N LG	LG = leaving groups (Cl, Br, SO_2CH_3, SO_2NH_2, CN)
β-Lactam	R, HN, O	R = any atom

Similarly, the β-lactams have also been used in the clinic despite their potential to acylate proteins and cause immune-mediated toxicity [1]. Some commonly used drugs that carry the β-lactam functionality are shown in Figure 5.4. Additional details on the mechanism of β-lactam pharmacology and toxicity are provided in Chapter 6.

Table 5.2 Reactions of the toxicophores with nucleophiles (Nu).

H—Nu: + R-X ⟶ Nu-R + XH	Alkylation reaction
	Alkylation reaction
	Alkylation reaction
	Acylation reaction
	Alkylation reaction
R-SH + HS—Protein ⟶ R-S-S-Protein	Oxidation reaction

R, any substituent; Nu, nucleophile; EWG, electron-withdrawing group; LG, leaving group.

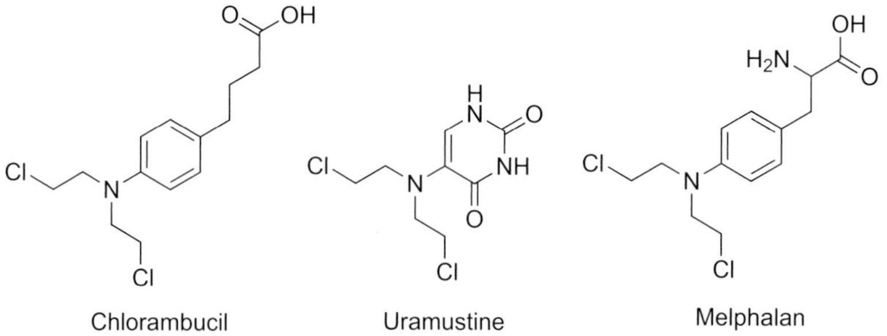

Figure 5.2 Structures of nitrogen mustards used in the clinic in chemotherapy.

5.2.2
Metal Complexing Functional Groups

This class of toxicophores comprises of structural motifs that are capable of complexing with metal ions (particularly the ones present in the active site of

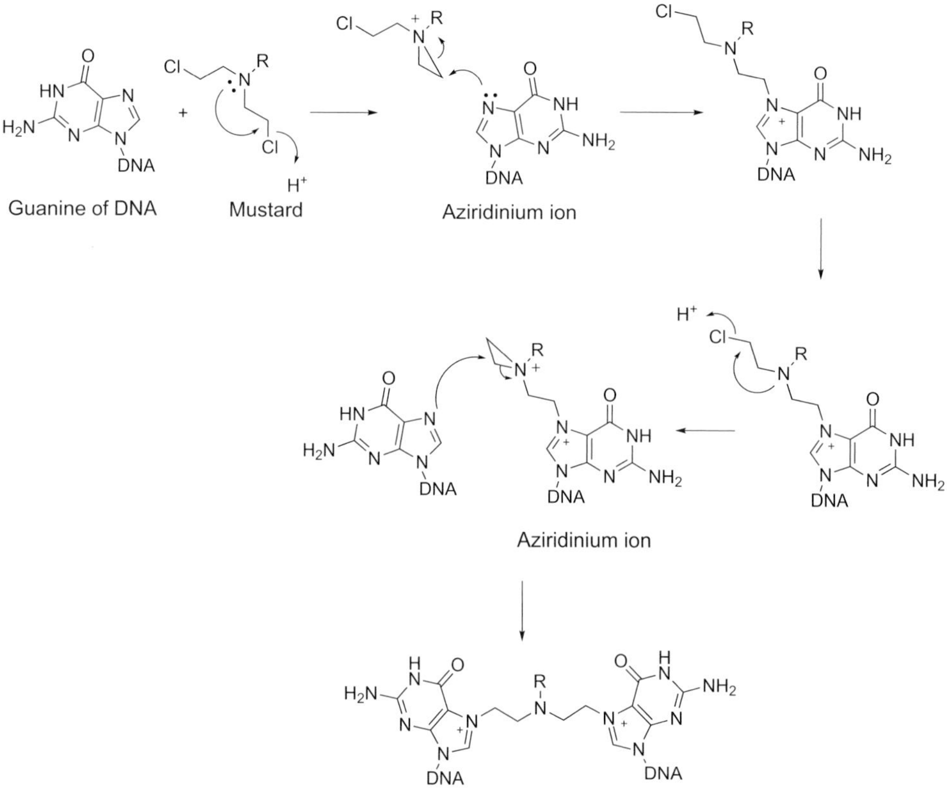

Figure 5.3 Alkylation of DNA by nitrogen mustards.

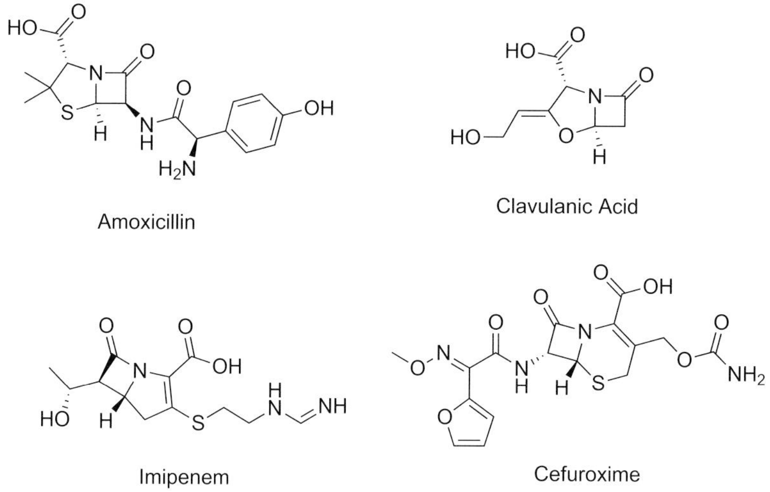

Figure 5.4 Structures of some of the β-lactam antibiotics used in the clinic.

enzymes and in hemoglobin). Compounds that possess metal chelating groups can bind to the lipophilic region of P450 and to the prosthetic heme iron simultaneously [2]. Complexation with heme iron makes such compounds potent inhibitors of P450 enzymes. The inhibitory potency of such compounds is governed by the strength of the bond between the lone pair of electrons present on the heteroatom and the prosthetic heme iron. Most nitrogen-containing heteroaromatic rings belong to this category (e.g., pyridine, imidazoles, etc.). Much work has been performed on imidazole and triazole ring-containing compounds. These agents are recognized as potent ligands of the heme iron atom in the P450 active site. For example, antifungal drugs such as fluconazole, ketoconazole, clotrimazole, and miconazole (Figure 5.5) are inhibitors of P450 and act by complexing with the heme iron [3]. These drugs have been frequently used both systemically and topically (depending on the particular agent) in the treatment of systemic *Candida* infections and mycoses.

Pyridines and pyrimidines are also known to bind directly to the heme iron as illustrated with metyrapone (Figure 5.5), a potent P450 inhibitor. The binding of inhibitors that are strong iron ligands gives rise to a type II difference spectrum. The heterocyclic nitrogen in these fragments displaces weak ligands (water) from the hexacoordinated heme group in P450 enzymes. This leads to the subsequent coordination to the pentacoordinated heme, resulting in the P450 shift from its high- to low-spin dominant form. This spin state change is accompanied by an increase in the redox potential of P450, which makes P450 reduction (by NADPH/P450 reductase) more difficult. Structure–activity relationship studies with HIV protease inhibitors containing a pyridine ring suggest that the substitution on the nitrogen-containing heterocycles and changes in the position of ring nitrogen play an important role in determining the

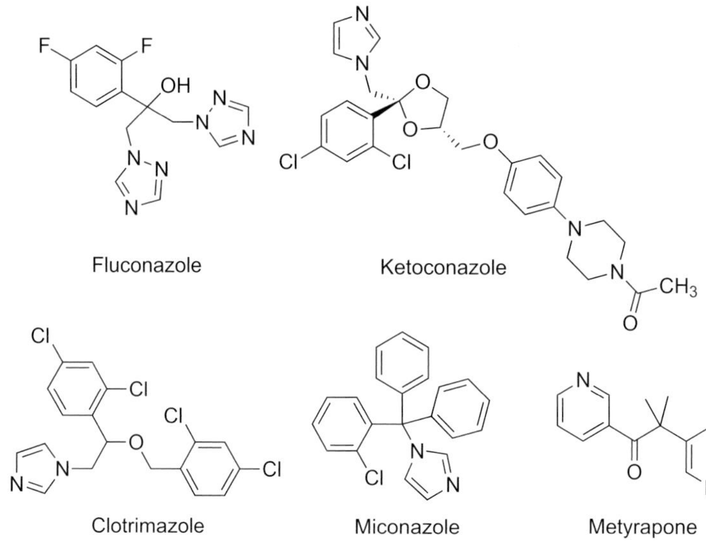

Figure 5.5 Drugs containing heteroaromatic rings that inhibit P450 via complexation with the heme prosthetic group.

manner of interaction with P450 and the concomitant magnitude of enzyme inhibition (Table 5.3) [4].

5.3
Toxicophores that Require Bioactivation to Reactive Metabolites

Most fragments that have been marked as structural alerts in medicinal chemistry belong to this class of toxicophores. Bioactivation of these relatively inert functional groups to reactive electrophilic intermediates is considered to be an obligatory event in the etiology of many drug-induced adverse reactions. Many of these fragments are also associated with higher incidence of mechanism-based inhibition of CYP enzymes. Even though the primary pathway leading to reactive metabolites is generally oxidative in nature, other reductive or conjugative pathways can also lead to reactive species.

5.3.1
Aromatic Amines (Anilines)

Aromatic amines or anilines have long been associated with chemical carcinogenesis, and reports have indicated that the genotoxicity of arylamines is tied to metabolic activation (also see Chapter 2) [5, 6]. The obligatory step in the bioactivation of all anilines involves *N*-hydroxylation on the primary amine nitrogen leading to the formation of the corresponding *N*-hydroxylamine derivatives [7].

Table 5.3 Effect of structural modifications on the type of P450 binding spectra and inhibitory potency against human P4503A4 [4].

Substitution (R)	P450 Binding Spectra	IC$_{50}$ (μM)
Indinavir	II	0.450
	II	0.873
	I	15.1
	I	8.70
	I	19.3

These N-hydroxylamine metabolites can undergo phase II conjugation to generate the more reactive N-O-sulfate and/or N-O-acetyl conjugates. The excellent leaving group tendency of the sulfonyloxy group and the acetoxy groups in the N-O-sulfate and/or N-O-acetyl conjugates [8] is thought to lead to a highly reactive nitrenium that may be the ultimate reactive intermediate involved in DNA adduct formation (Figure 5.6). Alternatively, the N-hydroxylamine intermediates can undergo a two-electron oxidation to an electrophilic nitroso intermediate that can covalently bind to sulfydryl groups in proteins (or with the endogenous antioxidant glutathione (GSH)) to give the corresponding sulfinamide derivative via the corresponding mercaptal intermediate [9]. It is important to note that heteroaromatic amines also undergo similar type of bioactivation reactions leading to formation of nitrenium ion and cause irreversible modification of macromolecules.

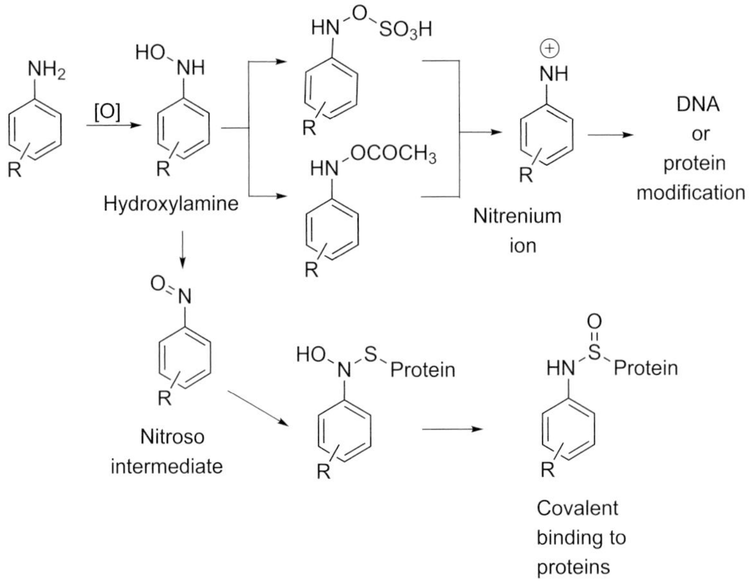

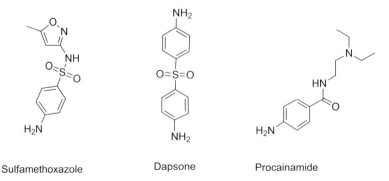

Figure 5.6 Metabolic activation of aromatic amines (anilines).

Noteworthy examples of aniline-containing drugs include the type IA antiarrhythmic agent procainamide, the sulfonamide antimicrobial sulfamethoxazole, used in combination with trimethoprim for the treatment of *Pneumocystis carinii* pneumonia in HIV-infected patients, and the sulfonamide dapsone, which remains the mainstay in leprosy treatment (Figure 5.7). The utility of all these drugs has been hampered by idiosyncratic adverse drug reactions including hypersensitivity reactions, hepatotoxicity, and/or agranulocytosis. Bioactivation of the aniline nitrogen to a reactive nitroso metabolite has been implicated as a causative factor in the toxicity associated with these drugs.

Sulfamethoxazole   Dapsone   Procainamide

Figure 5.7 Illustrations of aniline-based drugs, which are associated with idiosyncratic toxicity.

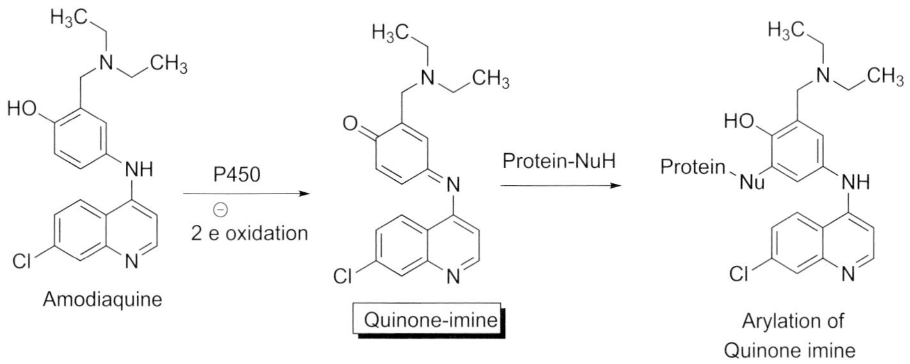

Figure 5.8 Metabolic activation of the antimalarial agent amodiaquine.

5.3.2
ortho- and *para*-Aminophenols

One of the most common pathways of reactive metabolite formation is via an enzymatic two-electron oxidation process on aromatic rings containing electron-rich functionalities in an *ortho* and/or *para* framework. Compounds containing *para*-hydroxyaniline groups are susceptible to oxidative biotransformation via two-electron oxidation to quinonoid species. These intermediates can undergo a Michael-type 1,4-addition with nucleophiles to yield immunogenic adducts that lead to hypersensitivity reactions or even hepatotoxicity. Some classic examples of drugs containing an aminophenol motif include acetaminophen, amodiaquine, and diclofenac. The two-electron bioactivation of acetaminophen by P450 to yield the electrophilic quinone imine intermediate is discussed in greater detail in Chapters 1 and 4. Amodiaquine is an antimalarial agent that is effective against chloroquine-resistant and -sensitive isolates of *P. falciparum*. However, life-threatening agranulocytosis and hepatotoxicity in ~1 in 2000 patients during prophylactic administration led to its withdrawal from commercial use [10]. The 4-aminophenol moiety in amodiaquine undergoes autoxidation or peroxidase-catalyzed two-electron oxidation to the corresponding quinone imine intermediate that can arylate proteins (Figure 5.8) [11, 12].

The nonsteroidal anti-inflammatory drugs diclofenac and lumiracoxib (Figure 5.9a and b) represent masked aniline derivatives that undergo P4503A4- and P4502C9-catalyzed metabolic activation via hydroxylated metabolites (hydroxylation occurs *para* to the nitrogen atom) [13–16]. These hydroxylated metabolites undergo a P450- or a MPO-catalyzed two-electron oxidation to the corresponding electrophilic quinone imine species, and this event is thought to contribute to their idiosyncratic hepatotoxicity in the clinic.

Clozapine, a drug used in the treatment of psychosis and depression [17], is another example of an aniline derivative that undergoes bioactivation via two-electron oxidation to form an iminium ion intermediate that can tautomerize to

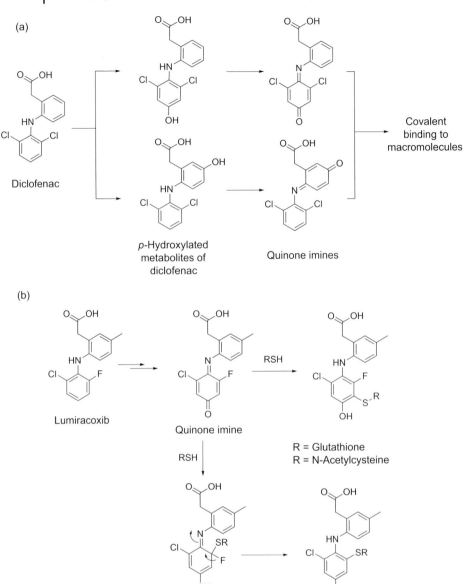

Figure 5.9 Metabolic activation of diclofenac (a) and lumiracoxib (b).

the nitrenium ion intermediate (Figure 5.10) [18]. These reactive intermediates are implicated in the hepatotoxicity and agranulocytosis that is associated with the benzodiazepine-based drug [19–21].

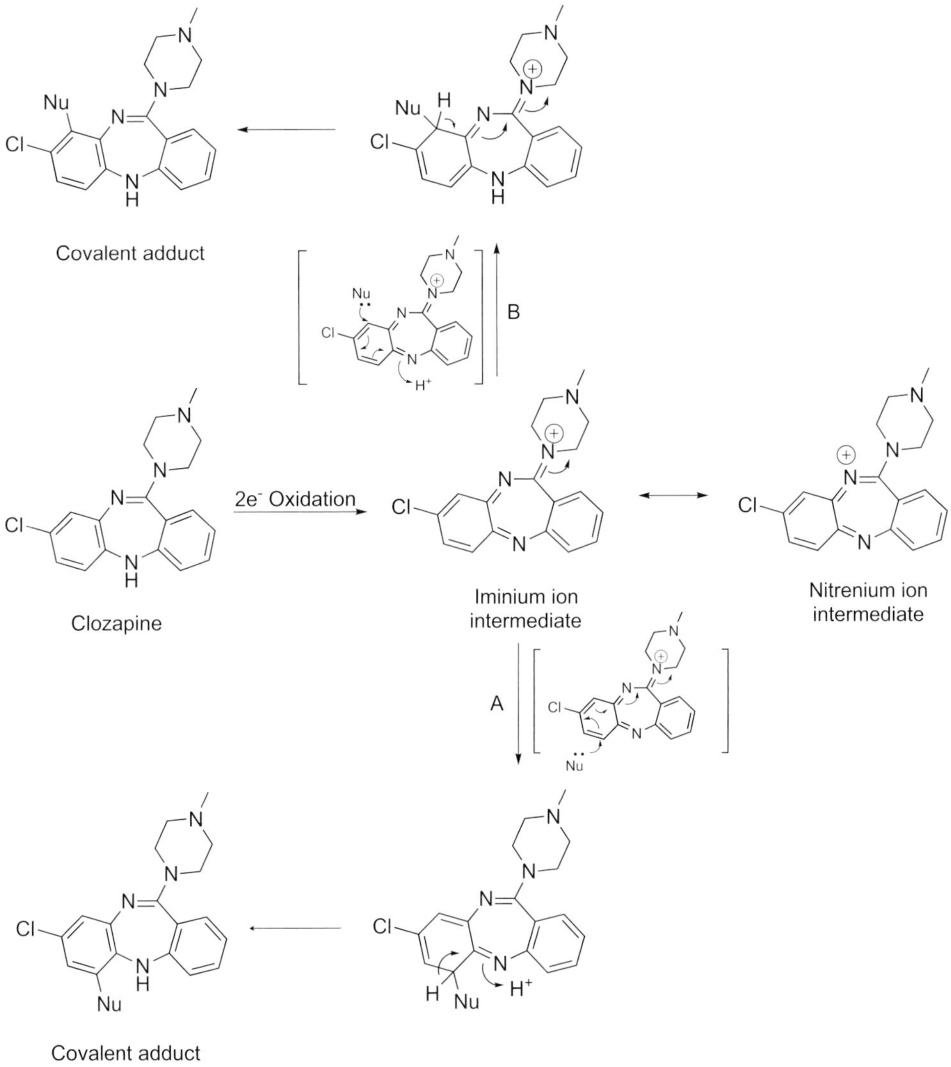

Figure 5.10 Metabolic activation of clozapine into a reactive iminium ion.

5.3.3
Nitroarenes

The toxicological properties of nitroarenes have been the subject of numerous investigations for the past 50 years [22]. A common metabolic fate of most nitro-aromatic compounds involves their six-electron reduction to the corresponding aniline metabolite, which is catalyzed by P450, xanthine oxidase, aldehyde oxidase, and quinone reductase (Figure 5.11) [23]. As described earlier, even

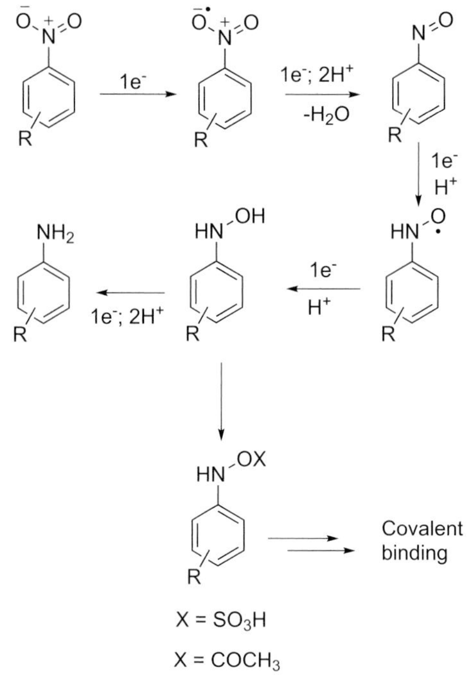

Figure 5.11 Reduction of nitroarenes to aromatic amines.

though covalent adduct formation arising from *N*-hydroxylamine and its *O*-sulfate derivative has been implicated in DNA adduct formation (Figure 5.6), several transient radical intermediates are formed along the way and can cause DNA damage in the form of DNA strand breaks. Some common drugs where reductive bioactivation of nitroarenes has been noted include chloramphenicol, nitrofurantoin, metronidazole, and tolcapone (Figure 5.12). Reductive

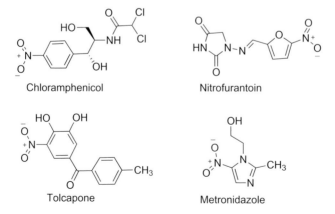

Figure 5.12 Chemical structures of drugs containing a nitro group.

metabolism of the nitro group to the corresponding reactive nitroso metabolite has also been proposed as an alternate mechanism of bioactivation leading to toxicity in the case of chloramphenicol [24].

5.3.4
Hydrazines

Drugs that contain a pendant hydrazine and/or hydrazide motif are potent P450, peroxidase, and monoamine oxidase inactivators and several are also associated with idiosyncratic hepatotoxicity [25–28]. The hydrazine group has been commonly used as an intermediate in the synthesis of a variety of pharmaceuticals including hydralazine (antihypertension), isoniazid (antituberculosis), iproniazid (antidepressant), phenelzine (antidepressant), and procarbazine (anticancer) (Figure 5.13).

Hydrazine-containing compounds undergo bioactivation via formation of diazenes or diazonium intermediates (Figure 5.14). Metabolism studies with phenylhydrazine have provided evidence for the formation of phenyldiazine, phenyldiazonium, and the putative phenyl radical as reactive intermediates. Spin trapping agents phenyl-*t*-butyl nitrone and 4-pyridyl-1-oxide-*t*-butyl nitrone were utilized to detect free radical species in isolated hepatocytes on incubation with isoniazid, iproniazid, and their respective metabolites *N*-acetyl-hydrazine and isopropyl-hydrazine [29, 30].

Hepatotoxicity associated with iproniazid and isoniazid is also linked to the bioactivation of the hydrazine group (Figure 5.15). Studies with isoniazid have shown that *N*-acetylhydrazine, a metabolite that is formed by *N*-acetylation followed by hydrolysis of the resulting *N*-acetylisoniazid, is the ultimate toxin [31–33]. The *N*-acetylhydrazine intermediate undergoes oxidation to form *N*-acetyldiazine that

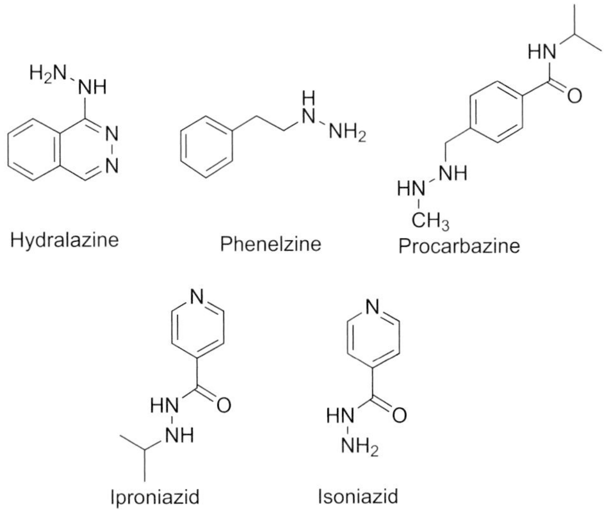

Figure 5.13 Structures of drugs containing a hydrazine/hydrazide motif.

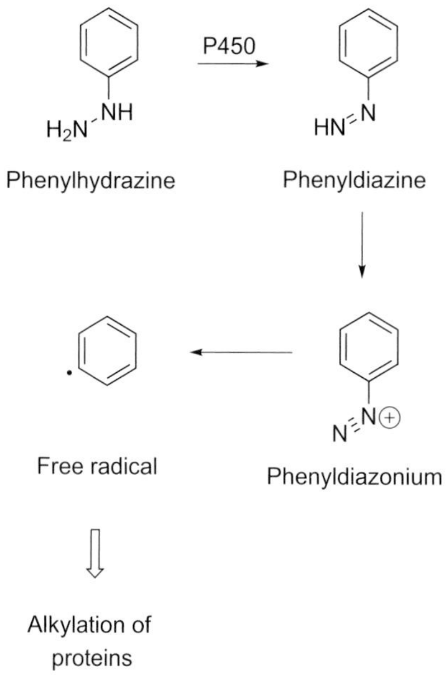

Figure 5.14 Metabolic activation of phenylhydrazine.

ultimately leads to an acetylating species (as either a free radical or an electrophilic acylium species) that can bind to proteins in the liver. Electron spin resonance studies have confirmed the formation of the acetyl free radical in incubations of isoniazid in perfused rat livers.

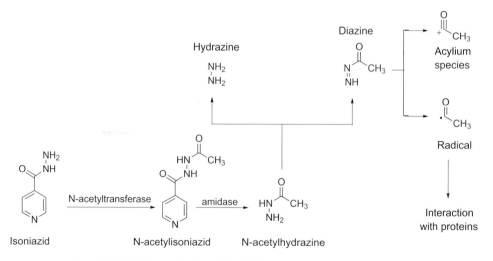

Figure 5.15 Metabolic activation of isoniazid.

5.3.5
Five-Membered Heteroaromatic Rings

Several five-membered heteroaromatic rings including thiophene, furans, and thiazoles have been marked as toxicophores. These heteroaromatic rings are metabolically activated to reactive metabolites that have been associated with liver, lung, and/or kidney necrosis [34, 35].

5.3.5.1 Furans
The importance of P450 in the bioactivation of furan ring has been substantiated by dosing furan or furan-containing compounds to rats pretreated with inhibitors or inducers that either alleviate or augment, respectively, their toxic effects [36]. Several furan-containing compounds such as ipomeanol, furosemide, menthofuran, and methoxsalen cause liver injury and renal necrosis in preclinical species and humans or in some cases form cross-links with DNA when irradiated with ultraviolet light (Figure 5.16) [37–44].

The predominant bioactivation pathway of furan involves its ring scission to α,β-unsaturated dicarbonyl metabolites (also see Chapter 2) [45]. These electrophilic dicarbonyl intermediates react with biological macromolecules via a 1,4-Michael addition across the α,β-unsaturated dicarbonyl moiety or via nucleophilic 1,2-addition to the aldehyde [42, 43, 46]. The mechanism of oxidative opening of furan rings to the corresponding α,β-unsaturated dicarbonyl or γ-ketoacid metabolites is thought to proceed via the initial formation of epoxide intermediate (Figure 5.35 47) [35, 47]. Indirect evidence for the formation of the epoxide intermediate has been reported for furosemide [44]. This epoxide directly rearranges to hydroxyfuran, which predominantly exists as the lactone tautomer. Hydrolysis of the lactone affords the γ-ketocarboxylic acid. The ring opening of the furanoyl epoxide can also lead to formation of γ-ketoenal. Oxidative ring opening of furan and irreversible protein binding of the corresponding substituted γ-ketoenals has been

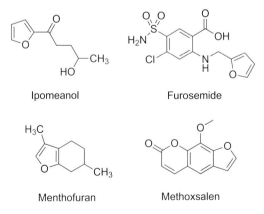

Ipomeanol	Furosemide
Menthofuran	Methoxsalen

Figure 5.16 Structures of furan-based xenobiotics.

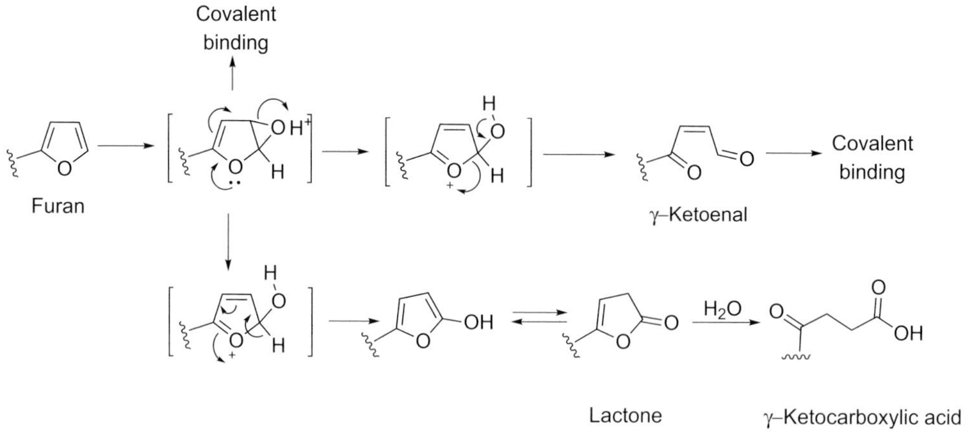

Figure 5.17 Metabolic activation of furans by P450.

reported during metabolism studies on many furan-containing biologically active compounds. Studies with the 5-lipooxygenase inhibitor L-739,010 and an experimental anti-HIV drug, L-754,394, have demonstrated the formation of O-methyloxime derivatives, respectively, suggesting furan ring opening (Figure 5.18) [47, 48].

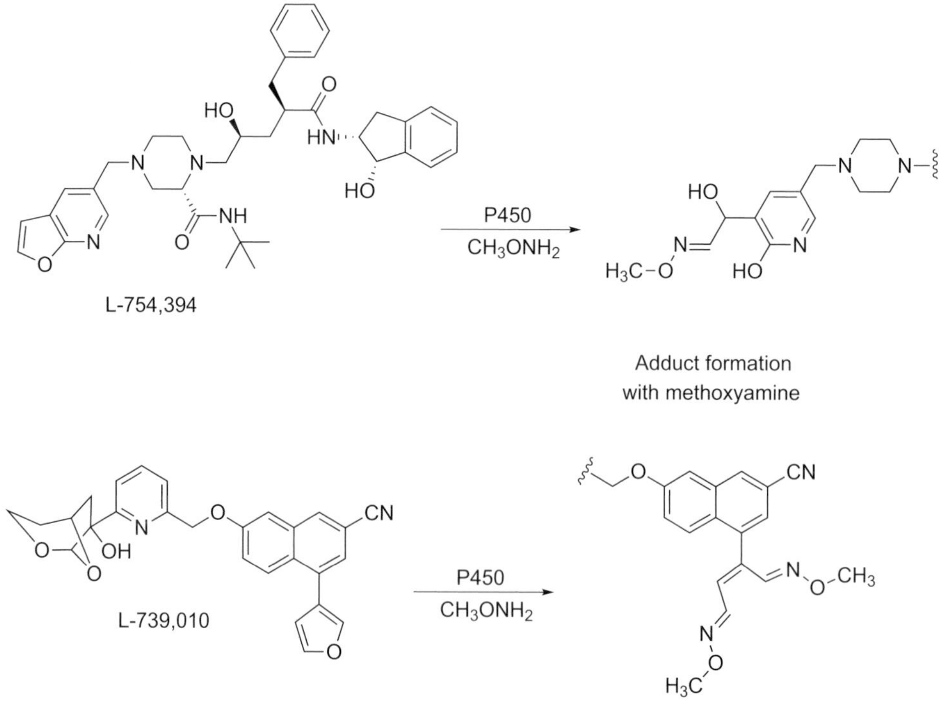

Figure 5.18 Metabolic activation of L-739,010 and L-754,394 and trapping of their corresponding γ-ketoenal intermediates.

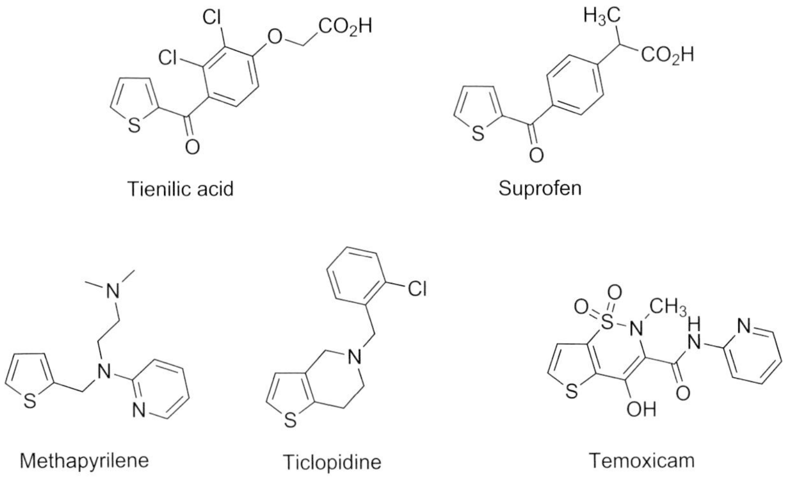

Figure 5.19 Drugs containing a thiophene ring.

5.3.5.2 Thiophenes

The thiophene nucleus is found in several commercially marketed and investigational drugs [49]. Thiophene rings have proven to be an attractive isosteric replacement for phenyl rings in the quest for improved potency and selectivity. However, several drugs containing this ring such as tienilic acid, suprofen, tenoxicam, ticlopidine, or methapyrilene (Figure 5.19) either elicit toxic effects or are mechanism-based inhibitors of P450s [28, 50].

As with furans, the metabolism of thiophenes is principally mediated by P450. In addition to formation of hydroxythiophenes via the obligatory thiophene 2.3-epoxide intermediate, thiophene rings also undergo a P450-catalyzed *S*-oxidation to the corresponding thiophene-*S*-oxide metabolite [51, 52]. This intermediate can form adducts with the sulfydryl residues in proteins via 1,4-Michael addition (Figure 5.20). The evidence for formation of the reactive *S*-oxide intermediate has been demonstrated by detection of the corresponding dimers that are formed via a cyclo-addition of the *S*-oxides, in *in vitro* and *in vivo* studies [51, 53]. In addition, a mercapturic acid conjugate of dihydrothiophene-*S*-oxide has been identified in the urine of rats treated with radiolabeled thiophene. The thiophene-*S*-oxide of tienilic acid has also been suggested as an intermediate in the inactivation of P4502C9. Consistent with P4502C9 inactivation process, antibodies directed to the acylated P4502C9 hapten were found circulating in the serum of individuals administered tienilic acid [54–57].

5.3.5.3 Thiazoles and 2-Aminothiazoles

Thiazoles and 2-aminothiazole groups predominantly undergo P450-catalyzed oxidative ring scission like the furans. In contrast to furans, however, the ring cleavage of substituted thiazoles results in the formation of α-dicarbonyl metabolites and thioamides or thioureas (Figure 5.21) [58–62].

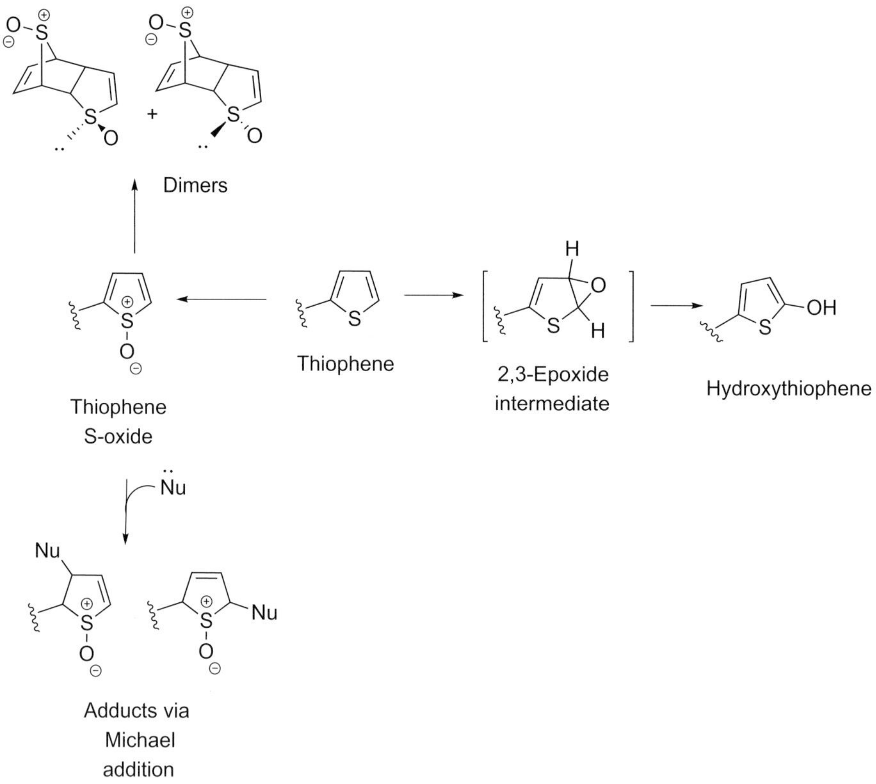

Figure 5.20 Bioactivation of thiophene.

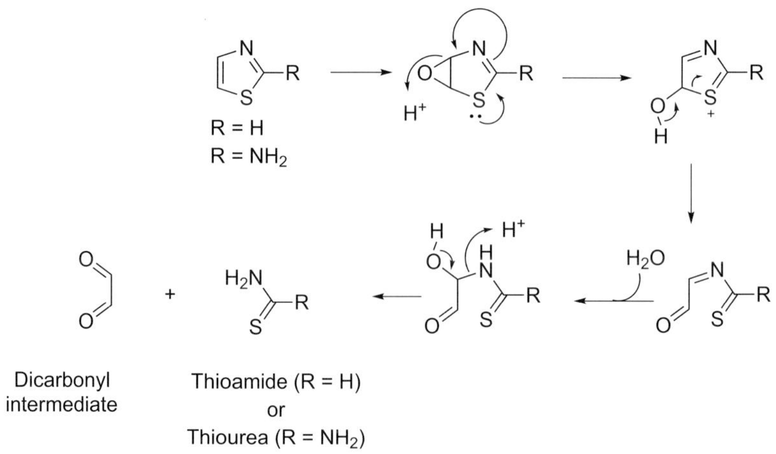

Figure 5.21 Oxidative ring scission of thiazole rings.

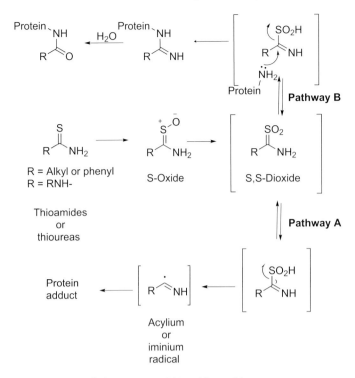

Figure 5.22 Metabolic activation of thioamides or thioureas.

It is well known that compounds containing a thiono functionality can exert various toxic effects, including liver and lung damage [63, 64]. The teratogenic properties of thioureas are also well characterized [65]. The adverse effects of thioamides are attributed to flavin monooxygenase or P450-catalyzed metabolic activation to reactive *S*-oxide (sulfenic acid) and subsequently to corresponding *S,S*-dioxide (sulfinic acid) intermediates that can modify proteins [66–69]. The mechanism involves decomposition of sulfinic acid, to either a carbon-centered acyl or iminium radical via C—S bond scission (Figure 5.22, pathway A) [70]. An alternative pathway involves acylation of the lysine residues in the proteins (Figure 5.22, pathway B) [68].

The well-established toxic properties of thioamides and thioureas have led to the speculation that thiazole toxicity is attributed to the P450-catalyzed cleavage of the heterocycle to the corresponding thioamide metabolites. The products obtained in studies with thiabendazole, a fungicide and antihelmintic agent, provide strong evidence of this ring scission. The primary metabolites following oxidative ring cleavage of thiabendazole include benzimidazol-2-ylglyoxal and thioformamide. The thioformamide thus formed is believed to be the proximate toxicant (Figure 5.23) [71]. Other examples of biologically active thiazoles that undergo ring cleavage to the corresponding thioamide derivatives include the immune-modulatory agent SM-8849, NSAID sudoxicam, and the hepatoprotective agent YH-439 (Figure 5.24) [72–75].

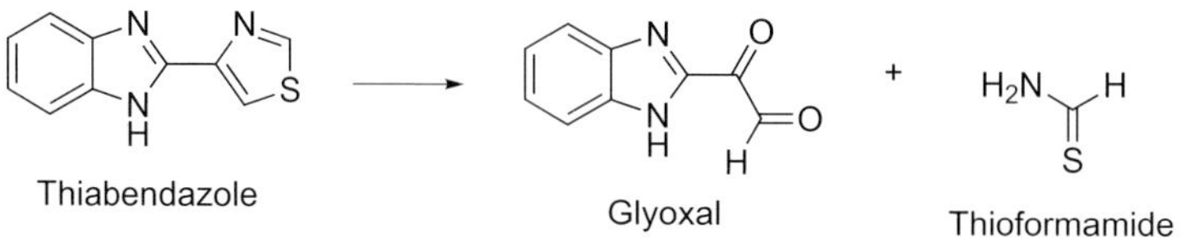

Figure 5.23 Metabolism of thiabendazole.

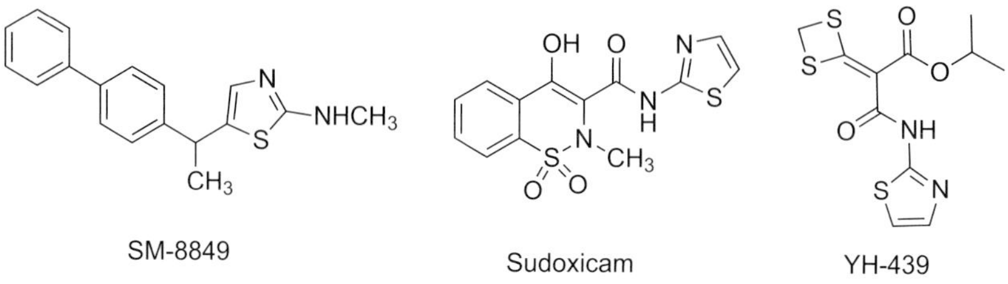

Figure 5.24 Compounds containing a thiazole ring.

5.3.5.4 3-Alkyl Pyrrole and 3-Alkylindole Derivatives

Compounds containing an alkyl group with at least one unsubstituted benzylic hydrogen atom at the C3 position of indole or pyrrole are susceptible to metabolic activation. For instance, 1,3,4-trisubstituted pyrrole analogues are bioactivated by P450 in the presence of NADPH to an iminium methide intermediate possibly via the dehydration of the alcohol (Figure 5.25) [76].

An alternative mechanism involves a P450-mediated two-electron oxidation via an initial hydrogen atom abstraction from the alkyl group followed by a single-electron oxidation that affords the imine-methide as depicted in the case of 3-methylindole (Figure 5.26) [77–81]. The corresponding imine-methide intermediate formed in both the cases can covalently bind to proteins and DNA [82–84]. An alternative pathway for metabolic activation involves epoxidation to 2,3-epoxy-3-methylindole intermediate that can also react covalently with macromolecules (Figure 5.26) [85].

Several 3-alkylindole-containing drugs such as zafirlukast, MK-0524, SPD-304, and L745,870 have been shown to undergo bioactivation by P450s through a similar dehydrogenation pathway (Figure 5.27) [86–89].

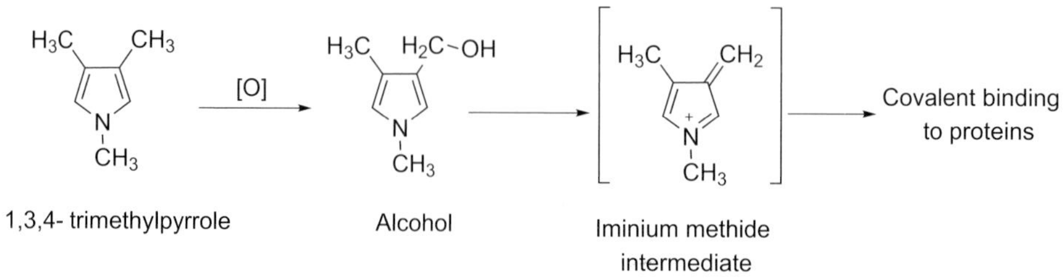

Figure 5.25 Activation of 3-alkylpyrroles.

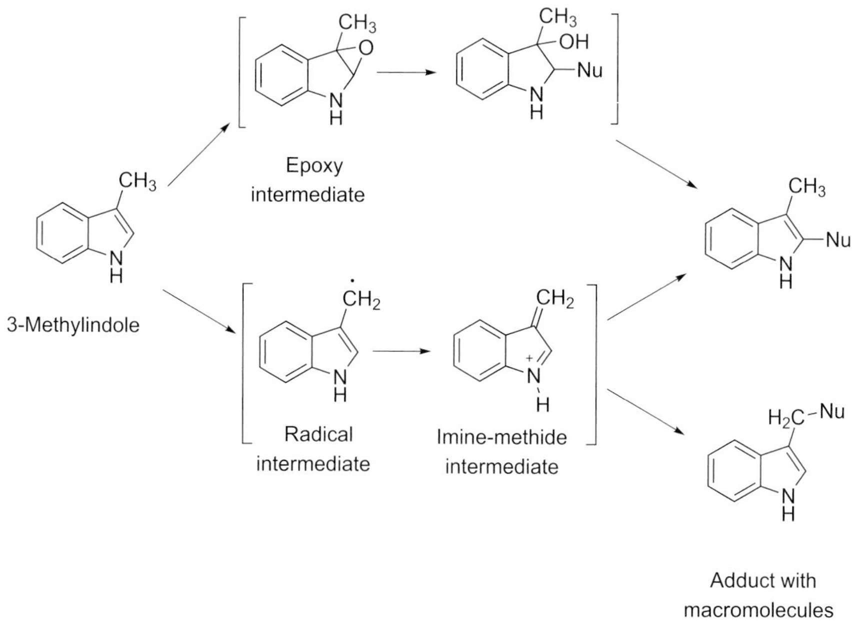

Figure 5.26 Metabolic activation of 3-methylindole.

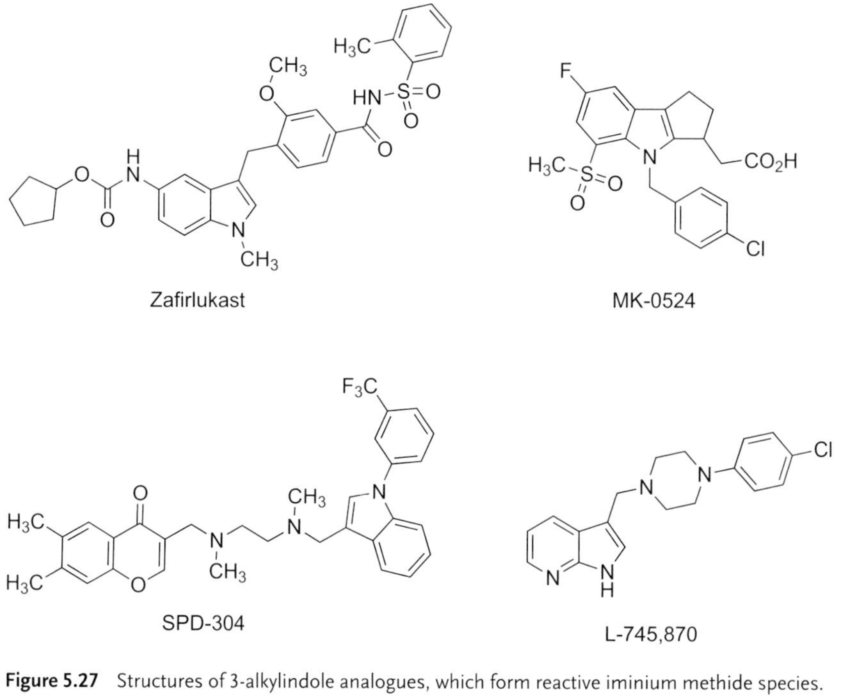

Zafirlukast

MK-0524

SPD-304

L-745,870

Figure 5.27 Structures of 3-alkylindole analogues, which form reactive iminium methide species.

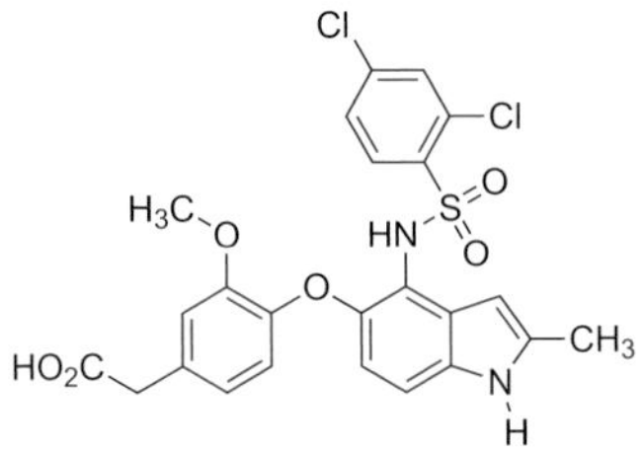

2-Methylindole derivative

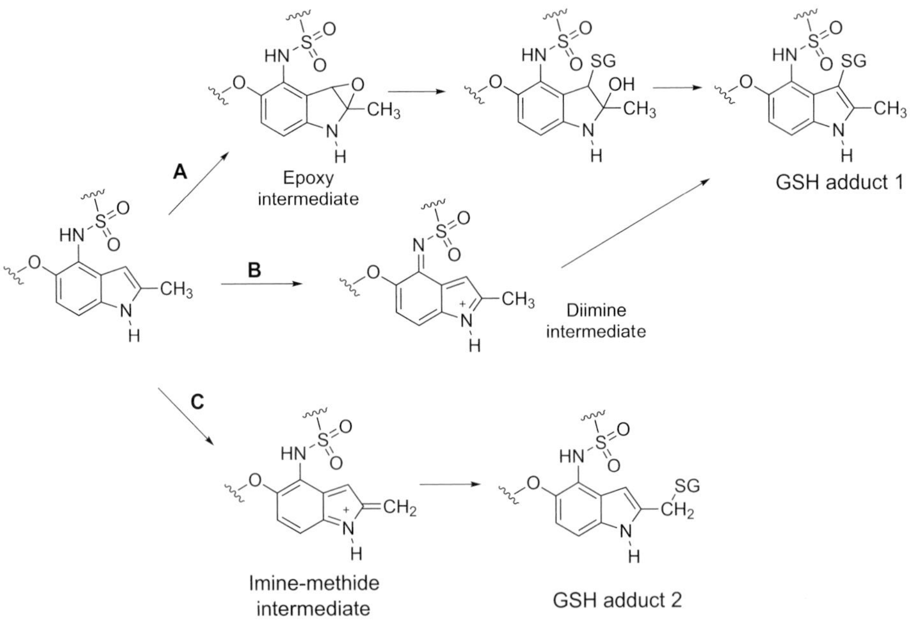

Figure 5.28 Metabolic activation of 2-methylindole derivative.

More recent studies have shown that a 2-methylsubstituted indole (Figure 5.28) also possesses the potential to form reactive metabolites capable of inactivating P450 and covalently binding to macromolecules in a manner similar to the 3-substituted congeners [90]. Two types of sulfydryl adducts have been detected in GSH- and NADPH-fortified microsomal incubation mixtures of the 2-methylindole analogue. Structural elucidation of adducts revealed three possible bioactivation pathways (Figure 5.28). The formation of GSH adduct 1 could be envisioned via epoxidation of the pyrrole ring of the 2-methylindole followed by ring opening of the corresponding epoxy intermediate (pathway A) or its formation via the diimine intermediate (pathway B). Alternatively, pathway C via the imine-methide intermediate would lead to GSH adduct 2 [90].

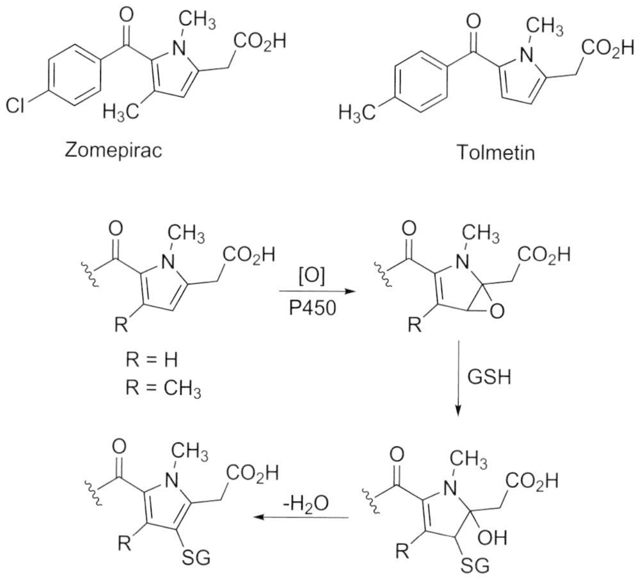

Figure 5.29 Chemical structures of zomepirac and tolmetin and their proposed metabolic activation [91].

The adduct formation via the pathway A (epoxide formation) has also been demonstrated for zomepirac and tolmetin (Figure 5.29) [91]. These 2-alkylpyrrole derivatives are bioactivated via an analogous mechanism involving an epoxide intermediate, and a GSH adduct has been identified with the glutathionyl moiety on the 3-position of the pyrrole ring (Figure 5.29).

5.3.5.5 1,3-Benzdioxole (Methylenedioxyphenyl) Motif

The 1,3-benzdioxole moiety is a common substituent found in natural products and synthetic medicinal agents (Figure 5.30). The functional group is considered to be a bioisostere of dialkoxyphenyl moieties and provides an electron-rich aromatic ring that is more resistant to oxidation relative to its catechol congeners.

As a consequence of its lipophilic nature, the 1,3-benzdioxole group is often a substrate for P450s [92]. The P450-catalyzed metabolism of the 1,3-benzdioxole moiety that leads to formation of catechol and formate metabolites has been well characterized (Figure 5.31) [93–97]. The resulting catechol metabolite is readily oxidized to an *ortho*-quinone that can undergo futile redox cycling resulting in reactive oxygen species. Alternatively, due to the electrophilic nature of *ortho*-quinones, these reactive intermediates have the potential of irreversibly binding to proteins and DNA [26, 98, 99]. The main liability of 1,3-benzdioxole-containing compounds is their potential to inactivate P450 enzymes via metabolic-intermediate complex (MI complex) formation with the enzyme (see Chapter 3) [100, 101]. Although the nature of the intermediate that complexes with the P450 Fe(II) form of the enzyme remains unclear, existing evidence points

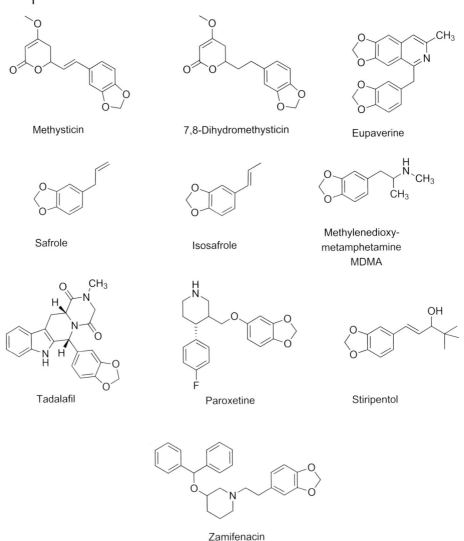

Figure 5.30 Chemical structures of xenobiotics and drugs containing the 1,3-benzdioxole (methylenedioxyphenyl) group.

toward a reactive carbene intermediate that is formed by hydrogen atom abstraction from the methylene carbon or by elimination of water from a hydroxymethylene intermediate. This is an intermediary step in the formation of the catechol metabolite (Figure 5.31).

Drugs that contain 1,3-benzdioxole group such as tadalafil, a phosphodiesterase-5 inhibitor, or paroxetine, a selective serotonin reuptake inhibitor, form MI complexes with human P4503A4 and P4502D6, resulting in the mechanism-based inactivation of these enzymes [102, 103]. The irreversible binding of *ortho*-quinones

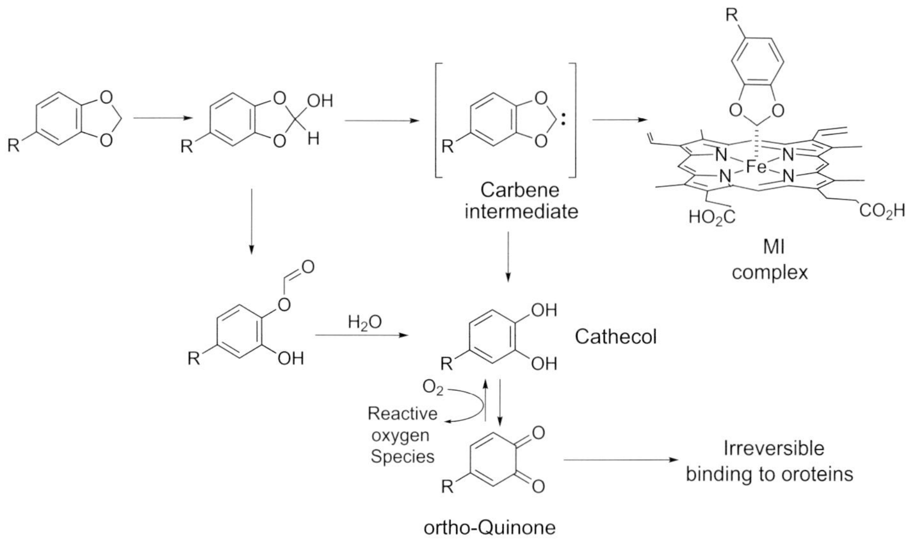

Figure 5.31 Metabolic activation of 1,3-benzdioxole (methylenedioxyphenyl) group.

to the active site of the enzyme has also been proposed as an alternate pathway leading to enzyme inactivation, as exemplified with methylenedioxymethamphetamine (ecstasy) and safrole [98, 99].

5.3.6
Terminal Alkenes and Alkynes

Drugs containing alkene and alkyne functional groups are prone to bioactivation by P450 and have been linked to porphyria. Numerous reports have documented the mechanism-based inactivation of P450 enzymes by alkene- and alkyne-containing compounds. P450-catalyzed oxidation of these functional groups leads to destruction of heme prosthetic group in the enzyme with concomitant formation of "green pigment" [104]. The terminal alkene and sedative hypnotic 2-allylisopropylacetamide (AIA) was one of the first recognized and perhaps the most widely studied irreversible inactivators of P450 [105]. Other examples include secobarbital and alclofenac (Figure 5.32).

Ortiz de Montellano and coworkers have elucidated the nature of the reactive metabolite that is formed by AIA and its allylation to the heme nitrogen (Figure 5.33). Initial studies have shown that this alkylation reaction affords a protoporphyrin IX with AIA bound to one of the nitrogen atoms [105–107].

Like AIA, P450 inactivation by secobarbital involves partitioning of the substrate between N-alkylation of the heme prosthetic group and alkylation of the apoprotein [108, 109]. Similarly, the allylic phenol derivative and nonsteroidal anti-inflammatory drug alclofenac exhibits mechanism-based inactivation of mouse liver microsomal P450 [110]. In this case, the inactivation of the enzyme is mediated by the

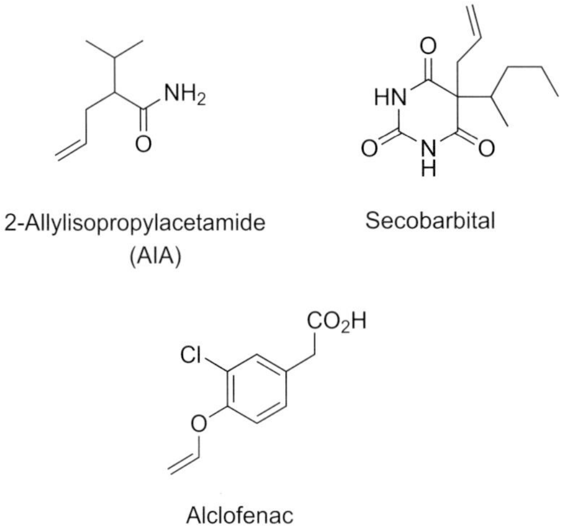

2-Allylisopropylacetamide (AIA)

Secobarbital

Alclofenac

Figure 5.32 Chemical structures of drugs with terminal alkenes as functional groups.

electrophilic epoxide metabolite (Figure 5.34) that is formed by oxidative metabolism of the alkene [111].

P450-catalyzed metabolism of an alkyne group also results in the formation of reactive metabolites that covalently modify the protein resulting in their

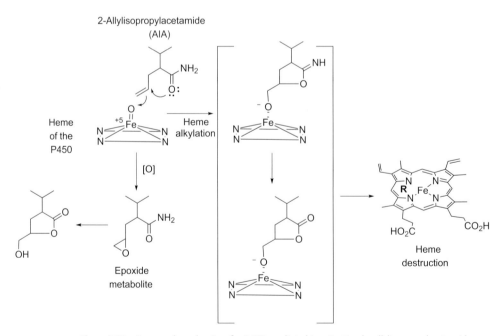

Figure 5.33 Proposed mechanism for P450-mediated inactivation by allylisopropylacetamide (AIA).

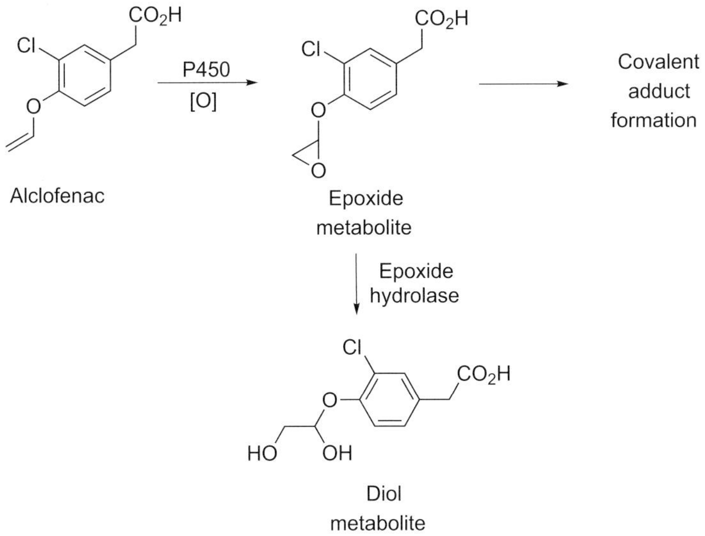

Figure 5.34 Metabolic activation of alclofenac.

inactivation [112]. Like in the case of the alkenes, the mechanism of P450 inactivation involves bioactivation of the alkyne moiety to a reactive species that can alkylate the heme prosthetic group or the apoprotein [113–118]. Two mechanisms for the inactivation process have been described with alkynes (Figure 5.35). In the case of terminal alkynes, oxygenation on the terminal carbon followed by a 1,2-hydrogen shift of the terminal hydrogen to the vicinal carbon is thought to

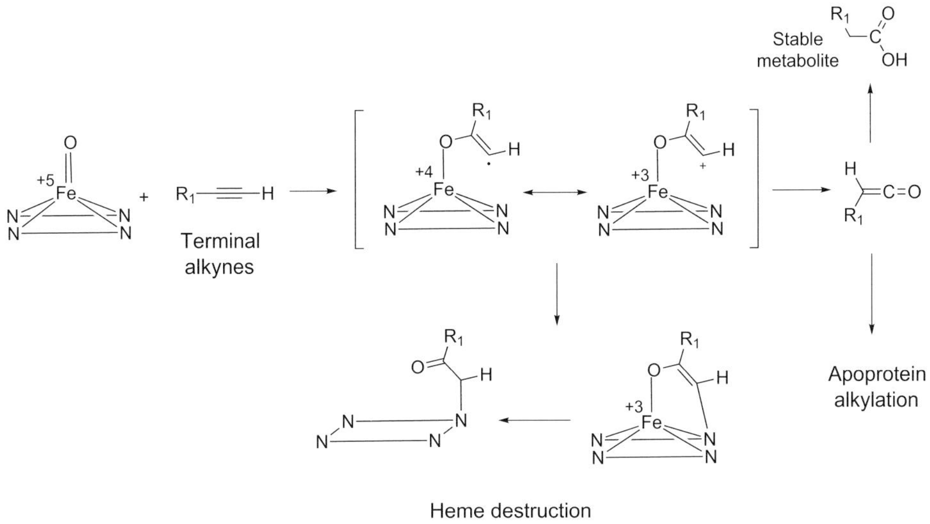

Figure 5.35 Bioactivation of terminal alkynes by P450.

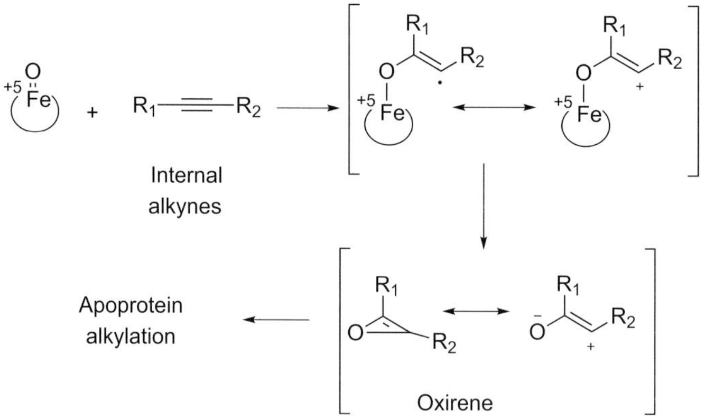

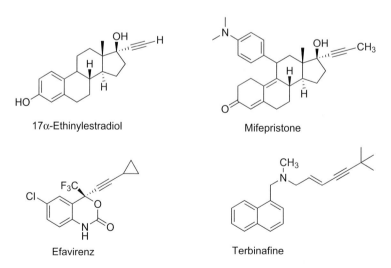

Figure 5.36 Bioactivation of internal alkynes by P450.

generate the reactive ketene intermediate [119]. The ketene can acylate nucleophilic residues within the P450 active site resulting in enzyme inactivation or undergo hydrolysis to the acetic acid metabolite detectable as the stable downstream product of terminal alkyne metabolism (Figure 5.35). With internal alkynes, oxidation on the internal carbon is followed by rearrangement to the oxirene, which then leads to heme or apoprotein alkylation (Figure 5.36) [114, 120].

Compounds that contain an alkyne moiety and are known to inactivate P450 include 17α-ethinylsteroids (e.g., norethindrone, 17α-ethinylestradiol) and the anti-progestin agent mifepristone (Figure 5.37).

Metabolism of 17α-ethinylestradiol by P450 results in irreversible inactivation of the responsible enzymes and destruction of the heme group via alkylation of the

17α-Ethinylestradiol

Mifepristone

Efavirenz

Terbinafine

Figure 5.37 Chemical structures of compounds with terminal and internal alkynes.

porphyrin ring nitrogens [121, 122]. Conversely, the mechanism-based inactivation of P450 with internal alkynes results in alkylation to the apoprotein and not the heme prosthetic group [123]. Efavirenz and terbinafine are other examples of compounds containing internal alkynes (Figure 5.37). Efavirenz produces renal tubular epithelial cell necrosis in rats but not in cynomolgus monkeys or humans. This species selectivity in nephrotoxicity is thought to result from a species-specific metabolism/bioactivation of efavirenz, since detailed comparison of efavirenz metabolites produced by rats, monkeys, and humans indicates that rats produce a unique GSH adduct derived from the bioactivation of the acetylenic group within the drug [124].

5.4
Concluding Remarks

This chapter highlights some of the common functional groups that have shown the propensity to undergo bioactivation to reactive species that can irreversibly bind to macromolecules. Although some groups are intrinsically reactive, others require metabolism to elicit their toxic effects. It is important for the medicinal chemist to be aware of structural features that have a higher than normal propensity for adverse outcomes. For certain structural fragments, there is a gathering weight of evidence that their incorporation into target molecules increases the risk of attrition. One strategy is to avoid these well-defined structural fragments that together represent only a small fraction of the huge diversity of chemical space. A number of excellent and comprehensive reviews have been published that catalog the literature evidence behind fragments of both classes [27, 28, 35, 50, 125–130].

References

1 Rolinson, G.N. (1986) Beta-lactam antibiotics. *Journal of Antimicrobial Chemotherapy*, **17** (1), 5–36.

2 Schenkman, J.B., Sligar, S.G., and Cinti, D.L. (1981) Substrate interaction with cytochrome P-450. *Pharmacology and Therapeutics*, **12** (1), 43–71.

3 Zhang, W., Ramamoorthy, Y., Kilicarslan, T., Nolte, H., Tyndale, R.F., and Sellers, E.M. (2002) Inhibition of cytochromes P450 by antifungal imidazole derivatives. *Drug Metabolism and Disposition*, **30** (3), 314–318.

4 Chiba, M., Jin, L., Neway, W., Vacca, J.P., Tata, J.R., Chapman, K., and Lin, J.H. (2001) P450 interaction with HIV protease inhibitors: relationship between metabolic stability, inhibitory potency, and P450 binding spectra. *Drug Metabolism and Disposition*, **29** (1), 1–3.

5 Hlavica F.P, Golly F.I, Lehnerer F.M, and Schulze F.J. (1997) Primary aromatic amines: their N-oxidative bioactivation. *Human and Experimental Toxicology*, **16** (8), 441–448.

6 Kim, D. and Guengerich, F.P. (2005) Cytochrome P450 activation of arylamines and heterocyclic amines. *Annual Reviews in Pharmacology and Toxicology*, **45**, 27–49.

7 Jones, C.R. and Sabbioni, G. (2003) Identification of DNA adducts using HPLC/MS/MS following in vitro and in vivo experiments with arylamines and

nitroarenes. *Chemical Research in Toxicology*, **16** (10), 1251–1263.

8 Turesky, R.J., Lang, N.P., Butler, M.A., Teitel, C.H., and Kadlubar, F.F. (1991) Metabolic activation of carcinogenic heterocyclic aromatic amines by human liver and colon. *Carcinogenesis*, **12** (10), 1839–1845.

9 Uetrecht, J.P. (1985) Reactivity and possible significance of hydroxylamine and nitroso metabolites of procainamide. *Journal of Pharmacology and Experimental Therapeutics*, **232** (2), 420–425.

10 Neftel, K.A., Woodtly, W., Schmid, M., Frick, P.G., and Fehr, J. (1986) Amodiaquine induced agranulocytosis and liver damage. *British Medical Journal (Clinical Research Edition)*, **292** (6522), 721–723.

11 Maggs, J.L., Tingle, M.D., Kitteringham, N.R., and Park, B.K. (1988) Drug–protein conjugates – XIV. Mechanisms of formation of protein-arylating intermediates from amodiaquine, a myelotoxin and hepatotoxin in man. *Biochemical Pharmacology*, **37** (2), 303–311.

12 Jewell, H., Maggs, J.L., Harrison, A.C., O'Neill, P.M., Ruscoe, J.E., and Park, B.K. (1995) Role of hepatic metabolism in the bioactivation and detoxication of amodiaquine. *Xenobiotica*, **25** (2), 199–217.

13 Tang, W., Stearns, R.A., Bandiera, S.M., Zhang, Y., Raab, C., Braun, M.P., Dean, D.C., Pang, J., Leung, K.H., Doss, G.A., Strauss, J.R., Kwei, G.Y., Rushmore, T.H., Chiu, S.H., and Baillie, T.A. (1999) Studies on cytochrome P-450-mediated bioactivation of diclofenac in rats and in human hepatocytes: identification of glutathione conjugated metabolites. *Drug Metabolism and Disposition*, **27** (3), 365–372.

14 Tang, W., Stearns, R.A., Wang, R.W., Chiu, S.H., and Baillie, T.A. (1999) Roles of human hepatic cytochrome P450s 2C9 and 3A4 in the metabolic activation of diclofenac. *Chemical Research in Toxicology*, **12** (2), 192–199.

15 Shen, S., Marchick, M.R., Davis, M.R., Doss, G.A., and Pohl, L.R. (1999) Metabolic activation of diclofenac by

human cytochrome P450 3A4: role of 5-hydroxydiclofenac. *Chemical Research in Toxicology*, **12** (2), 214–222.

16 Kang, P., Dalvie, D., Smith, E., and Renner, M. (2009) Bioactivation of lumiracoxib by peroxidases and human liver microsomes: identification of multiple quinone imine intermediates and GSH adducts. *Chemical Research in Toxicology*, **22** (1), 106–117.

17 Hummer, M., Kurz, M., Kurzthaler, I., Oberbauer, H., Miller, C., and Fleischhacker, W.W. (1997) Hepatotoxicity of clozapine. *Journal of Clinical Psychopharmacology*, **17** (4), 314–317.

18 Uetrecht, J.P. (1994) Metabolism of drugs by leukocytes. *Drug Metabolism and Drug Interactions*, **11** (4), 259–282.

19 Pirmohamed, M., Williams, D., Madden, S., Templeton, E., and Park, B.K. (1995) Metabolism and bioactivation of clozapine by human liver in vitro. *Journal of Pharmacology and Experimental Therapeutics*, **272** (3), 984–990.

20 Maggs, J.L., Williams, D., Pirmohamed, M., and Park, B.K. (1995) The metabolic formation of reactive intermediates from clozapine, a drug associated with agranulocytosis in man. *Journal of Pharmacology and Experimental Therapeutics*, **275** (3), 1463–1475.

21 Liu, Z.C. and Uetrecht, J.P. (1995) Clozapine is oxidized by activated human neutrophils to a reactive nitrenium ion that irreversibly binds to the cells. *Journal of Pharmacology and Experimental Therapeutics*, **275** (3), 1476–1483.

22 Rosenkranz, H.S. and Mermelstein, R. (1983) Mutagenicity and genotoxicity of nitroarenes. All nitro-containing chemicals were not created equal. *Mutation Research*, **114** (3), 217–267.

23 Boelsterli, U.A., Ho, H.K., Zhou, S., and Leow, K.Y. (2006) Bioactivation and hepatotoxicity of nitroaromatic drugs. *Current Drug Metabolism*, **7** (7), 715–727.

24 Wulferink, M., Dierkes, S., and Gleichmann, E. (2002) Cross-sensitization to haptens: formation of common haptenic metabolites, T cell recognition of cryptic peptides, and

true T cell cross-reactivity. *European Journal of Immunology*, **32** (5), 1338–1348.

25 Ortiz de Montellano, P.R. and Kerr, D.E. (1985) Inactivation of myoglobin by *ortho*-substituted arylhydrazines. Formation of prosthetic heme aryl-iron but not *N*-aryl adducts. *Biochemistry*, **24** (5), 1147–1152.

26 Nelson, S.D. (1982) Metabolic activation and drug toxicity. *Journal of Medicinal Chemistry*, **25** (7), 753–765.

27 Kalgutkar, A.S., Gardner, I., Obach, R.S., Shaffer, C.L., Callegari, E., Henne, K.R., Mutlib, A.E., Dalvie, D.K., Lee, J.S., Nakai, Y., O'Donnell, J.P., Boer, J., and Harriman, S.P. (2005) A comprehensive listing of bioactivation pathways of organic functional groups. *Current Drug Metabolism*, **6** (3), 161–225.

28 Kalgutkar, A.S. and Soglia, J.R. (2005) Minimising the potential for metabolic activation in drug discovery. *Expert Opinion in Drug Metabolism and Toxicology*, **1** (1), 91–142.

29 Tomasi, A., Albano, E., Botti, B., and Vannini, V. (1987) Detection of free radical intermediates in the oxidative metabolism of carcinogenic hydrazine derivatives. *Toxicology and Pathology*, **15** (2), 178–183.

30 Albano, E. and Tomasi, A. (1987) Spin trapping of free radical intermediates produced during the metabolism of isoniazid and iproniazid in isolated hepatocytes. *Biochemical Pharmacology*, **36** (18), 2913–2920.

31 Nelson, S.D., Mitchell, J.R., Snodgrass, W.R., and Timbrell, J.A. (1978) Hepatotoxicity and metabolism of iproniazid and isopropylhydrazine. *Journal of Pharmacology and Experimental Therapeutics*, **206** (3), 574–585.

32 Nelson, S.D., Mitchell, J.R., Timbrell, J.A., Snodgrass, W.R., and Corcoran, G.B. 3rd (1976) Isoniazid and iproniazid: activation of metabolites to toxic intermediates in man and rat. *Science*, **193** (4256), 901–903.

33 Timbrell, J.A., Mitchell, J.R., Snodgrass, W.R., and Nelson, S.D. (1980) Isoniazid hepatoxicity: the relationship between covalent binding and metabolism in vivo.

Journal of Pharmacology and Experimental Therapeutics, **213** (2), 364–369.

34 McMurtry, R.J. and Mitchell, J.R. (1977) Renal and hepatic necrosis after metabolic activation of 2-substituted furans and thiophenes, including furosemide and cephaloridine. *Toxicology and Applied Pharmacology*, **42** (2), 285–300.

35 Dalvie, D.K., Kalgutkar, A.S., Khojasteh-Bakht, S.C., Obach, R.S., and O'Donnell, J.P. (2002) Biotransformation reactions of five-membered aromatic heterocyclic rings. *Chemical Research in Toxicology*, **15** (3), 269–299.

36 Peterson, L.A. (2006) Electrophilic intermediates produced by bioactivation of furan. *Drug Metabolism Reviews*, **38** (4), 615–626.

37 Boyd, M.R. and Burka, L.T. (1978) In vivo studies on the relationship between target organ alkylation and the pulmonary toxicity of a chemically reactive metabolite of 4-ipomeanol. *Journal of Pharmacology and Experimental Therapeutics*, **207** (3), 687–697.

38 Boyd, M.R., Burka, L.T., Wilson, B.J., and Sasame, H.A. (1978) In vitro studies on the metabolic activation of the pulmonary toxin, 4-ipomeanol, by rat lung and liver microsomes. *Journal of Pharmacology and Experimental Therapeutics*, **207** (3), 677–686.

39 Sasame, H.A., Gillette, J.R., and Boyd, M.R. (1978) Effects of anti-NADPH-cytochrome c reductase and anti-cytochrome b5 antibodies on the hepatic and pulmonary microsomal metabolism and covalent binding of the pulmonary toxin 4-ipomeanol. *Biochemical and Biophysical Research Communications*, **84** (2), 389–395.

40 Mitchell, J.R., Nelson, W.L., Potter, W.Z., Sasame, H.A., and Jollow, D.J. (1976) Metabolic activation of furosemide to a chemically reactive, hepatotoxic metabolite. *Journal of Pharmacology and Experimental Therapeutics*, **199** (1), 41–52.

41 Thorgeirsson, S.S., Sasame, H.A., Mitchell, J.R., Jollow, D.J., and Potter, W.Z. (1976) Biochemical changes after hepatic injury from toxic doses of acetaminophen or furosemide. *Pharmacology*, **14** (3), 205–217.

42 Khojasteh-Bakht, S.C., Chen, W., Koenigs, L.L., Peter, R.M., and Nelson, S.D. (1999) Metabolism of (*R*)-(+)-pulegone and (*R*)-(+)-menthofuran by human liver cytochrome P-450s: evidence for formation of a furan epoxide. *Drug Metabolism and Disposition*, **27** (5), 574–580.

43 Khojasteh-Bakht, S.C., Nelson, S.D., and Atkins, W.M. (1999) Glutathione *S*-transferase catalyzes the isomerization of (*R*)-2-hydroxymenthofuran to mintlactones. *Archives of Biochemistry and Biophysics*, **370** (1), 59–65.

44 Wirth, P.J., Bettis, C.J., and Nelson, W.L. (1976) Microsomal metabolism of furosemide evidence for the nature of the reactive intermediate involved in covalent binding. *Molecular Pharmacology*, **12** (5), 759–768.

45 Chen, L.J., Hecht, S.S., and Peterson, L.A. (1995) Identification of *cis*-2-butene-1,4-dial as a microsomal metabolite of furan. *Chemical Research in Toxicology*, **8** (7), 903–906.

46 Chen, L.J., Hecht, S.S., and Peterson, L.A. (1997) Characterization of amino acid and glutathione adducts of *cis*-2-butene-1,4-dial, a reactive metabolite of furan. *Chemical Research in Toxicology*, **10** (8), 866–874.

47 Zhang, K.E., Naue, J.A., Arison, B., and Vyas, K.P. (1996) Microsomal metabolism of the 5-lipoxygenase inhibitor L-739,010: evidence for furan bioactivation. *Chemical Research in Toxicology*, **9** (2), 547–554.

48 Sahali-Sahly, Y., Balani, S.K., Lin, J.H., and Baillie, T.A. (1996) In vitro studies on the metabolic activation of the furanopyridine L-754,394, a highly potent and selective mechanism-based inhibitor of cytochrome P450 3A4. *Chemical Research in Toxicology*, **9** (6), 1007–1012.

49 Bohm, R. and Zeiger, G. (1980) Thiophene derivatives in pharmaceutical research. *Pharmazie*, **35**, 1–9.

50 Kalgutkar, A.S., Obach, R.S., and Maurer, T.S. (2007) Mechanism-based inactivation of cytochrome P450 enzymes: chemical mechanisms, structure–activity relationships and relationship to clinical drug–drug

interactions and idiosyncratic adverse drug reactions. *Current Drug Metabolism*, **8** (5), 407–447.

51 Dansette, P.M., Thang, D.C., el Amri, H., and Mansuy, D. (1992) Evidence for thiophene-*S*-oxide as a primary reactive metabolite of thiophene in vivo: formation of a dihydrothiophene sulfoxide mercapturic acid. *Biochemistry and Biophysical Research Communications*, **186** (3), 1624–1630.

52 Mansuy, D. (1997) Molecular structure and hepatotoxicity: compared data about two closely related thiophene compounds. *Journal of Hepatology*, **26** (Suppl. 2), 22–25.

53 Treiber, A., Dansette, P.M., and Mansuy, D. (2002) Mechanism of the aromatic hydroxylation of thiophene by acid-catalyzed peracid oxidation. *Journal of Organic Chemistry*, **67**, 7261–7266.

54 Dansette, P.M., Amar, C., Valadon, P., Pons, C., Beaune, P.H., and Mansuy, D. (1991) Hydroxylation and formation of electrophilic metabolites of tienilic acid and its isomer by human liver microsomes. Catalysis by a cytochrome P450 IIC different from that responsible for mephenytoin hydroxylation. *Biochemical Pharmacology*, **41** (4), 553–560.

55 Dansette, P.M., Bonierbale, E., Minoletti, C., Beaune, P.H., Pessayre, D., and Mansuy, D. (1998) Drug-induced immunotoxicity. *European Journal of Drug Metabolism and Pharmacokinetics*, **23** (4), 443–451.

56 Dansette, P.M., Bertho, G., and Mansuy, D. (2005) First evidence that cytochrome P450 may catalyze both *S*-oxidation and epoxidation of thiophene derivatives. *Biochemistry and Biophysical Research Communications*, **338** (1), 450–455.

57 Lopez-Garcia, M.P., Dansette, P.M., and Coloma, J. (2005) Kinetics of tienilic acid bioactivation and functional generation of drug–protein adducts in intact rat hepatocytes. *Biochemical Pharmacology*, **70** (12), 1870–1882.

58 Mizutani, T. and Suzuki, K. (1996) Relative hepatotoxicity of 2-(substituted phenyl)thiazoles and substituted thiobenzamides in mice: evidence for the involvement of thiobenzamides as ring cleavage metabolites in the hepatotoxicity of 2-phenylthiazoles. *Toxicological Letters*, **85** (2), 101–105.

59 Mizutani, T., Suzuki, K., Murakami, M., Yoshida, K., and Nakanishi, K. (1996) Nephrotoxicity of thioformamide, a proximate toxicant of nephrotoxic thiazoles, in mice depleted of glutathione. *Research Communications in Molecular Pathology and Pharmacology*, **94** (1), 89–101.

60 Mizutani, T., Yoshida, K., and Ito, K. (1992) Nephrotoxicity of thiazoles structurally related to thiabendazole in mice depleted of glutathione by treatment with buthionine sulfoximine. *Research Communications in Chemical Pathology and Pharmacology*, **75** (1), 29–38.

61 Mizutani, T., Yoshida, K., Ito, K., and Kawazoe, S. (1992) Sex difference in the nephrotoxicity of thiabendazole in mice depleted of glutathione by treatment with DL-buthionine sulphoximine. *Food and Chemical Toxicology*, **30** (3), 247–250.

62 Mizutani, T., Yoshida, K., and Kawazoe, S. (1994) Formation of toxic metabolites from thiabendazole and other thiazoles in mice. Identification of thioamides as ring cleavage products. *Drug Metabolism and Disposition*, **22** (5), 750–755.

63 Chilakapati, J., Shankar, K., Korrapati, M.C., Hill, R.A., and Mehendale, H.M. (2005) Saturation toxicokinetics of thioacetamide: role in initiation of liver injury. *Drug Metabolism and Disposition*, **33** (12), 1877–1885.

64 Neal, R.A. and Halpert, J. (1982) Toxicology of thiono-sulfur compounds. *Annual Reviews in Pharmacology and Toxicology*, **22**, 321–339.

65 Teramoto, S., Kaneda, M., Aoyama, H., and Shirasu, Y. (1981) Correlation between the molecular structure of *N*-alkylureas and *N*-alkylthioureas and their teratogenic properties. *Teratology*, **23** (3), 335–342.

66 Hanzlik, R.P. and Cashman, J.R. (1983) Microsomal metabolism of thiobenzamide and thiobenzamide S-oxide. *Drug Metabolism and Disposition*, **11** (3), 201–205.

67 Hanzlik, R.P., Cashman, J.R., and Traiger, G.J. (1980) Relative hepatotoxicity of substituted thiobenzamides and thiobenzamide-S-oxides in the rat. *Toxicology and Applied Pharmacology*, **55** (2), 260–272.

68 Ji, T., Ikehata, K., Koen, Y.M., Esch, S.W., Williams, T.D., and Hanzlik, R.P. (2007) Covalent modification of microsomal lipids by thiobenzamide metabolites in vivo. *Chemical Research in Toxicology*, **20** (4), 701–708.

69 Henderson, M.C., Krueger, S.K., Stevens, J.F., and Williams, D.E. (2004) Human flavin-containing monooxygenase form 2 S-oxygenation: sulfenic acid formation from thioureas and oxidation of glutathione. *Chemical Research in Toxicology*, **17** (5), 633–640.

70 Nishida, C.R. and Ortiz de Montellano, P.R. (2011) Bioactivation of antituberculosis thioamide and thiourea prodrugs by bacterial and mammalian flavin monooxygenases. *Chemico-Biological Interactions*, **192** (1–2), 21–25.

71 Coulet, M., Eeckhoutte, C., Larrieu, G., Sutra, J.F., Alvinerie, M., Mace, K., Pfeifer, A., Zucco, F., Stammati, A.L., De Angelis, I., Vignoli, A.L., and Galtier, P. (2000) Evidence for cytochrome P4501A2-mediated protein covalent binding of thiabendazole and for its passive intestinal transport: use of human and rabbit derived cells. *Chemico-Biological Interactions*, **127** (2), 109–124.

72 Yabuki, M., Shimakura, J., Ito, M., Kanamaru, H., Iba, K., and Nakatsuka, I. (1997) Metabolism of 4-[1-(2-fluoro-4-biphenylyl)ethyl]-2-methylaminothiazole (SM-8849) in rats. *European Journal of Drug Metabolism and Pharmacokinetics*, **22** (1), 25–33.

73 Hobbs, D.C. and Twomey, T.M. (1977) Metabolism of sudoxicam by the rat, dog, and monkey. *Drug Metabolism and Disposition*, **5** (1), 75–81.

74 Yoon, W.H., Yoo, J.K., Lee, J.W., Shim, C.K., and Lee, M.G. (1998) Simultaneous determination of a new hepatoprotective agent, YH439, and its metabolites, M4, M5, and M7 in plasma and urine by high-performance liquid chromatography. *Research*

Communications in Molecular Pathology and Pharmacology, **99** (1), 117–124.

75 Yoon, W.H., Yoo, J.K., Lee, J.W., Shim, C.K., and Lee, M.G. (1998) Species differences in pharmacokinetics of a hepatoprotective agent, YH439, and its metabolites, M4, M5, and M7, after intravenous and oral administration to rats, rabbits, and dogs. *Drug Metabolism and Disposition*, **26** (2), 152–163.

76 Guengerich, F.P. and Mitchell, M.B. (1980) Metabolic activation of model pyrroles by cytochrome P-450. *Drug Metabolism and Disposition*, **8** (1), 34–38.

77 Bray, T.M., Carlson, J.R., and Nocerini, M.R. (1984) In vitro covalent binding of 3-[14C]methylindole metabolites in goat tissues. *Proceedings of the Society for Experimental Biology and Medicine*, **176**, 48–53.

78 Nocerini, M.R., Carlson, J.R., and Yost, G.S. (1984) Electrophilic metabolites of 3-methylindole as toxic intermediates in pulmonary oedema. *Xenobiotica*, **14** (7), 561–564.

79 Skiles, G.L. and Yost, G.S. (1996) Mechanistic studies on the cytochrome P450-catalyzed dehydrogenation of 3-methylindole. *Chemical Research in Toxicology*, **9** (1), 291–297.

80 D'Agostino, J., Zhuo, X., Shadid, M., Morgan, D.G., Zhang, X., Humphreys, W.G., Shu, Y.Z., Yost, G.S., and Ding, X. (2009) The pneumotoxin 3-methylindole is a substrate and a mechanism-based inactivator of CYP2A13, a human cytochrome P450 enzyme preferentially expressed in the respiratory tract. *Drug Metabolism and Disposition*, **37** (10), 2018–2027.

81 Weems, J.M., Cutler, N.S., Moore, C., Nichols, W.K., Martin, D., Makin, E., Lamb, J.G., and Yost, G.S. (2009) 3-Methylindole is mutagenic and a possible pulmonary carcinogen. *Toxicological Sciences*, **112** (1), 59–67.

82 Regal, K.A., Laws, G.M., Yuan, C., Yost, G.S., and Skiles, G.L. (2001) Detection and characterization of DNA adducts of 3-methylindole. *Chemical Research in Toxicology*, **14** (8), 1014–1024.

83 Thornton-Manning, J., Appleton, M.L., Gonzalez, F.J., and Yost, G.S. (1996)

Metabolism of 3-methylindole by vaccinia-expressed P450 enzymes: correlation of 3-methyleneindolenine formation and protein-binding. *Journal of Pharmacology and Experimental Therapeutics*, **276** (1), 21–29.

84 Lanza, D.L. and Yost, G.S. (2001) Selective dehydrogenation/oxygenation of 3-methylindole by cytochrome p450 enzymes. *Drug Metabolism and Disposition*, **29** (7), 950–953.

85 Yost, G.S. (2001) Bioactivation of toxicants by cytochrome p450-mediated dehydrogenation mechanisms. *Advances in Experimental Medicine and Biology*, **500**, 53–62.

86 Kassahun, K., Skordos, K., McIntosh, I., Slaughter, D., Doss, G.A., Baillie, T.A., and Yost, G.S. (2005) Zafirlukast metabolism by cytochrome P450 3A4 produces an electrophilic alpha,beta-unsaturated iminium species that results in the selective mechanism-based inactivation of the enzyme. *Chemical Research in Toxicology*, **18** (9), 1427–1437.

87 Dean, B.J., Chang, S., Silva Elipe, M.V., Xia, Y.Q., Braun, M., Soli, E., Zhao, Y., Franklin, R.B., and Karanam, B. (2007) Metabolism of MK-0524, a prostaglandin D2 receptor 1 antagonist, in microsomes and hepatocytes from preclinical species and humans. *Drug Metabolism and Disposition*, **35** (2), 283–292.

88 Levesque, J.F., Day, S.H., Chauret, N., Seto, C., Trimble, L., Bateman, K.P., Silva, J.M., Berthelette, C., Lachance, N., Boyd, M., Li, L., Sturino, C.F., Wang, Z., Zamboni, R., Young, R.N., and Nicoll-Griffith, D.A. (2007) Metabolic activation of indole-containing prostaglandin D2 receptor 1 antagonists: impacts of glutathione trapping and glucuronide conjugation on covalent binding. *Bioorganic Medicinal Chemistry Letters*, **17** (11), 3038–3043.

89 Zhang, K.E., Kari, P.H., Davis, M.R., Doss, G., Baillie, T.A., and Vyas, K.P. (2000) Metabolism of A dopamine D(4)-selective antagonist in rat, monkey, and humans: formation of A novel mercapturic acid adduct. *Drug Metabolism and Disposition*, **28** (6), 633–642.

90 Wong, S.G., Fan, P.W., Subramanian, R., Tonn, G.R., Henne, K.R., Johnson, M.G., Tadano Lohr, M., and Wong, B.K. (2010) Bioactivation of a novel 2-methylindole-containing dual chemoattractant receptor-homologous molecule expressed on T-helper type-2 cells/D-prostanoid receptor antagonist leads to mechanism-based CYP3A inactivation: glutathione adduct characterization and prediction of in vivo drug–drug interaction. *Drug Metabolism and Disposition*, **38** (5), 841–850.

91 Chen, Q., Doss, G.A., Tung, E.C., Liu, W., Tang, Y.S., Braun, M.P., Didolkar, V., Strauss, J.R., Wang, R.W., Stearns, R.A., Evans, D.C., Baillie, T.A., and Tang, W. (2006) Evidence for the bioactivation of zomepirac and tolmetin by an oxidative pathway: identification of glutathione adducts in vitro in human liver microsomes and in vivo in rats. *Drug Metabolism and Disposition*, **34** (1), 145–151.

92 Kumagai, Y., Lin, L.Y., Hiratsuka, A., Narimatsu, S., Suzuki, T., Yamada, H., Oguri, K., Yoshimura, H., and Cho, A.K. (1994) Participation of cytochrome P450-2B and -2D isozymes in the demethylenation of methylenedioxymethamphetamine enantiomers by rats. *Molecular Pharmacology*, **45** (2), 359–365.

93 Haddock, R.E., Johnson, A.M., Langley, P.F., Nelson, D.R., Pope, J.A., Thomas, D.R., and Woods, F.R. (1989) Metabolic pathway of paroxetine in animals and man and the comparative pharmacological properties of its metabolites. *Acta Psychiatrica Scandinavica. Supplementum*, **350**, 24–26.

94 Kaye, C.M., Haddock, R.E., Langley, P.F., Mellows, G., Tasker, T.C., Zussman, B.D., and Greb, W.H. (1989) A review of the metabolism and pharmacokinetics of paroxetine in man. *Acta Psychiatrica Scandinavica. Supplementum*, **350**, 60–75.

95 Marquardt, G.M. and DiStefano, V. (1974) The hepatic microsomal metabolism of beta-3,4-methylenedioxyamphetamine (MDA). *Life Sciences*, **15** (9), 1603–1610.

96 Casida, J.E., Engel, J.L., Essac, E.G., Kamienski, F.X., and Kuwatsuka, S. (1966) Methylene-C14-dioxyphenyl compounds: metabolism in relation to their synergistic action. *Science*, **153** (740), 1130–1133.

97 Yu, L.S., Wilkinson, C.F., and Anders, M.W. (1980) Generation of carbon monoxide during the microsomal metabolism of methylenedioxyphenyl compounds. *Biochemical Pharmacology*, **29** (8), 1113–1122.

98 Wu, D., Otton, S.V., Inaba, T., Kalow, W., and Sellers, E.M. (1997) Interactions of amphetamine analogs with human liver CYP2D6. *Biochemical Pharmacology*, **53** (11), 1605–1612.

99 Bolton, J.L., Acay, N.M., and Vukomanovic, V. (1994) Evidence that 4-allyl-*o*-quinones spontaneously rearrange to their more electrophilic quinone methides: potential bioactivation mechanism for the hepatocarcinogen safrole. *Chemical Research in Toxicology*, **7** (3), 443–450.

100 Murray, M. (2000) Mechanisms of inhibitory and regulatory effects of methylenedioxyphenyl compounds on cytochrome P450-dependent drug oxidation. *Current Drug Metabolism*, **1** (1), 67–84.

101 Fukuto, J.M., Kumagai, Y., and Cho, A.K. (1991) Determination of the mechanism of demethylenation of (methylenedioxy)phenyl compounds by cytochrome P450 using deuterium isotope effects. *Journal of Medicinal Chemistry*, **34** (9), 2871–2876.

102 Bertelsen, K.M., Venkatakrishnan, K., Von Moltke, L.L., Obach, R.S., and Greenblatt, D.J. (2003) Apparent mechanism-based inhibition of human CYP2D6 in vitro by paroxetine: comparison with fluoxetine and quinidine. *Drug Metabolism and Disposition*, **31** (3), 289–293.

103 Ring, B.J., Patterson, B.E., Mitchell, M.I., Vandenbranden, M., Gillespie, J., Bedding, A.W., Jewell, H., Payne, C.D., Forgue, S.T., Eckstein, J., Wrighton, S.A., and Phillips, D.L. (2005) Effect of tadalafil on cytochrome P450 3A4-mediated clearance: studies in vitro and

in vivo. *Clinical Pharmacology and Therapeutics*, **77** (1), 63–75.

104 Testa, B. and Jenner, P. (1981) Inhibitors of cytochrome P-450s and their mechanism of action. *Drug Metabolism Reviews*, **12** (1), 1–117.

105 Ortiz de Montellano, P.R. and Mico, B.A. (1981) Destruction of cytochrome P-450 by allylisopropylacetamide is a suicidal process. *Archives of Biochemistry and Biophysics*, **206** (1), 43–50.

106 Silber, B., Mico, B.A., Ortiz de Montellano, P.R., Dols, D.M., and Riegelman, S. (1981) In vivo effects of the cytochrome P-450 suicide substrate 2-isopropyl-4-pentenamide (allylisopropylacetamide) on the disposition and metabolic pattern of propranolol. *Journal of Pharmacology and Experimental Therapeutics*, **219** (1), 125–133.

107 Ortiz de Montellano, P.R., Yost, G.S., Mico, B.A., Dinizo, S.E., Correia, M.A., and Kumbara, H. (1979) Destruction of cytochrome P-450 by 2-isopropyl-4-pentenamide and methyl 2-isopropyl-4-pentenoate: mass spectrometric characterization of prosthetic heme adducts and nonparticipation of epoxide metabolites. *Archives of Biochemistry and Biophysics*, **197** (2), 524–533.

108 Levin, W., Jacobson, M., Sernatinger, E., and Kuntzman, R. (1973) Breakdown of cytochrome P-450 heme by secobarbital and other allyl-containing barbiturates. *Drug Metabolism and Disposition*, **1** (1), 275–285.

109 Lunetta, J.M., Sugiyama, K., and Correia, M.A. (1989) Secobarbital-mediated inactivation of rat liver cytochrome P-450b: a mechanistic reappraisal. *Molecular Pharmacology*, **35** (1), 10–17.

110 Brown, L.M. and Ford-Hutchinson, A.W. (1982) The destruction of cytochrome P-450 by alclofenac: possible involvement of an epoxide metabolite. *Biochemical Pharmacology*, **31** (2), 195–199.

111 Slack, J.A. and Ford-Hutchinson, A.W. (1980) Determination of a urinary epoxide metabolite of alclofenac in man. *Drug Metabolism and Disposition*, **8** (2), 84–86.

112 Ortiz de Montellano, P.R. and Kunze, K.L. (1980) Self-catalyzed inactivation of hepatic cytochrome P-450 by ethynyl substrates. *Journal of Biological Chemistry*, **255** (12), 5578–5585.

113 Roberts, E.S., Hopkins, N.E., Zaluzec, E.J., Gage, D.A., Alworth, W.L., and Hollenberg, P.F. (1994) Identification of active-site peptides from 3H-labeled 2-ethynylnaphthalene-inactivated P450 2B1 and 2B4 using amino acid sequencing and mass spectrometry. *Biochemistry*, **33** (12), 3766–3771.

114 Roberts, E.S., Hopkins, N.E., Foroozesh, M., Alworth, W.L., Halpert, J.R., and Hollenberg, P.F. (1997) Inactivation of cytochrome P450s 2B1, 2B4, 2B6, and 2B11 by arylalkynes. *Drug Metabolism and Disposition*, **25** (11), 1242–1248.

115 Ortiz de Montellano, P.R., Mico, B.A., Mathews, J.M., Kunze, K.L., Miwa, G.T., and Lu, A.Y. (1981) Selective inactivation of cytochrome P-450 isozymes by suicide substrates. *Archives of Biochemistry and Biophysics*, **210** (2), 717–728.

116 Ortiz de Montellano, P.R. and Kunze, K.L. (1981) Cytochrome P-450 inactivation: structure of the prosthetic heme adduct with propyne. *Biochemistry*, **20** (25), 7266–7271.

117 Correia, M.A., Farrell, G.C., Olson, S., Wong, J.S., Schmid, R., Ortiz de Montellano, P.R., Beilan, H.S., Kunze, K.L., and Mico, B.A. (1981) Cytochrome P-450 heme moiety. The specific target in drug-induced heme alkylation. *Journal of Biological Chemistry*, **256** (11), 5466–5470.

118 Ortiz de Montellano, P.R., Kunze, K.L., Yost, G.S., and Mico, B.A. (1979) Self-catalyzed destruction of cytochrome P-450: covalent binding of ethynyl sterols to prosthetic heme. *Proceedings of the National Academy of Sciences of the United States of America*, **76** (2), 746–749.

119 Ortiz de Montellano, P.R. and Komives, E.A. (1985) Branchpoint for heme alkylation and metabolite formation in the oxidation of arylacetylenes by cytochrome P-450. *Journal of Biological Chemistry*, **260** (6), 3330–3336.

120 Foroozesh, M., Primrose, G., Guo, Z., Bell, L.C., Alworth, W.L., and Guengerich, F.P. (1997) Aryl acetylenes as mechanism-based inhibitors of cytochrome P450-dependent monooxygenase enzymes. *Chemical Research in Toxicology*, **10** (1), 91–102.

121 Lin, H.L., Kent, U.M., and Hollenberg, P.F. (2002) Mechanism-based inactivation of cytochrome P450 3A4 by 17 alpha-ethynylestradiol: evidence for heme destruction and covalent binding to protein. *Journal of Pharmacology and Experimental Therapeutics*, **301** (1), 160–167.

122 Guengerich, F.P. (1988) Oxidation of 17 alpha-ethynylestradiol by human liver cytochrome P-450. *Molecular Pharmacology*, **33** (5), 500–508.

123 He, K., Woolf, T.F., and Hollenberg, P.F. (1999) Mechanism-based inactivation of cytochrome P-450-3A4 by mifepristone (RU486). *Journal of Pharmacology and Experimental Therapeutics*, **288** (2), 791–797.

124 Mutlib, A.E., Gerson, R.J., Meunier, P.C., Haley, P.J., Chen, H., Gan, L.S., Davies, M. H., Gemzik, B., Christ, D.D., Krahn, D.F., Markwalder, J.A., Seitz, S.P., Robertson, R. T., and Miwa, G.T. (2000) The species-dependent metabolism of efavirenz produces a nephrotoxic glutathione conjugate in rats. *Toxicology and Applied Pharmacology*, **169** (1), 102–113.

125 Williams, D.P. and Park, B.K. (2003) Idiosyncratic toxicity: the role of toxicophores and bioactivation. *Drug Discovery Today*, **8** (22), 1044–1050.

126 Kalgutkar, A.S. and Didiuk, M.T. (2009) Structural alerts, reactive metabolites, and protein covalent binding: how reliable are these attributes as predictors of drug toxicity? *Chemistry and Biodiversity*, **6** (11), 2115–2137.

127 Kalgutkar, A.S., Fate, G., Didiuk, M.T., and Bauman, J. (2008) Toxicophores, reactive metabolites and drug safety: when is it a cause for concern. *Expert Reviews in Clinical Pharmacology*, **1** (1), 515–531.

128 Kalgutkar, A.S. (2011) Handling reactive metabolite positives in drug discovery: what has retrospective structure–toxicity analyses taught us? *Chemico-Biological Interactions*, **192** (1–2), 46–55.

129 Stepan, A.F., Walker, D.P., Bauman, J., Price, D.A., Baillie, T.A., Kalgutkar, A.S., and Aleo, M.D. (2011) Structural alert/reactive metabolite concept as applied in medicinal chemistry to mitigate the risk of idiosyncratic drug toxicity: a perspective based on the critical examination of trends in the top 200 drugs marketed in the United States. *Chemical Research in Toxicology*, **24** (9), 1345–1410.

130 Shu, Y.Z., Johnson, B.M., and Yang, T.J. (2008) Role of biotransformation studies in minimizing metabolism-related liabilities in drug discovery. *AAPS Journal*, **10** (1), 178–192.

6
Intrinsically Electrophilic Compounds as a Liability in Drug Discovery

Abbreviations

GSH Glutathione
GST Glutathione transferase
SAR Structure–activity relationship

6.1
Introduction

Electrophilic compounds represent a significant liability in drug discovery and development because they often possess chemical reactivity similar to affinity labeling agents such as *N*-substituted maleimides and/or alkyl halides (e.g., iodoacetamide), which have been utilized extensively to label active site cysteines in proteins [1, 2]. Intrinsically electrophilic compounds can indiscriminately alkylate amino acid residues in proteins, DNA bases, and/or the endogenous antioxidant glutathione (GSH), leading to a toxicological outcome [3–8]. Because of the potential safety concerns, electrophilic functional groups (e.g., alkyl halides, Michael acceptors, etc.) are generally avoided in drug design as outlined in chapters 5 and 13.

6.2
Intrinsic Electrophilicity of β-Lactam Antibiotics as a Causative Factor in Toxicity

The bacteriocidal action of β-lactam antibiotics such as amoxicillin (Figure 6.1) is directly attributable to their ability to react with the serine-type D-ala-D-ala carboxypeptidase [9]. This enzyme is a serine protease involved in the bacterial synthesis of the peptidoglycan layer in the cell wall. All β-lactam antibacterial agents irreversibly acylate the active site serine forming a serine ester–linked adduct (Figure 6.1) [10]. Although β-lactam drugs are generally well tolerated, they are also frequently associated with allergic and anaphylactic reactions. For instance, amoxicillin treatment

Reactive Drug Metabolites, First Edition. Amit S. Kalgutkar, Deepak Dalvie, R. Scott Obach, and Dennis A. Smith.
© 2012 Wiley-VCH Verlag GmbH & Co. KGaA. Published 2012 by Wiley-VCH Verlag GmbH & Co. KGaA.

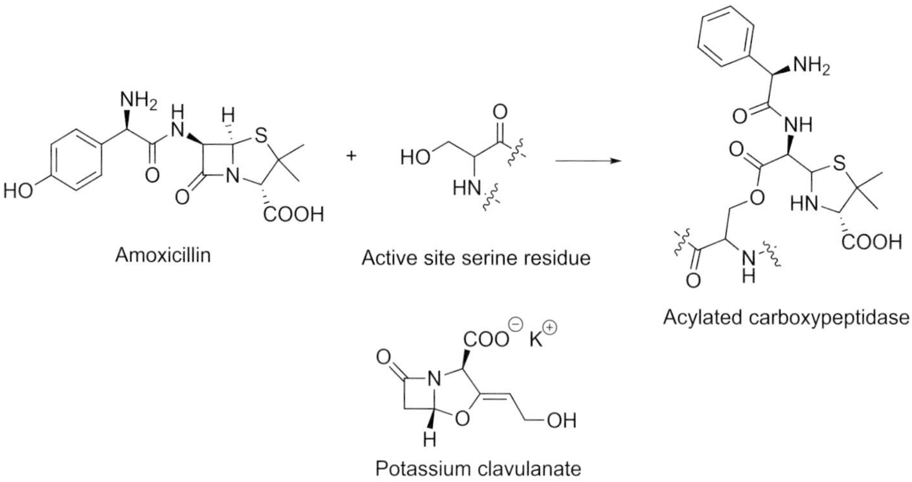

Figure 6.1 Irreversible acylation of serine-type D-ala-D-ala carboxypeptidase by amoxicillin.

is often associated with a very low rate of mild hepatocellular and cholestatic injury [11]. The acute nature of antibiotic therapy most likely aids the tolerability, considering that the daily doses of β-lactam antibiotics are very high (>1000 mg). The adverse events associated with β-lactam antibacterial agents have been studied in much detail. The β-lactam ring is intrinsically electrophilic, and in some patients, acylation of free amino and sulfydryl groups on proteins via a nonenzymatic β-lactam ring scission leads to an immune response against the penicillin–protein adduct. If the antibody response generates sufficient IgE antibodies, a severe allergic reaction such as anaphylaxis can occur [12–15]. In fact, one of the principal metabolites of amoxicillin in humans is derived from the hydrolysis of the β-lactam ring [16]. While the rate of hepatic injury with amoxicillin is very low, it is interesting to note that combination with the β-lactamase inhibitor potassium clavulanate (see Figure 6.1) increases this risk [11]. Potassium clavulanate is used in conjunction with amoxicillin (combination sold as augmentin) to destroy penicillin-resistant strains of bacteria. By itself, clavulanate does not possess antibacterial activity. Bacteria produce the serine hydrolase β-lactamase to hydrolyze carboxypeptidase inhibitors, forming a hydrolytically labile serine ester–linked adduct [17]. Reactions between the catalytic serine residue in β-lactamase and specific β-lactamase inhibitors such as clavulanate result in the formation of stable adducts derived from β-lactam ring opening, functionally inactivating the bacterial resistance mechanism [17]. Evidence that clavulanate is principally responsible for hepatotoxicity stems from the observation that clavulanate combined with other β-lactams can also lead to liver injury [18]. A genetic basis for amoxicillin/clavulanate hepatotoxicity has been identified with linkage to the human leukocyte antigen haplotype suggesting that the toxicity has an immunological component [19]. Furthermore, individuals with glutathione transferase (GST) null genotypes are known to be at an increased risk of amoxicillin–clavulanate hepatotoxicity, a finding that is consistent with a deficiency in clavulanate detoxification by GSH [20].

6.3
Intrinsically Electrophilic Compounds in Drug Discovery

While avoidance of structural alerts is a common practice in drug design, examination of medicinal chemistry literature reveals several examples of seemingly "chemically inert" compounds, which are prone to nucleophilic addition/displacement by GSH and/or amino acid residues on proteins. Because metabolism is not required for this type of reactivity, such compounds will usually lie outside the scope of currently used structural alerts. In most instances, reaction with GSH can occur under nonenzymatic (pH 7.4 phosphate buffer, 37 °C) and/or enzymatic conditions [21–30]. In the case of enzyme-assisted reactions, GSH conjugation to electrophilic centers is mediated by microsomal, cytosolic, and/or mitochondrial glutathione transferases (GSTs) [31–34]. From a structure–activity relationship (SAR) perspective, a recurring structural theme in these examples is the presence of the methyl sulfone/sulfonamide and/or halide leaving group, which is attached to an electron-deficient aromatic (e.g., cyano- and nitrobenzene) heteroaromatic ring systems (e.g., pyridine, pyridone, benzothiazole, thiadiazole, benzofuran, indole, etc.) (Figure 6.2). The electrophilicity of heterocyclic sulfonamides was first demonstrated with the carbonic anhydrase inhibitor benzothiazole-2-sulfonamide (**1**) (Figure 6.2) [21, 22]. Although **1** demonstrates potent inhibition of carbonic anhydrase activity *in vitro*, the compound is devoid of *in vivo* pharmacological activity in preclinical species even after administration at high doses. The absence of **1** in circulation and/or urine after administration of ^{35}S-radiolabeled material appears to provide a rational argument for the *in vitro–in vivo* pharmacology disconnect. While >80% of the radioactivity was eliminated in the urine, none of the characterized metabolites (e.g., benzothiazole-2-mercapturic acid (3)) were radioactive implicating the loss of the ^{35}S label [22]. The proposed mechanism, which collectively accounted for these observations, involves a quantitative nucleophilic displacement of the 2 in the 2-sulfonamide group in the parent compound by the endogenous pool of GSH in the mammal to yield GSH conjugate 2, ^{35}SO$_2$, and ammonia. The demonstration that all urinary radioactivity was due to inorganic sulfate confirms the nucleophilic displacement of the sulfonamide group by GSH. Subsequent enzymatic breakdown of **2** affords the mercapturic acid conjugate **3**. The overall displacement mechanism for sulfonamides is similar to the one described for GST-catalyzed nucleophilic aromatic substitution reactions (see Figure 6.2 for an illustration) and involves nucleophilic attack by the thiolate anion of GSH across the electrophilic center to yield the negatively charged σ-complex or Meisenheimer complex followed by elimination of the appropriate leaving group (see Figure 6.2) [31–37]. Accordingly, the chemical reactivity of electrophiles with GSH can be governed by steric and/or electronic factors that are predetermined by the nature and position of heteroaromatic substituents.

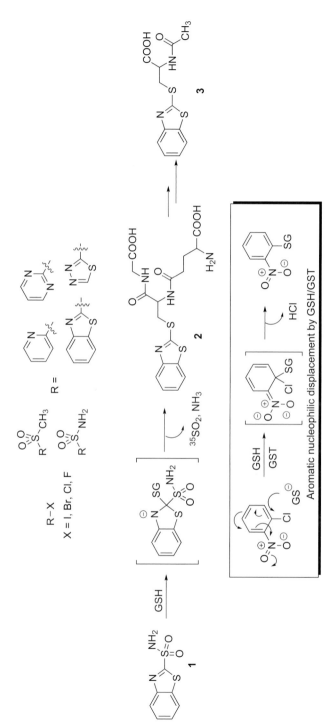

Figure 6.2 Reaction of intrinsically electrophilic sulfonamides/methyl sulfones with GSH.

6.3.1
Linking Innate Electrophilicity with Drug Toxicity

An illustration associating a toxicological outcome with the biochemical reactivity of an electrophilic compound is evident in structure–toxicity relationships with a series of heterocyclic sulfonamide-based carbonic anhydrase inhibitors. The clinical development of 2-sulfamoylbenzo[*d*]thiazol-6-yl pivalate (**4**), a prodrug form of 6-hydroxybenzothiazole-2-sulfonamide (**5**) (Figure 6.3), was suspended due a significant incidence of allergy in a three-month ocular safety study in rabbits [24]. Subsequent evaluation in a guinea pig model for dermal sensitization potential revealed that the compounds were potent allergens. A number of related 6-substituted benzothiazole-2-sulfonamides (Figure 6.3) were found to share this attribute [24]. It was presumed that the allergic reactions were likely mediated via protein arylation resulting in an immune response since the sulfonamide moiety in these derivatives was readily displaced (half-life <1 h) by GSH (Figure 6.3) under physiological conditions (pH 7.4 phosphate buffer, 37 °C) [24, 25]. Support for this hypothesis was evident from analogous studies with the corresponding deaza analogues of benzothiazoles, that is, benzothiophene-2-sulfonamides, which were practically inert toward reaction with GSH (Figure 6.3) and were also devoid of allergic side reactions in animals [24]. In contrast with the observation on benzothiophene-2-sulfonamides, the corresponding benzofuran- and indole-2-sulfonamide derivatives were found to react with GSH (Figure 6.3), at a threefold to sevenfold greater rate than the corresponding benzothiophene-2-sulfonamides [26].

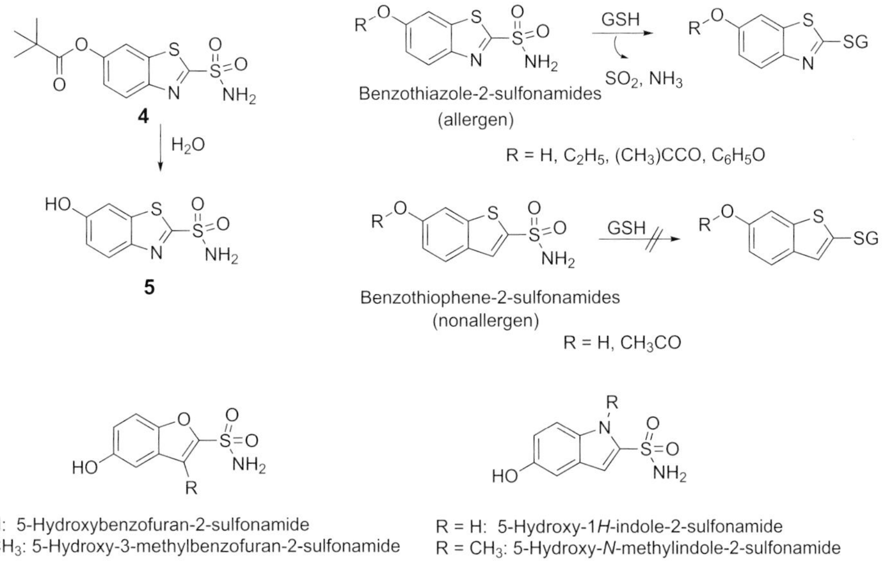

Figure 6.3 Relationship between GSH reactivity and adverse reactions of heterocyclic sulfonamides.

Consistent with the *in vitro* findings on GSH reactivity, representative members of the benzofuran- and indole-2-sulfonamide series also elicited moderate to strong allergic responses in the guinea pig dermal sensitization assay [26]. While a straightforward linear correlation between GSH reactivity and sensitization potential was not apparent in these studies, it seems clear that a compound is likely to induce an allergic response if some threshold level of electrophilicity is exceeded. From a SAR perspective, it is of interest to note that the *N*-methyl- and 3-methyl-substituted derivatives of the indole- and benzofuran-2-sulfonamides were considerably more reactive toward GSH than the desmethyl compounds (Figure 6.3), suggesting that the mechanism of GSH substitution reaction is not a simple addition–elimination process [26]. A further indication of the possible mechanistic complexity of the GSH displacement reaction in the SAR studies was the unusual substituent effect on GSH reactivity in the benzofuran series: electron-donating substituents on the six-membered ring either did not affect or accelerate the rate of the displacement reaction. This stands in contrast to the benzothiazole series where a 6-amino or 6-hydroxy substituent markedly reduced the electrophilicity of the system.

6.4
Serendipitous Identification of Intrinsically Electrophilic Compounds in Drug Discovery

The first illustration of the serendipitous characterization of "nonobvious" electrophiles in drug discovery is depicted with the 4-sulfonyl-2-pyridone-based glucokinase activators as potential antidiabetic agents (Figure 6.4) [35, 36]. In the course of SAR studies, a unique metabolic liability of the 4-sulfonyl-2-pyridone scaffold in the lead compound **6** was identified wherein the heterocycle readily adducted with GSH in pH 7.4 phosphate buffer to a derivative that was unambiguously identified to be the GSH adduct **8** (Figure 6.5). Nucleophilic displacement by GSH led to an increase in yield of **8** when incubations were conducted in liver microsomes, liver cytosol, and placental GSTs highlighting the role of enzyme catalysis. The identification of **8** in circulation following intravenous administration of **6** to rats confirmed the relevance of the *in vitro* findings [36]. The general mechanism for the formation of **8** involves nucleophilic attack by the thiolate anion of GSH at the electrophilic center on the pyridone ring to give the addition product **7** followed by elimination of the methylsulfonyl group. Under identical experimental conditions, GSH was devoid of reactivity with the parent 2-pyridone moiety (compound **9**) or the methyl sulfone regioisomers of **6**, that is, compounds **10** (R = 3-SO₂CH₃) and **11** (R = 5-SO₂CH₃) (Figure 6.5) [36]. The 4-bromo-2-pyridone derivative **12** is less electrophilic at position C4 compared to **6** (Br is less electron-withdrawing than SO₂CH₃) and therefore possesses a significantly diminished reactivity toward nucleophilic displacement by GSH under nonenzymatic conditions [36]. Interestingly, incubation of **12** with GSH in the presence of human liver

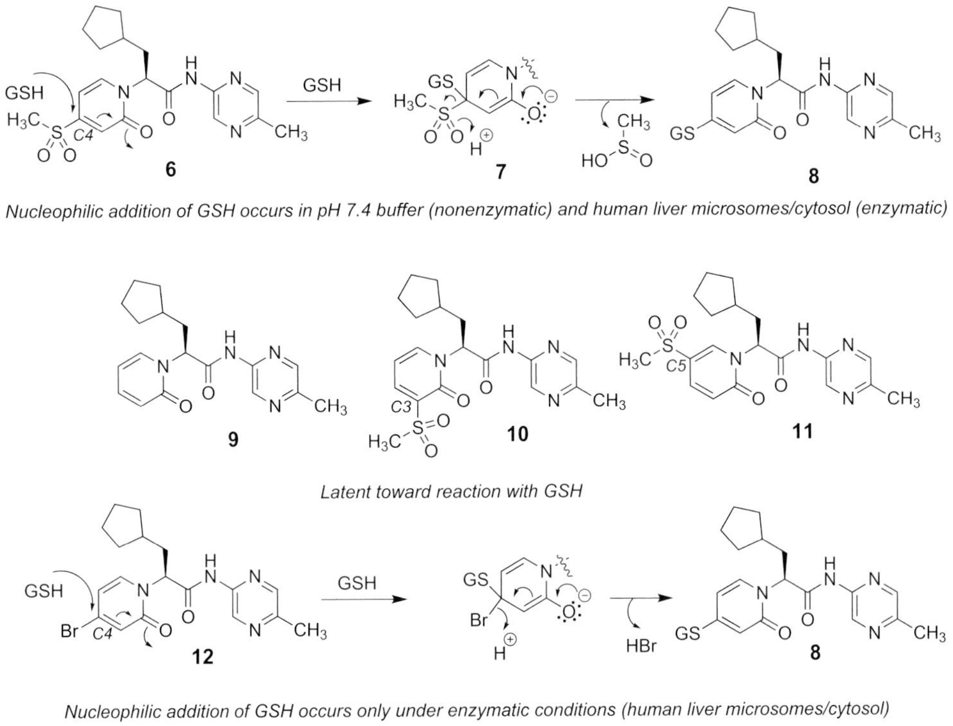

Nucleophilic addition of GSH occurs in pH 7.4 buffer (nonenzymatic) and human liver microsomes/cytosol (enzymatic)

Latent toward reaction with GSH

Nucleophilic addition of GSH occurs only under enzymatic conditions (human liver microsomes/cytosol)

Figure 6.4 Intrinsic electrophilicity of the 4-methylsulfonyl-2-pyridone scaffold.

cytosol led to the formation of **8** in a quantitative fashion. Lack of similar reactivity on replacement of liver cytosol with liver microsomes implied the selective role of cytosolic GSTs in facilitating the nucleophilic displacement reaction between thiol and compound **12** [36].

The second illustration of the *in vitro* and *in vivo* reactivity of GSH with activated sulfonamides is evident with the HIV-1 protease inhibitor PNU-10912 (Figure 6.5) [28, 29]. From a SAR perspective, PNU-140690 that is obtained by exchanging the cyanopyridinyl motif in PNU-10912 with a trifluoromethylpyridinyl moiety was latent toward reactivity with GSH *in vitro* and *in vivo* animal studies (Figure 6.5). A role of GSTs isozymes in the nucleophilic displacement reaction was also demonstrated in the course of these studies. Additional SAR studies on pyridine-2-sulfonamides further confirmed the requirement of the electrophilic center (e.g., pyridine nitrogen) α to the sulfonyl group for reaction with GSH. Sulfonamide displacement by GSH was not dependent on the substituents attached to the nitrogen; however, pyridine ring substituents markedly influenced the process. Thus, *ortho* and *para* ring substituents capable of withdrawing sufficient electron density from the carbon atom α to the sulfonyl group were the critical requirement for the GST-mediated sulfonamide displacement (Figure 6.5).

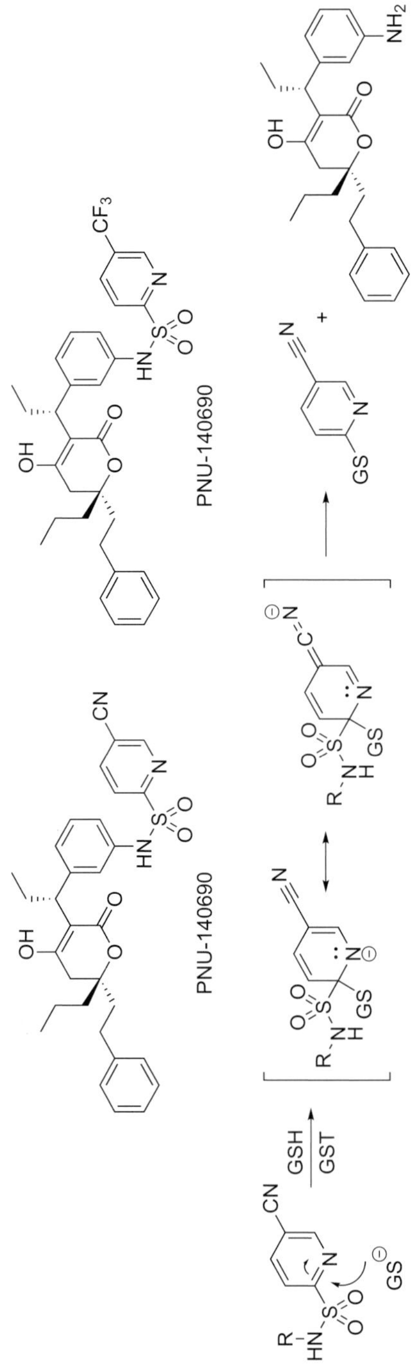

Figure 6.5 SAR studies on the nucleophilic displacement reaction on pyridine-2-sulfonamides by GSH.

The third example of unanticipated innate electrophilicity in a lead chemical series is illustrated with 6-(2-methylpyridinyloxy)-5-cyanopyrimidine derivatives exemplified by compound **13** [37]. Compound **13** was shown to undergo a nucleophilic displacement reaction with GSH under nonenzymatic conditions (pH 7.4 phosphate buffer) to yield adduct **15** (Figure 6.6). The rate of formation of **15** was substantially increased on inclusion of liver microsomes, liver cytosol, and semipurified GST enzymes implicating their role in facilitating the nucleophilic displacement reaction. The mechanism for the formation of **15** can be rationalized as follows: first, nucleophilic GSH attacks the C6 pyrimidine carbon in **13** that is attached to a 2-methylpyridinyl group via an ether linkage (Figure 6.6). This center is activated toward nucleophilic attack due to the presence of electron-withdrawing substituents (pyrimidine nitrogens in positions 1 and 3 and the cyano group attached to C5). These electron-withdrawing groups also stabilize the transition state of the reaction (intermediate **14**) via the Meisenheimer complex. Elimination then occurs in **14** to generate metabolite **15** and the corresponding 2-methylpyridinylphenol derivative. This elimination reaction is possible due to the good leaving group ability of the phenol (low pK_a of ~8.0). Replacement of the 5-cyano group in **13** with a 5-methyl group results in compound **16** (see Figure 6.6) that does not undergo the analogous displacement reaction with GSH under nonenzymatic and enzymatic conditions. The observation suggests that the combined electron-withdrawing potential of the cyano group and pyrimidine nitrogens is essential for the nucleophilic displacement to occur.

The final example of an innately electrophilic compound is evident in the mechanistic studies by Teffera *et al.* [38] on the oncology clinical candidate 1-(2-hydroxy-2-methylpropyl)-*N*-[5-(7-methoxyquinolin-4-yloxy)pyridine-2-yl]-5-methyl-3-oxo-2-phenyl-2,3-dihydro-1*H*-pyrazole-4-carboxamide (AMG 458) (Figure 6.7), which was found to covalently bind to liver microsomal proteins in the absence of NADPH. Subsequent incubations of [^{14}C]-AMG 458 in phosphate buffer (pH 7.4) or rat liver microsomes fortified with sulfydryl nucleophiles (e.g., GSH and *N*-acetylcysteine) led to the identification of sulfydryl conjugates derived from a nucleophilic displacement to yield a quinoline thioether metabolite (Figure 6.7). The mechanism most likely involves protonation of the lone pair on the quinoline nitrogen (under physiological conditions) leading to the increased electrophilicity at position C4 (occupied by the pyridinyloxy motif), which activates this center toward nucleophilic attack. The thioether adducts were also detected in bile and urine of bile duct–cannulated rats dosed with [^{14}C]-AMG 458. Insights gained from the characterization of sulfydryl conjugates of AMG 458 led to the design of analogues that were devoid of the displacement reaction liability (Figure 6.7). Overall, the findings of Teffera *et al.* are very interesting considering that quinolines substituted with electron-donating groups are not considered chemically reactive and are often used in drug design.

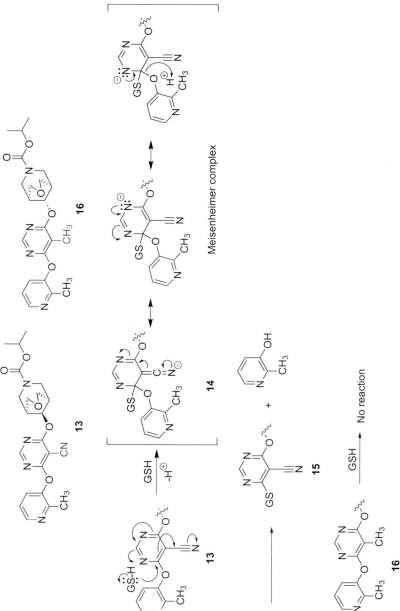

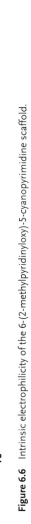

Figure 6.6 Intrinsic electrophilicity of the 6-(2-methylpyridinyloxy)-5-cyanopyrimidine scaffold.

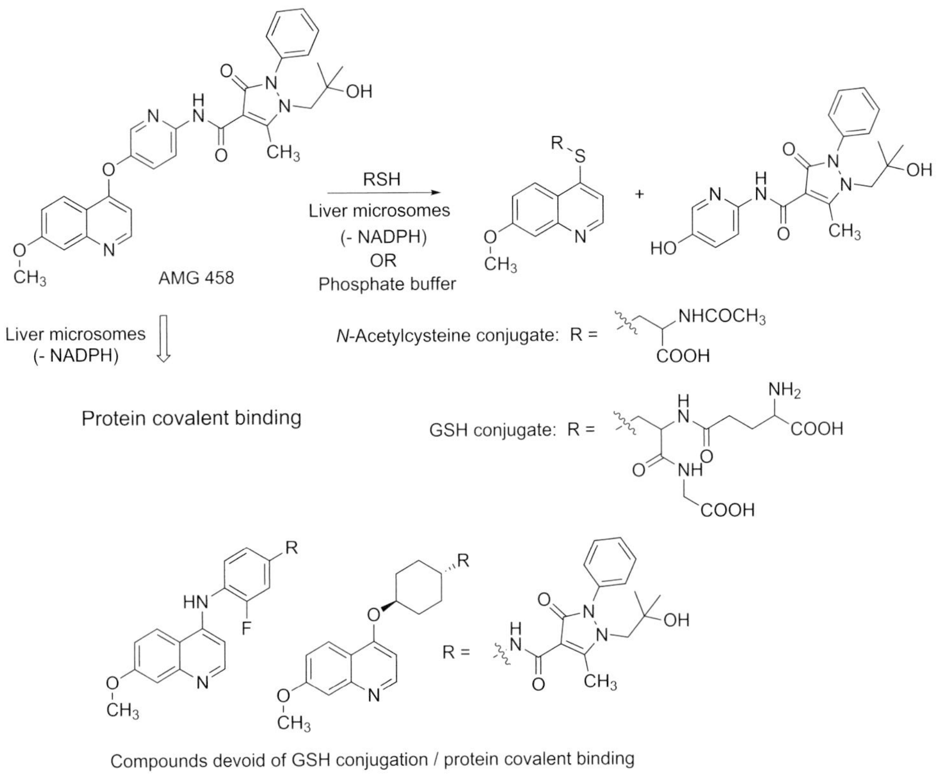

Figure 6.7 Chemical reactivity of a methoxy 4-*O*-aryl quinoline derivative (AMG 458) with GSH.

References

1 Kennedy, T.A., Smith, C.J., and Marnett, L.J. (1994) Investigation of the role of cysteines in catalysis by prostaglandin endoperoxide synthase. *Journal of Biological Chemistry*, **269** (44), 27357–27364.

2 Boja, E.S. and Fales, H.M. (2001) Overalkylation of a protein digest with iodoacetamide. *Analytical Chemistry*, **73** (15), 3576–3582.

3 Guengerich, F.P. (2005) Principles of covalent binding of reactive metabolites and examples of activation of bis-electrophiles by conjugation. *Archives of Biochemistry and Biophysics*, **433** (2), 369–378.

4 Liebler, D.C. (2008) Protein damage by reactive electrophiles: targets and consequences. *Chemical Research in Toxicology*, **21** (1), 117–128.

5 Anders, M.W. (2004) Glutathione-dependent bioactivation of haloalkanes and haloalkenes. *Drug Metabolism Reviews*, **36** (3–4), 583–594.

6 Anders, M.W. (2008) Chemical toxicology of reactive intermediates formed by the glutathione-dependent bioactivation of halogen-containing compounds. *Chemical Research in Toxicology*, **21** (1), 145–159.

7 Marnett, L.J. (1999) Chemistry and biology of DNA damage by malondialdehyde. *IARC Scientific Publications*, **150**, 17–27.

8 Guengerich, F.P. (2005) Activation of alkyl halides by glutathione transferases. *Methods in Enzymology*, **401**, 342–353.

9 Potashman, M.H. and Duggan, M.E. (2009) Covalent modifiers: an orthogonal approach to drug design. *Journal of Medicinal Chemistry*, **52** (5), 1231–1246.

10 Lu, W.P., Kincaid, E., Sun, Y., and Bauer, M.D. (2001) Kinetics of beta-lactam interactions with penicillin-susceptible and -resistant penicillin-binding protein 2x proteins from *Streptococcus pneumoniae*. Involvement of acylation and deacylation in beta-lactam resistance. *Journal of Biological Chemistry*, **276** (34), 31494–31501.

11 Fontana, R.J., Shakil, A.O., Greenson, J.K., Boyd, I., and Lee, W.M. (2005) Acute liver failure due to amoxicillin and amoxicillin clavulanate. *Digestive Diseases and Sciences*, **50** (10), 1785–1790.

12 Zhao, Z., Baldo, B.A., and Rimmer, J. (2002) beta-Lactam allergenic determinants: fine structural recognition of a cross-reacting determinant on benzylpenicillin and cephalothin. *Clinical and Experimental Allergy*, **32** (11), 1644–1650.

13 Levine, B.B. (1960) Formation of D-penicillamine-cysteine mixed disulfide by reaction of D-benzylpenicilloic acid with cysteine. *Nature*, **187**, 940–941.

14 Levine, B.B. and Ovary, Z. (1961) Studies on the mechanism of the formation of the penicillin antigen. III. The *N*-(D-alpha-benzylpenicilloyl) group as an antigenic determinant responsible for hypersensitivity to penicillin G. *The Journal of Experimental Medicine*, **114**, 875–904.

15 Levine, B.B. (1960) Studies on the mechanism of the formation of the penicillin antigen. I. Delayed allergic cross-reactions among penicillin G and its degradation products. *The Journal of Experimental Medicine*, **112**, 1131–1156.

16 Connor, S.C., Everett, J.R., Jennings, K.R., Nicholson, J.K., and Woodnut, G. (1994) High resolution ^{1}H NMR spectroscopic studies of the metabolism and excretion of ampicillin in rats and amoxicillin in rats and man. *Journal of Pharmacy and Pharmacology*, **46** (2), 128–134.

17 Drawz, S.M. and Bonomo, R.A. (2010) Three decades of beta-lactamase inhibitors. *Clinical Microbiology Reviews*, **23** (1), 160–201.

18 Van der Auwerea, P. and Legrand, J.C. (1985) Ticarcillin clavulanic acid therapy in severe infections. *Drugs under Experimental Clinical Research*, **11** (11), 805–813.

19 Hautekeete, M.L., Horsmans, Y., Van Waeyenberge, C., Demanet, C., Henrion, J., Verbist, L., Brenard, R., Sempoux, C., Michielsen, P.P., Yap, P.S., Rahier, J., and Geubel, A.P. (1999) HLA association of amoxicillin–clavulanate induced hepatitis. *Gastroenterology*, **117** (5), 1181–1186.

20 Lucena, M.I., Andrade, R.J., Martinez, C., Ulzurrun, E., Garcia-Martin, E., Borraz, Y., Fernandez, M.C., Romero-Gomez, M., Castiella, A., Planas, R., Costa, J., Anzola, S., and Agundez, J.A.G. (2008) Glutathione *S*-transferase M1 and T1 null genotypes increase susceptibility to idiosyncratic drug-induced liver injury. *Hepatology*, **48** (2), 588–596.

21 Clapp, J.W. (1956) A new metabolic pathway for a sulfonamide group. *Journal of Biological Chemistry*, **233** (1), 207–214.

22 Colucci, D.F. and Buyske, D.A. (1965) The biotransformation of a sulfonamide to a mercaptan and to a mercapturic acid and glucuronide conjugate. *Biochemical Pharmacology*, **14**, 457–466.

23 Conroy, C.W., Schwam, H., and Maren, T.H. (1984) The nonenzymatic displacement of the sulfamoyl group from different classes of aromatic compounds by glutathione and cysteine. *Drug Metabolism and Disposition*, **12** (5), 614–618.

24 Graham, S.L., Shepard, K.L., Anderson, P.S., Baldwin, J.J., Best, D.B., Christy, M.E., Freedman, M.B., Gautheron, P., Habecker, C.N., Hoffman, J.M., Lyle, P.A., Michelson, S.R., Ponticello, G.S., Robb, C.M., Schwam, H., Smith, A.M., Smith, R.L., Sondey, J.M., Strohmaier, K.M., Sugrue, M.F., and Varga, S.L. (1989) Topically active carbonic anhydrase inhibitors. 2. Benzo[*b*] thiophenesulfonamide derivatives with ocular hypotensive activity. *Journal of Medicinal Chemistry*, **32** (12), 2548–2554.

25 Woltersdorf, O.W. Jr., Schwam, H., Bicking, J.B., Brown, S.L., deSolms, S.J.,

Fishman, D.R., Graham, S.L., Gautheron, P.D., Hoffman, J.M., Larson, R.D., Lee, W.S., Michelson, S.R., Robb, C.M., Share, N.N., Shepard, K.L., Smith, A.M., Smith, R.L., Sondey, J.M., Strohmaier, K.M., Sugrue, M.F., and Viader, M.P. (1989) Topically active carbonic anhydrase inhibitors. 1. *O*-Acyl derivatives of 6-hydroxybenzothiazole-2-sulfonamide. *Journal of Medicinal Chemistry*, **32** (11), 2486–2492.

26 Graham, S.L., Hoffman, J.M., Gautheron, P., Michelson, S.R., Scholz, T.H., Schwam, H., Shepard, K.L., Smith, A.M., Smith, R.L., Sondey, J.M., and Sugrue, M.F. (1990) Topically active carbonic anhydrase inhibitors. 3. Benzofuran- and indole-2-sulfonamides. *Journal of Medicinal Chemistry*, **33** (2), 749–754.

27 Kishida, K., Akaki, Y., Sasabe, T., Yamamoto, C., and Manabe, R. (1990) Glutathione conjugation of methazolamide and subsequent reactions in the ciliary body in vitro. *Journal of Pharmaceutical Sciences*, **79** (7), 638–642.

28 Koeplinger, K.A., Zhao, Z., Peterson, T., Leone, J.W., Schwende, F.S., Heinrikson, R.L., and Tomasselli, A.G. (1999) Activated sulfonamides are cleaved by glutathione-*S*-transferases. *Drug Metabolism and Disposition*, **27** (9), 986–991.

29 Zhao, Z., Koeplinger, K.A., Peterson, T., Conradi, R.A., Burton, P.S., Suarato, A., Heinrikson, R.L., and Tomasselli, A.G. (1999) Mechanism, structure–activity studies, and potential applications of glutathione *S*-transferase-catalyzed cleavage of sulfonamides. *Drug Metabolism and Disposition*, **27** (9), 992–998.

30 Inoue, K., Ohe, T., Mori, K., Sagara, T., Ishii, Y., and Chiba, M. (2009) Aromatic substitution reaction of 2-chloropyridines catalyzed by microsomal glutathione *S*-transferase 1. *Drug Metabolism and Disposition*, **37** (9), 1797–1800.

31 Habig, W.H., Pabst, M.J., and Jakoby, W.B. (1974) Glutathione *S*-transferases. *Journal of Biological Chemistry*, **249** (22), 7130–7139.

32 Armstrong, R.N. (1991) Glutathione *S*-transferases: reaction mechanism, structure, and function. *Chemical Research in Toxicology*, **4** (2), 131–140.

33 Armstrong, R.N. (1997) Structure, catalytic mechanism, and evolution of the glutathione transferases. *Chemical Research in Toxicology*, **10** (1), 2–18.

34 Patskovsky, Y., Patskovska, L., Almo, S.C., and Listowsky, I. (2006) Transition state model and mechanism of nucleophilic aromatic substitution reactions catalyzed by human glutathione *S*-transferase M1a-1a. *Biochemistry*, **45** (12), 3852–3862.

35 Pfefferkorn, J.A., Lou, J., Minich, M.L., Filipski, K.J., He, M., Zhou, R., Ahmed, S., Benbow, J., Perez, A.G., Tu, M., Litchfield, J., Sharma, R., Metzler, K., Bourbonais, F., Huang, C., Beebe, D.A., and Oates, P.J. (2009) Pyridones as glucokinase activators: identification of a unique metabolic liability of the 4-sulfonyl-2-pyridone heterocycle. *Bioorganic Medicinal Chemistry Letters*, **19** (12), 3247–3252.

36 Litchfield, J., Sharma, R., Atkinson, K., Filipski, K.J., Wright, S.W., Pfefferkorn, J.A., Tan, B., Kosa, R.E., Stevens, B., Tu, M., and Kalgutkar, A.S. (2010) Intrinsic electrophilicity of the 4-methylsulfonyl-2-pyridone scaffold in glucokinase activators: role of glutathione-*S*-transferases and in vivo quantitation of a glutathione conjugate in rats. *Bioorganic Medicinal Chemistry Letters*, **20** (21), 6262–6267.

37 Kalgutkar, A.S., Mascitti, V., Sharma, R., Walker, G.W., Ryder, T., McDonald, T.S., Chen, Y., Preville, C., Basak, A., McClure, K.F., Kohrt, J.T., Robinson, R.P., Munchhof, M.J., and Cornelius, P. (2011) Intrinsic electrophilicity of a 4-substituted-5-cyano-6-(2-methylpyridin-3-yloxy) pyrimidine derivative: structural characterization of glutathione conjugates in vitro. *Chemical Research in Toxicology*, **24** (2), 269–278.

38 Teffera, Y., Colletti, A.E., Harmange, J.C., Hollis, L.J., Albrecht, B.K., Boezio, A.A., Liu, J., and Zhao, Z. (2008) Chemical reactivity of methoxy 4-*O*-aryl quinolines: identification of glutathione displacement products in vitro and in vivo. *Chemical Research in Toxicology*, **21** (11), 2216–2222.

7
Role of Reactive Metabolites in Pharmacological Action

Abbreviations

MTIC   5-[3-Methyl-1-triazenyl]imidazole-4-carboxamide
P450   Cytochrome P450

7.1
Introduction

While the role of reactive metabolites in drug toxicity is widely recognized, it is also important to note that in some cases, conversion of drugs to reactive metabolites and the subsequent covalent binding of these reactive metabolites to macromolecules are required for primary pharmacology. Various classes of anticancer agents belong to this category. Activation of these compounds to reactive metabolites can be mediated enzymatically or nonenzymatically. Enzymatically, these compounds may undergo oxidative or reductive bioactivation. This chapter discusses examples of drugs and natural products that require bioactivation to reactive species as the rate-limiting step for beneficial pharmacological action.

7.2
Drugs Activated Nonenzymatically and by Oxidative Metabolism

7.2.1
Proton Pump Inhibitors

Substituted benzimidazoles, such as omeprazole, lansoprazole, and pantoprazole (Figure 7.1), represent a novel class of compounds that inhibit acid secretion that is mediated by H^+/Na^+-ATPase, the gastric proton pump [1].

This class of compounds does not interact directly with the pump. However, in the acidic environment of the stomach, they are converted to relatively nonselective reactive intermediates, which react with essential thiol groups on the pump (Figure 7.2). Studies

Reactive Drug Metabolites, First Edition. Amit S. Kalgutkar, Deepak Dalvie, R. Scott Obach, and Dennis A. Smith.
© 2012 Wiley-VCH Verlag GmbH & Co. KGaA. Published 2012 by Wiley-VCH Verlag GmbH & Co. KGaA.

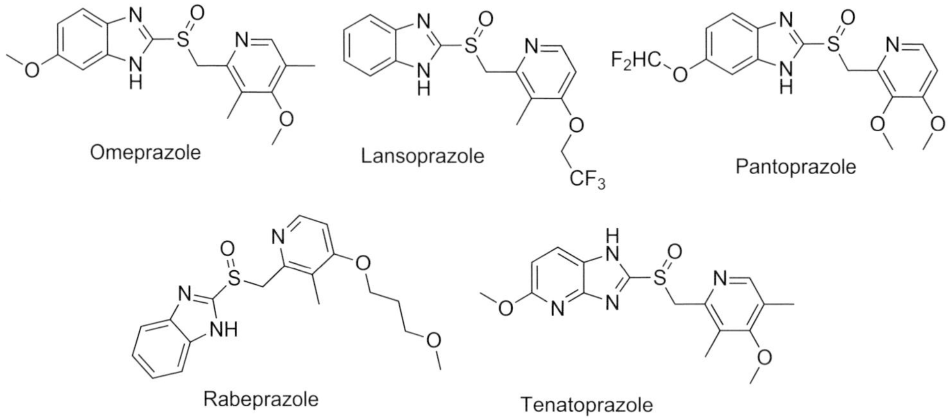
Omeprazole
Lansoprazole
Pantoprazole
Rabeprazole
Tenatoprazole

Figure 7.1 Structures of proton pump inhibitors.

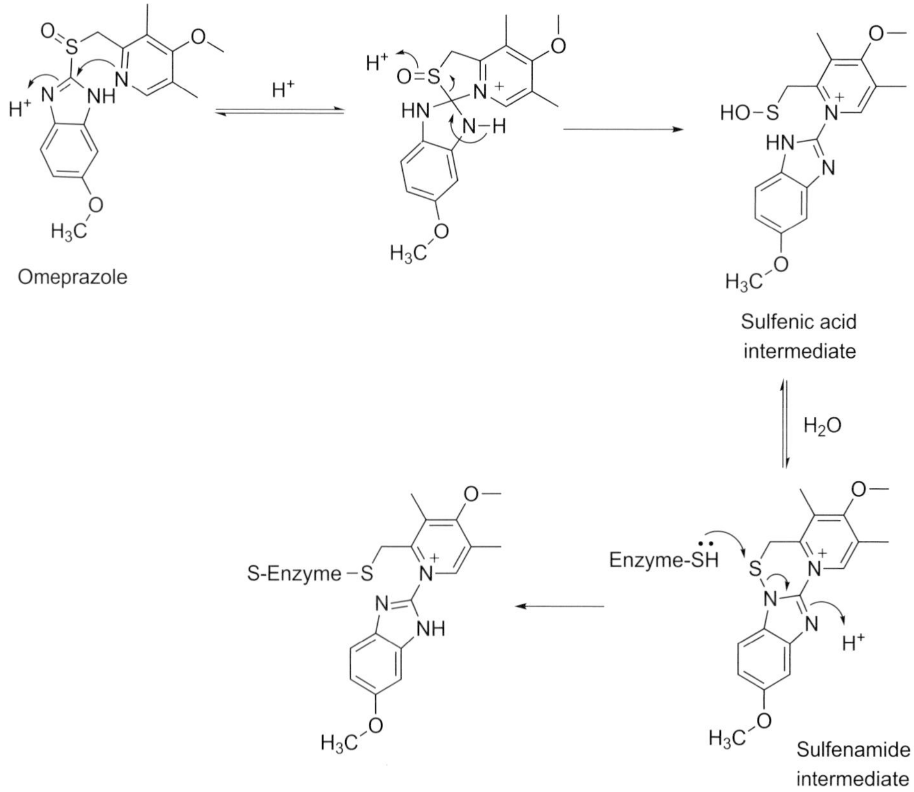
Omeprazole
Sulfenic acid intermediate
Enzyme-SH
S-Enzyme
Sulfenamide intermediate

Figure 7.2 Acid-catalyzed bioactivation of omeprazole.

indicate that the reactive intermediate derived from omeprazole, and related compounds of this type, is a rearranged cyclic sulfenamide [2–4].

7.2.2
Nitrosoureas

Nitrosoureas are important bifunctional antitumor agents that have demonstrated activity against a wide spectrum of human malignancies [5–7]. Bis(2-chloroethyl) nitrosourea (carmustine), a prototypical nitrosourea in this class, has been used as an antineoplastic agent in the treatment of Hodgkin's lymphoma, multiple myeloma, and primary or metastatic brain tumors [8–10]. Nitrosoureas can cross the blood–brain barrier due to their lipophilic nature and are therefore considered in the treatment of brain tumors [6, 11, 12]. Several other nitrosoureas have since been introduced, which include *N*-(2-chloroethyl)-*N*-cyclohexyl-*N*-nitrosourea (lomustine), *N*-(2-chloroethyl)-*N*-(4-methylcyclohexyl)-*N*-nitrosourea (semustine), streptozocin, and chlorozotocin (Figure 7.3) [13, 14].

It is generally assumed that all nitrosoureas exert their cytotoxicity via a base-catalyzed degradation that leads to the liberation of an alkylating chloroethyl moiety and a carbamoylating isocyanate moiety, as shown for carmustine in Figure 7.4 [15–17].

The 2-chloroethyl moiety is a strong electrophile and is capable of alkylating guanine, cytidine, and adenine bases in DNA resulting in intrastrand or

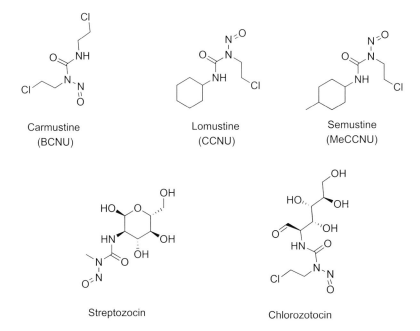

Figure 7.3 Structures of nitrosoureas.

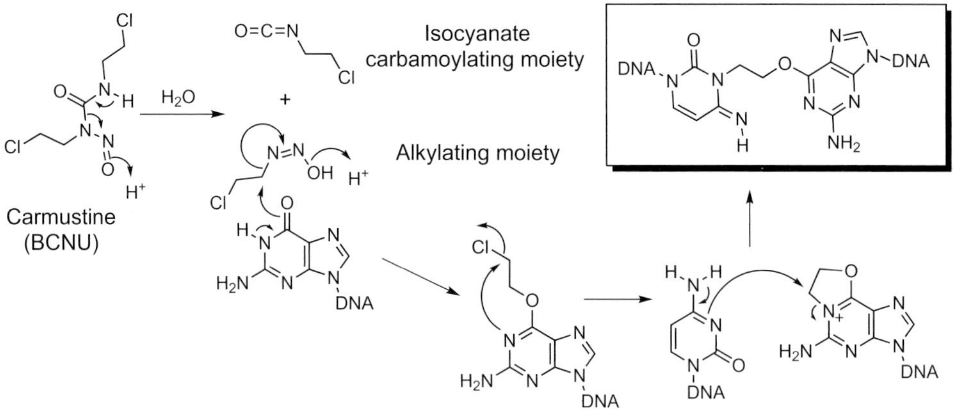

Figure 7.4 Proposed mechanism of activation of nitrosoureas to a DNA alkylating moiety.

interstrand DNA cross-links. The mechanism involves chloroethylation of the O^6 position in guanine followed by intramolecular cyclization to a highly electrophilic species, which is trapped by N-3 of the Watson–Crick paired cytosine to yield the interstrand cross-linked base pair [18–20]. The alkylating action of the compound has been suggested to be responsible for its therapeutic effects. The organic isocyanate, on the other hand, carbamoylates lysine residues of proteins, and this reaction may inactivate some DNA repair enzymes. This carbamoylation of proteins is also believed to be responsible for the toxic effects of these compounds. Of these five nitrosoureas, chlorozotocin and streptozotocin have low carbamoylating activity.

7.2.3
Imidazotriazenes

The utility of imidazotriazenes as antitumor agents has received a lot of attention owing to the alkylating activity of these compounds following chemical or enzymatic degradation [21–24]. Three compounds, mitozolomide, dacarbazine, temozolomide (Figure 7.5), in this class have been extensively studied. Among these,

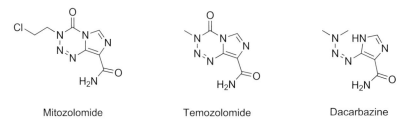

Mitozolomide   Temozolomide   Dacarbazine

Figure 7.5 Structures of triazene derivatives.

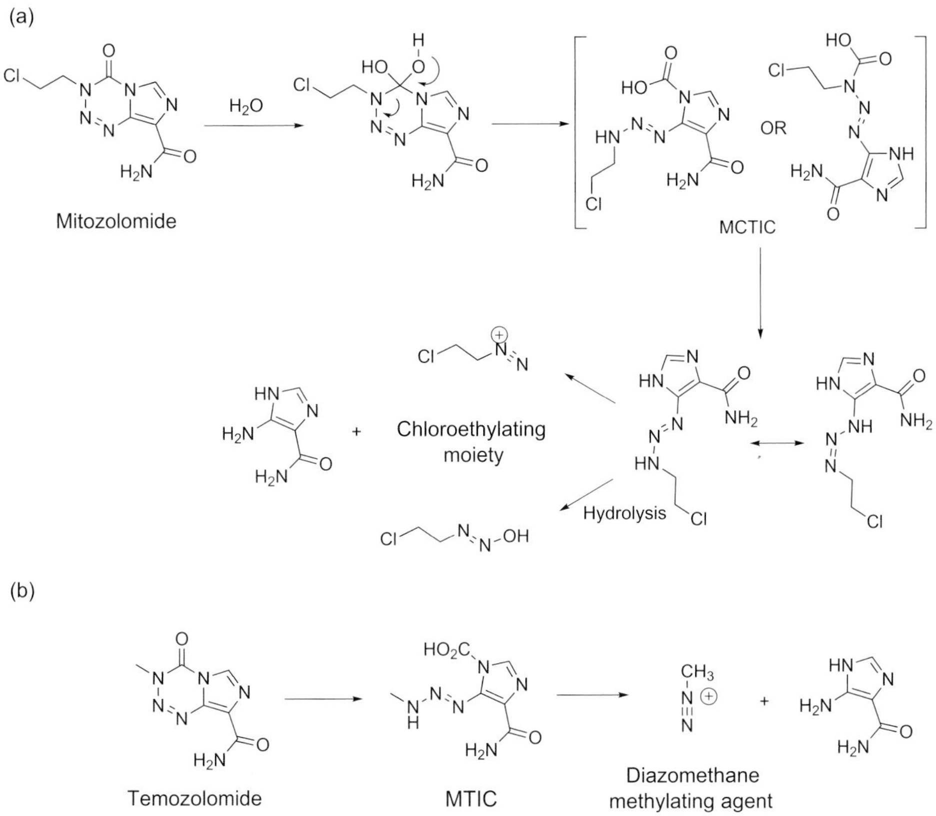

(a)

Mitozolomide

MCTIC

Chloroethylating
moiety

Hydrolysis

(b)

Temozolomide

MTIC

Diazomethane
methylating agent

Figure 7.6 Decomposition of mitozolomide and temozolomide.

dacarbazine and temozolomide are used clinically in the treatment of various cancers including malignant melanoma and gliomas, Hodgkin lymphoma, and sarcoma [25–29].

Although the anticancer mechanism of triazenes is not fully understood, these compounds presumably exert their effect by forming interstrand cross-links with DNA [30, 31]. A minor structural difference between the three agents yields major differences in the manner in which the agents exert their cytotoxic effects. Studies with mitozolomide and temozolomide have demonstrated that these compounds undergo nonenzymatic degradation and spontaneous decarboxylation by an attack of a hydroxyl group at the C4 position to the corresponding cytotoxic triazene intermediates 5-[3-(2-chloroethyl)-1-triazenyl]imidazole-4-carboxamide (MCTIC) and 5-[3-methyl-1-triazenyl]imidazole-4-carboxamide (MTIC), respectively (Figure 7.6) [24, 32, 33]. This intermediate undergoes spontaneous decomposition to yield diazomethane, which in turn is capable of methylating the N7 position of guanine.

In contrast to temozolomide, the rate-limiting step in DNA alkylation by dacarbazine is dependent on a cytochrome P450 (P450)–mediated oxidative

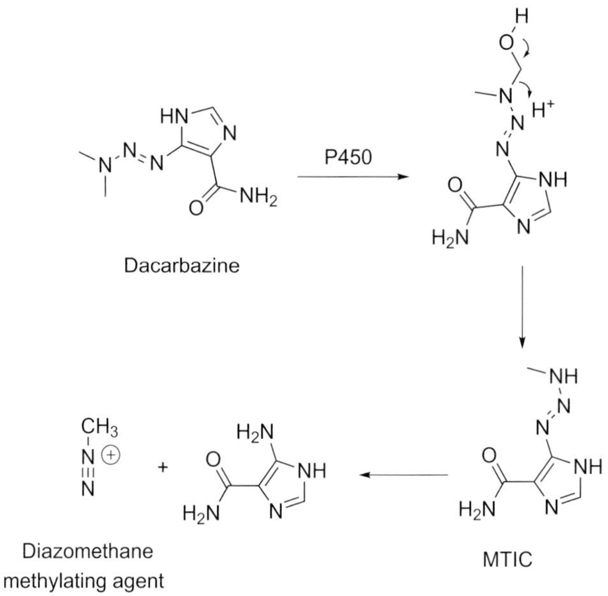

Figure 7.7 Metabolic activation of dacarbazine by P450.

N-demethylation (Figure 7.7) [34–37]. The initial product of P450-catalyzed oxidation, which is a carbinolamine, produces MTIC after elimination of formaldehyde. Rapid decomposition of MTIC gives the carboxamide and the reactive diazomethane, which produces molecular nitrogen and a methyl carbocation believed to be the methylating species. The formation of diazomethane in this case has been confirmed by detection of the carboxamide metabolite in the plasma and urine of mouse following an intraperitoneal dose of [^{14}C-methyl] dacarbazine [37].

7.2.4
Thienotetrahydropyridines

Thienotetrahydropyridines such as ticlopidine, clopidogrel, and prasugrel are antithrombotic agents that inhibit platelet aggregation and require oxidative metabolic activation to an active moiety before they can exert their pharmacological effect [38]. The metabolic activation occurs in two steps (Figure 7.8) [39–41]. The first step is a classical P4502C19-catalyzed monooxygenation of the thiophene ring that leads to the thiolactone metabolite. The second step involves sulfoxidation of the thiolactone that undergoes spontaneous cleavage to the corresponding sulfenic acid intermediate. This highly reactive intermediate forms a covalent S–S bridge with a thiol group in platelet ADP receptors, thereby causing their long-lasting inactivation.

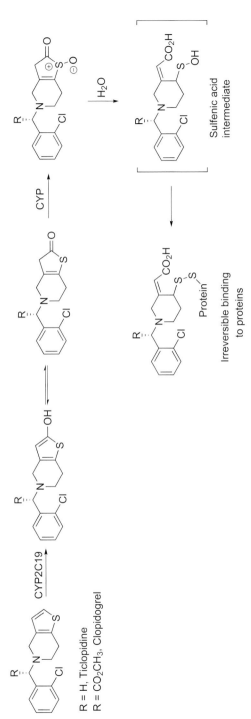

Figure 7.8 Bioactivation of ticlopidine and clopidogrel.

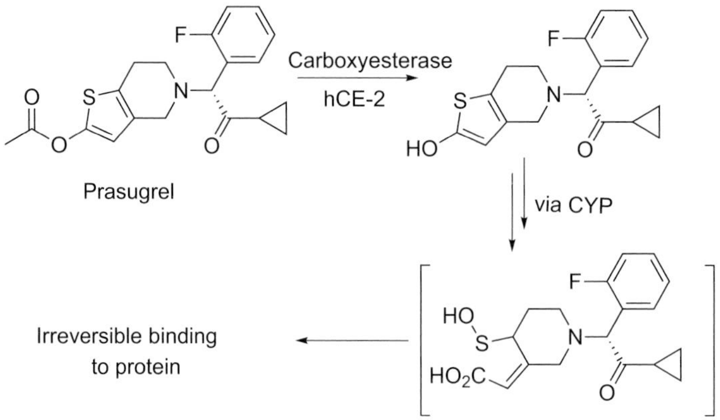

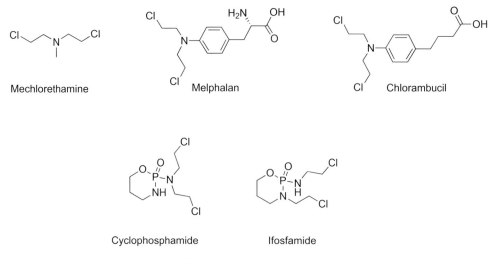

Figure 7.9 Metabolic activation of prasugrel.

On the other hand, prasugrel, which is the newest member of this class of drugs, is first hydrolyzed by human carboxyesterase 2 (hCE2) to the thiolactone (Figure 7.9) [38, 42–44]. The thiolactone is then activated to sulfenic acid via a P450-mediated pathway that is similar to the one described for clopidogrel and ticlopidine.

7.2.5
Oxazaphosphorines

The oxazaphosphorine classes of cytotoxic agents were designed as prodrugs of nitrogen mustards (e.g., mechlorethamine, melphalan, or chlorambucil) (Figure 7.10). The rationale was to mask the reactivity of the mustard group or use properties specific to the cancerous cells to increase the selectivity (versus normal

Mechlorethamine   Melphalan   Chlorambucil

Cyclophosphamide   Ifosfamide

Figure 7.10 Structures of nitrogen mustards used clinically.

tissue). The two primary drugs that belong to this class are cyclophosphamide and ifosfamide (Figure 7.10) [45]. These drugs are frequently employed either as a single agent or in combination with other chemotherapeutics.

Both agents require enzymatic bioactivation to manifest cytostatic activity [46, 47]. The mechanism of bioactivation involves P450-mediated oxidation to 4-hydroxycyclophosphamide or 4-hydroxyifosfamide (Figure 7.11) [46, 48–50]. The 4-hydroxymetabolite readily diffuses into the cells where it undergoes spontaneous and reversible ring opening to afford aldophosphamide [51, 52]. A subsequent, nonenzymatic elimination of the phosphoryl group from aldophosphamide yields active phosphoramide mustard and the side product, acrolein [53]. The former is responsible for the generation of interstrand DNA cross-links, therefore inhibiting its replication and causing cell death by apoptosis, while acrolein results in additional DNA lesions [54–56].

It is important to note that the presence of the 2-chloroethyl moiety on the two secondary nitrogens in ifosfamide provides a very different chemical reactivity profile relative to cyclophosphamide. In contrast to the aziridinium ion intermediate that is responsible for the formation of interstrand DNA cross-links with cyclophosphamide, ifosfamide bioactivation leads to an aziridine moiety (Figure 7.12). The aziridine species is ~4 times less reactive compared to the aziridinium ion intermediate, which in turn affects the toxicity profile of the compound. Several other phosphoramide derivatives have been synthesized and advanced to clinical trials since then (see Figure 7.12c).

7.2.6
N,N,N',N',N',N'-Hexamethylmelamine

Hexamethylmelamine (Figure 7.13) is an antitumor agent shown to be effective against metastatic breast cancer, lymphoma, and cervical, bladder, and ovarian cancers [57]. The biochemical basis for its pharmacological action is bioactivation by P450. The first step involves oxidation of N,N-dimethylamino group to a carbinolamine followed by spontaneous dehydration to an iminium ion intermediate, a potent electrophile, which is likely the active species responsible for DNA alkylation (Figure 7.13) [58]. Similarly, a second iminium ion intermediate formation followed by DNA alkylation can lead to interstrand or intrastrand DNA cross-linking (Figure 7.13). This elucidation of mechanism of activation has led to the design of N^2,N^4,N^6-trimethylmelamine (trimelamol), a "preactivated" analogue of the parent, which is more water soluble than its predecessor and circumvents the necessity for oxidative activation (Figure 7.13) [58].

7.3
Bioreductive Activation of Drugs

Bioreduction of drugs yields reactive intermediates in the form of free radicals or electrophilic intermediates that can alkylate macromolecules such as DNA and other proteins. Some classes of drugs that belong to this category are described below.

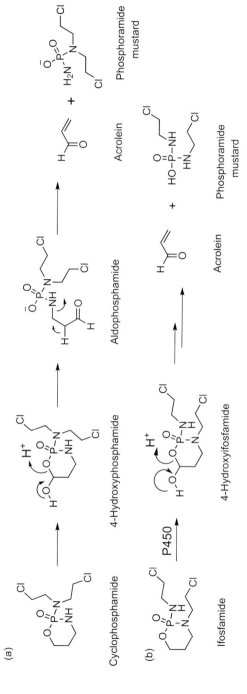

Figure 7.11 Metabolic activation of cyclophosphamide (a) and ifosfamide (b).

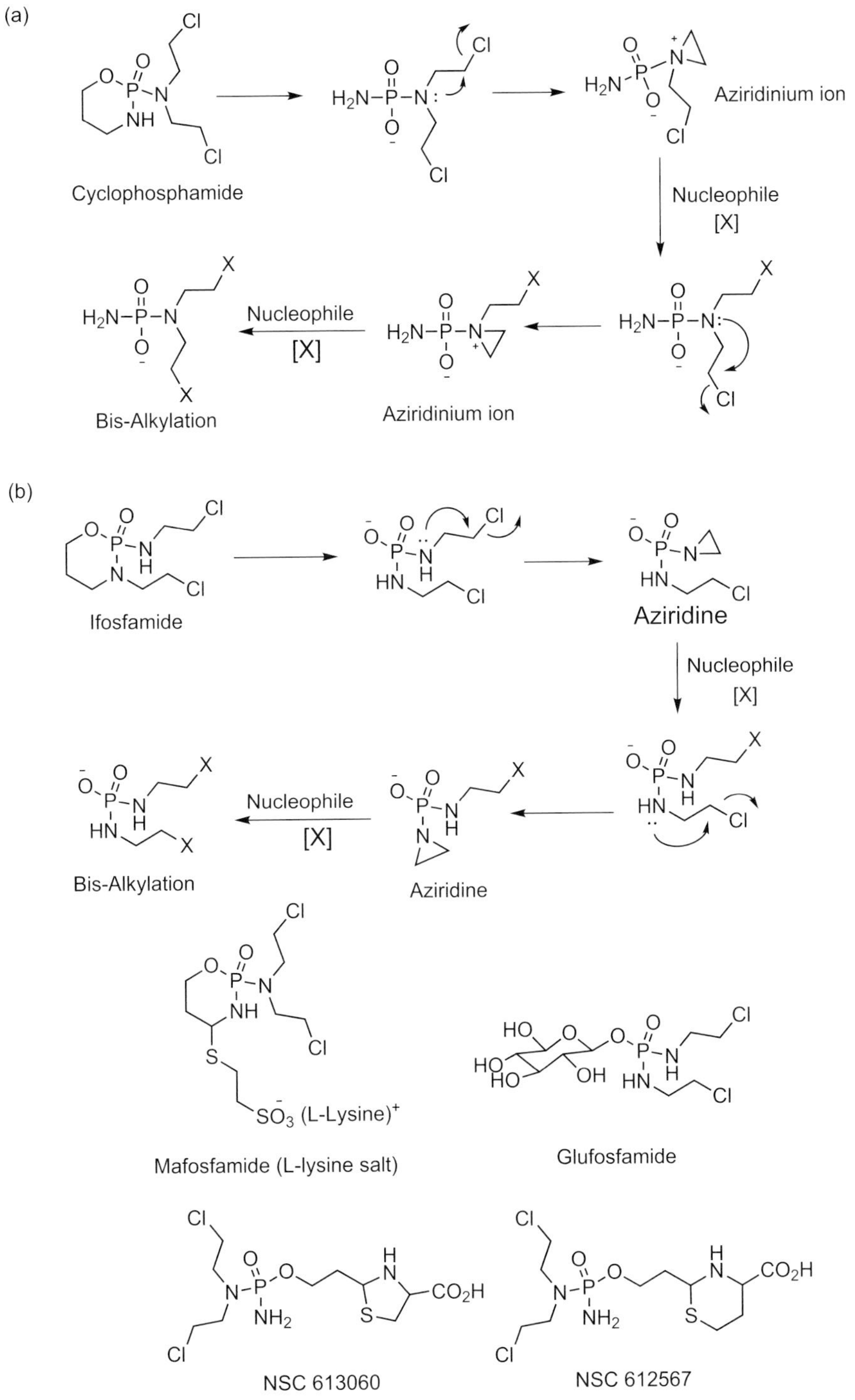

Figure 7.12 Bioactivation of (a) cyclophosphamide, (b) ifosfamide and (c) structures of related phosphoramide derivatives in the clinic.

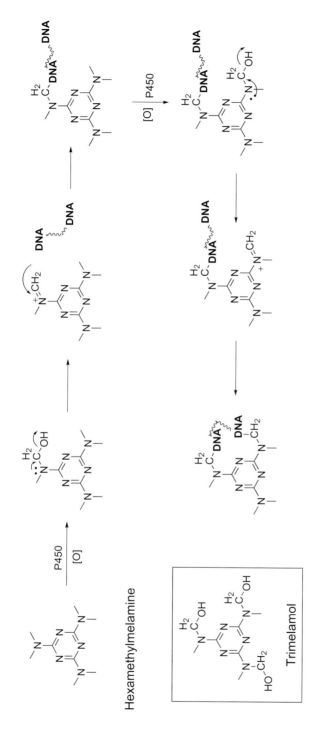

Figure 7.13 Metabolic activation of hexamethylmelamine.

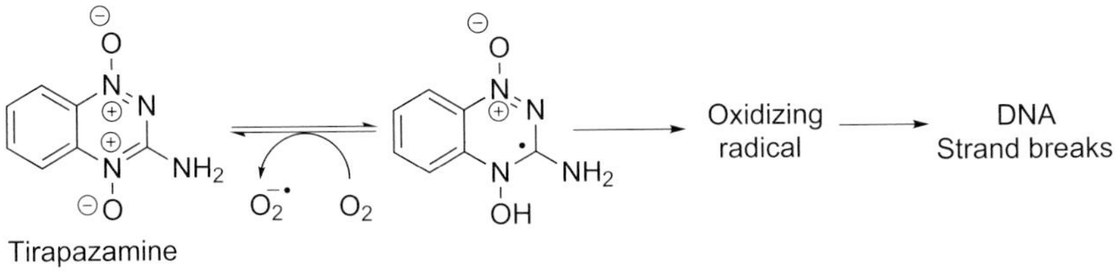

Tirapazamine

Figure 7.14 Bioreductive activation of tirapazamine.

7.3.1
Bioreduction to Radical Intermediates

7.3.1.1 Tirapazamine
Perhaps the best-known bioreductive prodrug, which undergoes P450 or P450 reductase one-electron reduction to the corresponding oxidizing radical of undetermined structure, is tirapazamine (Figure 7.14) [59]. Tirapazamine is very selective (100- to 200-fold) for hypoxic cells and generates radicals in DNA, which result in cytotoxic DNA breaks [60]. Although it forms a single radical species only, tirapazamine causes a high proportion of (relatively lethal) double-strand DNA breaks, possibly by generating high local concentrations of radicals in the vicinity of the DNA. This compound has been extensively studied in clinical trials, both as a single agent and in combination with radiation and with cisplatin [61, 62].

7.3.1.2 Anthracyclines
The anthracycline class of antitumor antibiotics represents the largest class of clinically useful quinonoid-based antitumor agents. These drugs are characterized by their tetracyclic quinone nucleus. The tetracyclic ring of anthracycline core is generally linked to a mono-, di-, and trisaccharide carbohydrate chain. Some clinically important anthracycline antibiotics are daunorubicin, doxorubicin, epirubicin, and idarubicin (Figure 7.15) [63]. The pharmacological activity of this class of compounds can be attributed in part to the reductive activation of the quinone functionality to free radicals that lead to DNA damage or lipid peroxidation in tumor cells.

Anthracyclines undergo flavoenzyme-catalyzed one-electron reduction to a semiquinone species that regenerates parent quinone by reducing molecular oxygen to a reactive oxygen species such as the superoxide anion ($O_2^{-\bullet}$), hydrogen peroxide (H_2O_2), or the hydroxyl radical ($OH^\bullet$) (Figure 7.16). This futile cycle is supported by a number of NAD(P)H-oxidoreductases (e.g., P450 or -b5 reductases, mitochondrial NADH dehydrogenase, xanthine dehydrogenase, and the reductase domain of the endothelial nitric oxide synthase) [64]. During this cycle, the semiquinone can result in reductive deglycosidation and formation of 7-deoxyaglycone. Alternatively, it could yield a carbon-centered radical, which along with the reactive oxygen species can oxidize lipids that could yield DNA adducts (Figure 7.16). Due to their increased lipid solubility, aglycones can intercalate into biological membranes and form reactive oxygen species in the closest proximity to sensitive targets [63, 64].

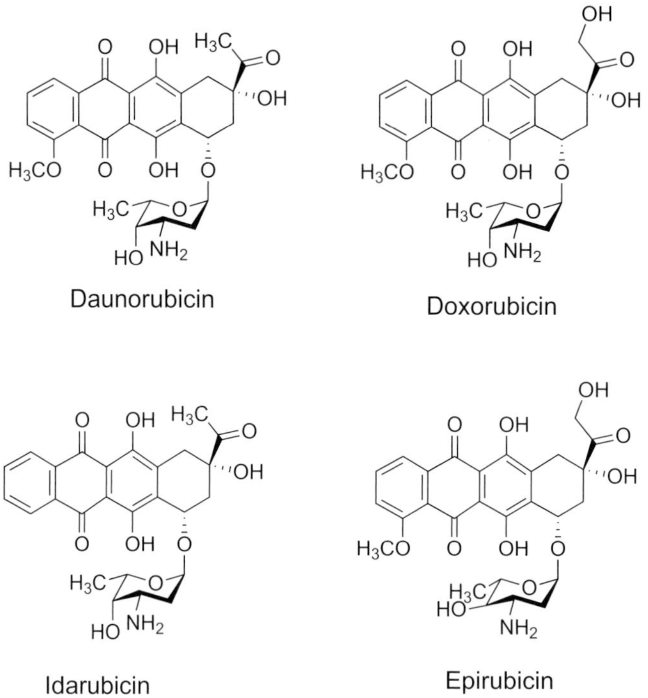

Figure 7.15 Structures of important clinically useful anthracycline antibiotics.

7.3.1.3 Enediynes

The enediyne class of antibiotics is a family of natural products and has been of great interest not only because of its unique molecular architecture but also because of its biochemical mode of action [65, 66]. Enediynes are structurally characterized by an unsaturated core of two acetylenic groups conjugated to a double bond or incipient double bond and are subdivided into two subfamilies. One class contains 9-membered cyclic enediyne chromophores such as neocarzinostatin [67], kedarcidin [68], and lidamycin [69], while others have a 10-membered ring system such as calicheamicins γ_1 [70], esperamicins A_1 [71], and dynemicin A [72] (Figure 7.17).

Both 9- and 10-membered enediyne chromophores require bioactivation for biological activity. The primary mechanism involves electronic rearrangement to form a benzenoid diradical (via a Bergman rearrangement) (Figure 7.18) [73]. These functionalities undergo reductive activation and result in cycloaromatization of the enediyne and generation of the highly reactive diradical intermediate. This diradical produces single- or double-stranded DNA lesions (and, in some cases, RNA lesions) via abstraction of hydrogen atoms from the sugar moiety of the DNA or RNA. The DNA damage in turn causes a significant decrease in DNA replication competency and ultimately leads to cell death.

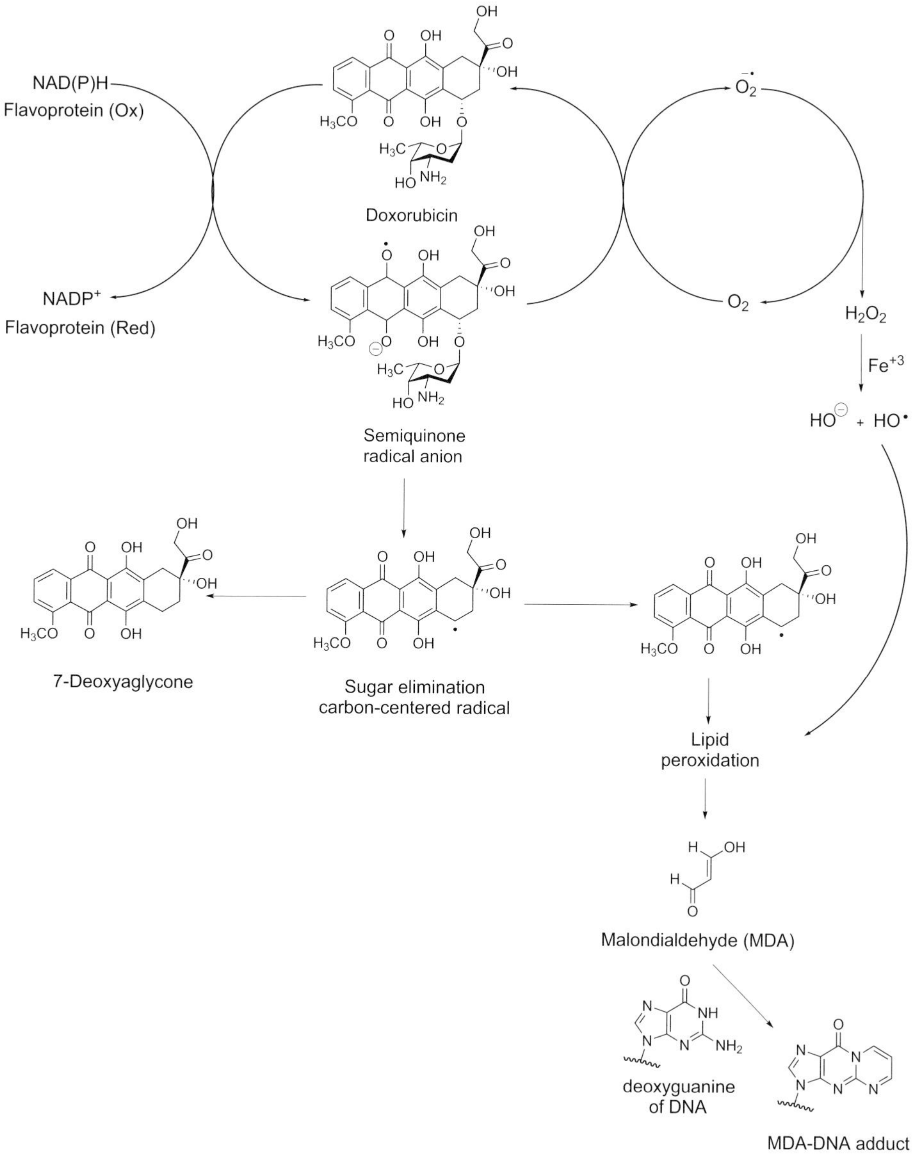

Figure 7.16 Reductive activation of anthracyclines to carbon-centered free radicals and reactive oxygen species.

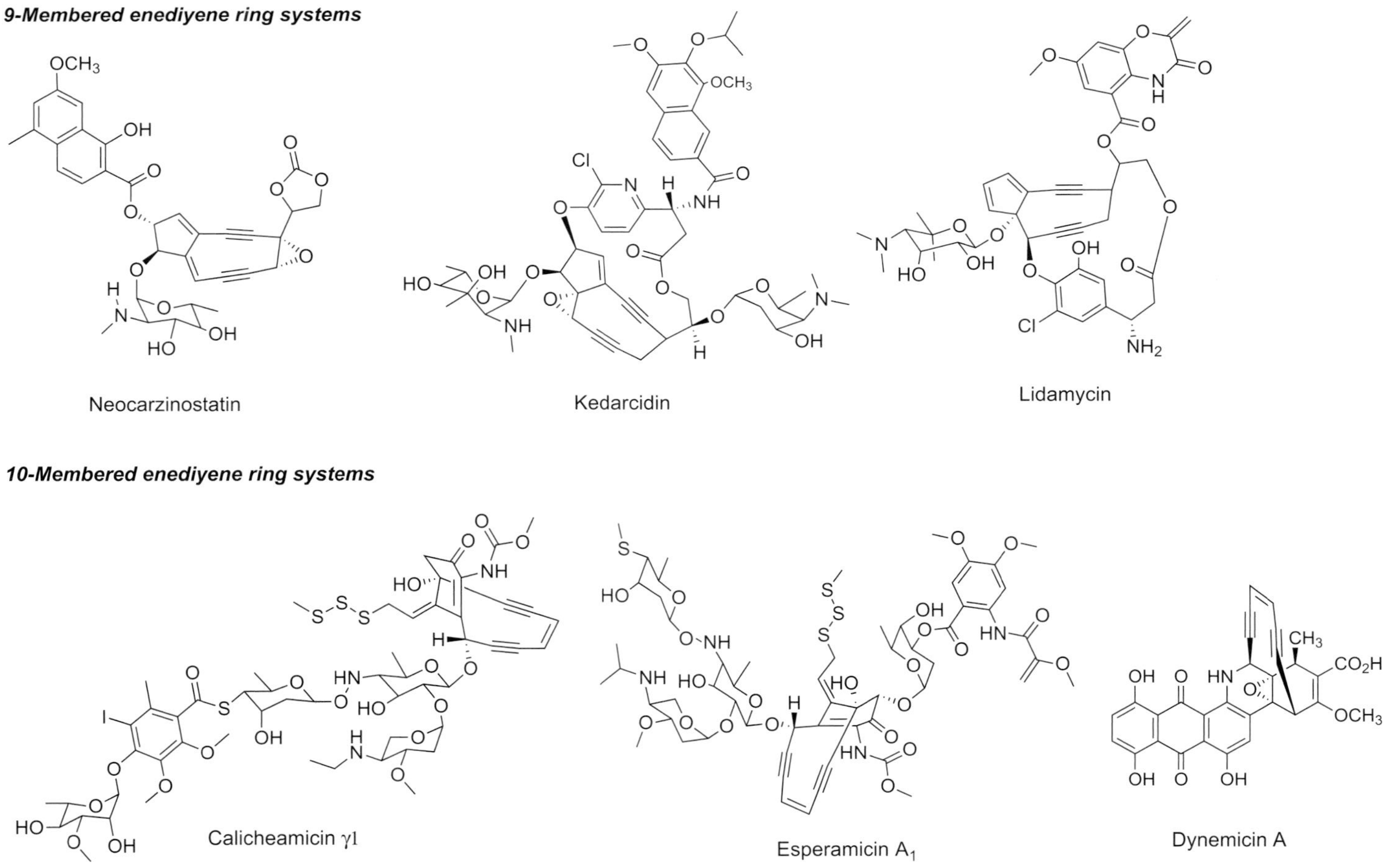

9-Membered enediyene ring systems

Lidamycin

Kedarcidin

Neocarzinostatin

Dynemicin A

Esperamicin A₁

10-Membered enediyene ring systems

Calicheamicin γ1

Figure 7.17 Structures of enediyne anticancer agents.

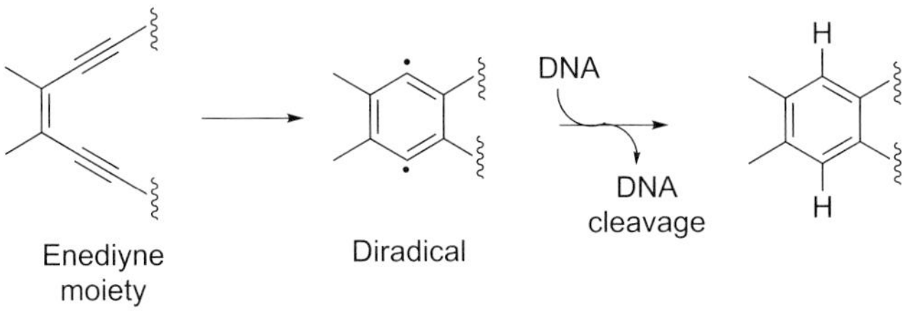

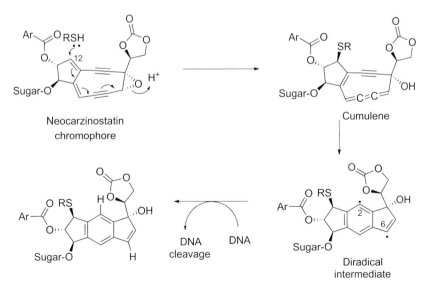

Figure 7.18 Cycloaromatization of the enediyne system.

The mechanism of activation of the neocarzinostatin chromophore was first suggested in 1987 (Figure 7.19) [74]. According to this mechanism, the DNA damage is initiated by a stereospecific nucleophilic attack at C(12) followed by a rearrangement of the ring skeleton with epoxide opening and formation of a cumulene intermediate. This highly strained reactive intermediate then undergoes a rapid cycloaromatization to form a diradical intermediate. This free radical abstracts a hydrogen atom from the 5′- or 4′-position of the carbon atom of deoxyribose in DNA to form a carbon-centered radical that in the presence of O_2 undergoes subsequent reactions leading to strand break (Figure 7.20) [75]. Thiols and UV radiation greatly enhance the DNA-cleaving properties of the neocarzinostatin chromophore [76].

In the case of calicheamicins, a nucleophile such as glutathione attacks the central sulfur atom of the trisulfide group yielding a thiol intermediate, which adds intramolecularly to the proximal α,β-unsaturated ketone embedded within the framework of the aglycone. The high strain caused by the intramolecular attack results in Bergmann rearrangement and cycloaromatization generating a

Figure 7.19 Bioactivation mechanism of the neocarzinostatin chromophore.

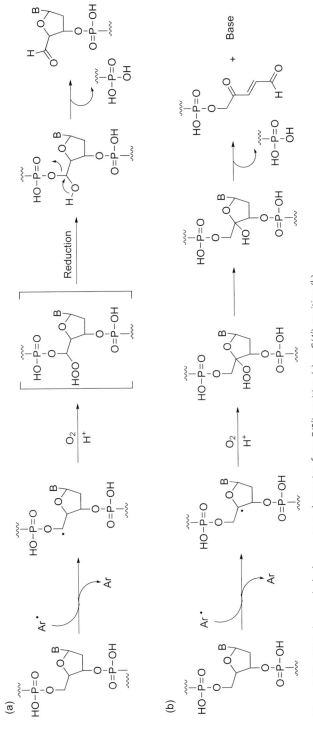

Figure 7.20 DNA cleavage by hydrogen atom abstraction from C(5′) position (a) or C(4′) position (b).

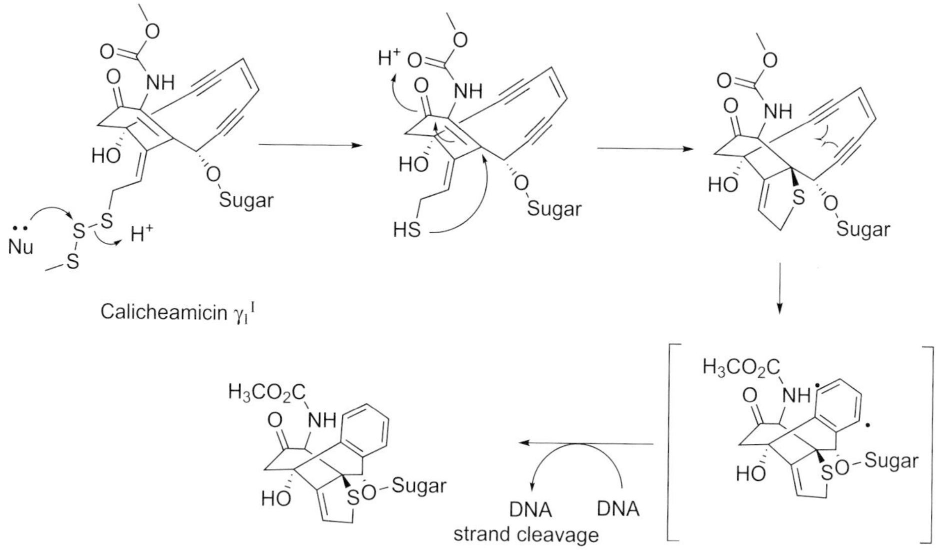

Figure 7.21 Activation of calicheamicin γ_1.

reactive diradical (similar to the one proposed in the activation of neocarzinostatin) (Figure 7.21). The esperamicins are thought to exert their biological action through cleavage of DNA in an almost identical manner to the calicheamicins [66].

In contrast, dynemicins, which contain an anthraquinone moiety in addition to the enediyne warhead, cleave DNA via reduction of the quinone moiety (Figure 7.22). It is suggested that the intercalation of the anthraquinone portion of the molecule is the first step in the activation [77]. The anthraquinone then undergoes bioreduction (Figure 7.22) to give the anthraquinol. The electron-rich anthraquinol generates a quinone methide intermediate via epoxide ring opening. The resulting quinone methide is trapped water (pathway A) or protonated (pathway B), to yield the corresponding alcohols. Opening the epoxide introduces a great deal of strain into the system, which is rapidly relieved by the molecule undergoing the cycloaromatization reaction to generate a 1,4-benzenoid diradical species that abstracts hydrogen atoms from the DNA, resulting in its cleavage (Figure 7.22) [78–80].

Even though enediynes are used clinically (e.g., neocarzinostatin in the treatments of gastric carcinoma and pancreatic adenocarcinoma), direct use of these compounds as antitumor agents is generally limited due to lack of tumor cell specificity and extreme cytotoxicity. To overcome this, most enediynes are generally modified by conjugation with various polymers or antibodies. For instance, conjugation of neocarzinostatin with polystyrene-co-maleic acid or its various alkyl esters has dramatically improved the uptake and overall toxicological profile, and, as a consequence, the polymer-conjugated derivative of neocarzinostatin has been used to treat hepatocellular carcinoma in Japan since 1994 [81–83]. One promising approach to compensate for cytotoxicity has been to conjugate 10-membered

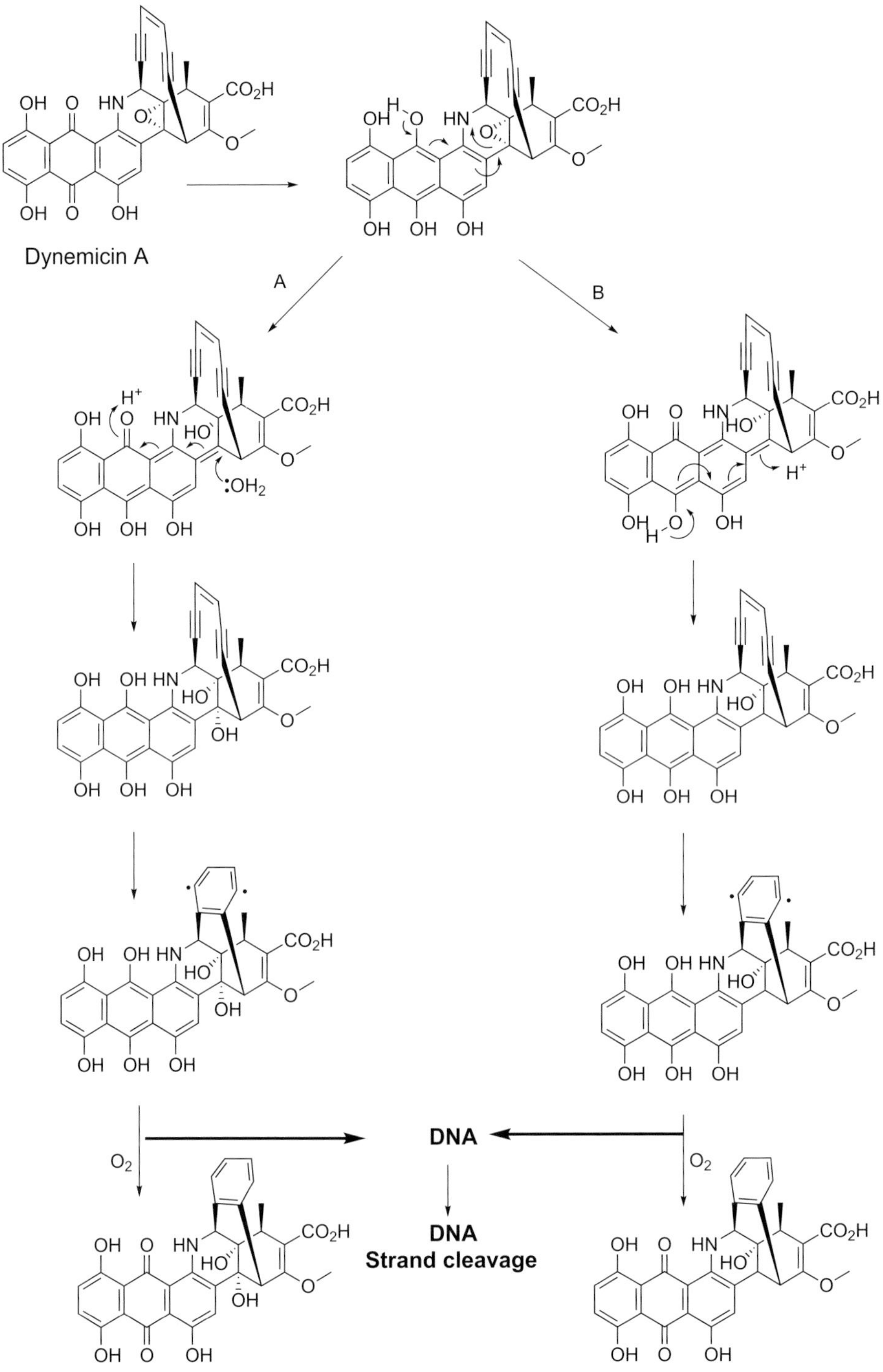

Figure 7.22 Bioactivation of dynemicin A.

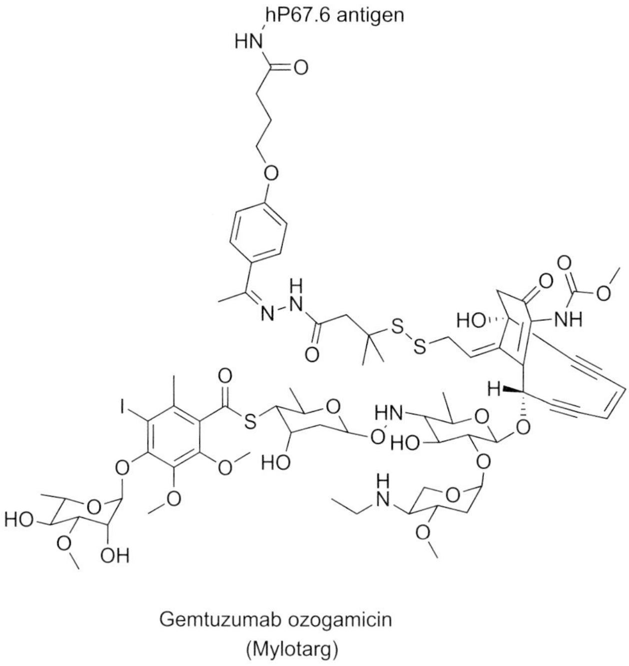

Gemtuzumab ozogamicin
(Mylotarg)

Figure 7.23 Structure of gemtuzumab ozogamicin.

enediynes to tumor-directed monoclonal antibodies (mABs). Such antibody-targeted chemotherapy is heavily dependent on the specific delivery of the enediyne to tumor cells via the tumor-associated antigen-mAb recognition to provide a localized exposure to the cytotoxic agent. For example, the 10-membered enediyne calicheamicin has been conjugated with humanized mAB (HuM195) specific for the antigen CD33, to reduce general cytotoxicity (Figure 7.23) [84–88]. The drug is covalently coupled to a humanized mAb via an immunoconjugate linker. The antibody HuM195 binds to the antigen CD33, a glycosylated transmembrane protein with an expression pattern that is confined to the hematopoietic system and results in endocytosis of the antibody–drug complex. Lysosomal acid hydrolysis of the linker in the mAb–CAL conjugate efficiently releases the 10-membered enediyne inside the cell. This anti-CD33 antibody–calicheamicin conjugate was named gemtuzumab ozogamicin and was sold under the trade name of Mylotarg to treat acute myeloid leukemia (AML) until recently (http://www.fda.gov/Safety/MedWatch/SafetyInformation/SafetyAlertsforHumanMedicalProducts/ucm216458.htm) [89, 90]. The patients treated with Mylotarg exhibited far less toxicity than patients who received standard chemotherapy. A similar conjugate inotuzumab ozogamicin, a CD22-specific immunoconjugate of CAL and mAb that binds to CD22 with high affinity and causes potent cytotoxic activity against malignant $CD22^+$ B cells, is being evaluated in clinical trials in Phase III [91, 92].

7.3.1.4 **Artemisinin Derivatives**

Artemisinin is a sesquiterpene trioxane lactone containing an endoperoxide bridge that represents a new class of antimalarial agents (Figure 7.24) [93–97]. Artemisinin and its derivatives are toxic to malarial parasites at nanomolar concentrations, but micromolar concentrations are required for toxicity to mammalian cells [98, 99].

The endoperoxide motif has been shown to be important for biological activity since an artemisinin derivative lacking this group is devoid of antimalarial activity. The selectivity of artemisinin toward parasite-infected erythrocytes over normal erythrocytes has been rationalized by heme Fe(II)-dependent bioactivation of the endoperoxide bridge to generate cytotoxic radical species in the infected erythrocytes [99]. Two pathways of bioactivation of the endoperoxide motif have been suggested [93, 94]. One pathway involves an initial heme Fe(II)-induced (or other sources of ferrous iron within the malaria parasite) reductive scission of the peroxide bridge to oxygen-centered radicals (Figure 7.25). These radicals can subsequently rearrange into one or both of two distinctive carbon-centered radical species. Association of Fe(II) with oxygen (O1) of the endoperoxide (Figure 7.25) provides an oxy radical that goes on to produce a primary carbon-centered radical. Alternatively, association with oxygen provides an oxy radical species, which, via a 1,5-H shift, can produce a secondary carbon-centered radical. The presence of the ring-contracted tetrahydrofuran derivative and 4-hydroxydeoxyartemisinin acts as surrogate markers for these two radical intermediates [94, 100, 101]. Alkylation of macromolecules (such as heme, specific proteins, and other targets), by these reactive radical intermediates, results in the death of malaria parasites [101]. PfATP6, the sarco/endoplasmic reticulum Ca^{2+}-ATPase, has been shown to be a specific target for artemisinin derivatives [102]. Alternatively, these radicals induce lipid peroxidation and this phenomenon provides access to downstream reactive oxygen species such as hydroxyl radicals and the superoxide anion that in turn leads to oxidative damage to receptors and enzymes located in the vicinity of the lipid bilayer of the cell membrane. Biomimetic studies by Berman and Adams have demonstrated a sixfold increase in heme-mediated lipid membrane damage [103].

The alternative pathway proposes the hydroperoxide to act as a masked source of hydroperoxide [93, 94]. In this pathway, Fe^{2+} acts as a Lewis acid to facilitate ionic,

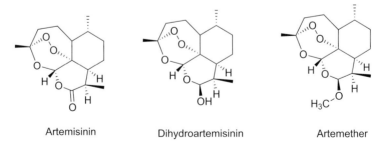

Artemisinin   Dihydroartemisinin   Artemether

Figure 7.24 Artemisinin and its derivatives.

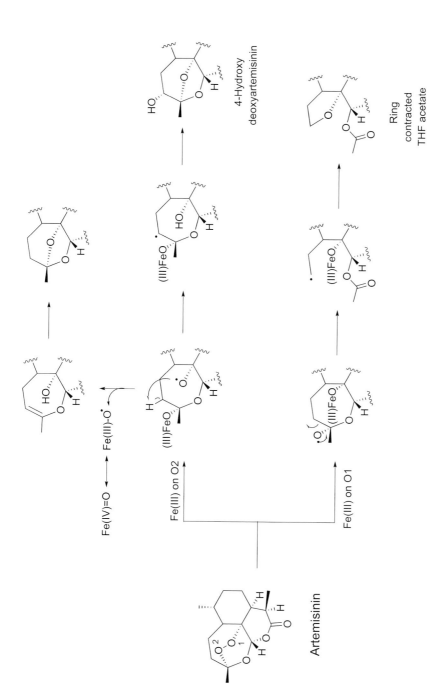

Figure 7.25 Bioactivation of artemisinin via reductive scission.

rather than radical, bioactivation of the artemisinins [101, 104, 105]. The endoperoxide bridge can undergo heterolytic cleavage via a zwitterion intermediate to yield a hydroxyl hydroperoxide moiety (A) or an unsaturated hydroperoxide moiety (B) (Figure 7.26). Subsequent Fenton-like degradation of either hydroperoxide intermediate can produce hydroxyl radicals that could oxidize target amino acid residues and irreversibly modify proteins by direct oxidation.

Artemisinin derivatives have also been shown to possess some antitumor activity as a consequence of their bioactivation to reactive oxygen species or carbon-centered radicals. These can play an important role in DNA damage, mitochondrial depolarization, or apoptosis [106].

7.3.2
Bioreductive Activation to Electrophilic Intermediates

The concept of bioreductive alkylation was developed by Sartorelli and coworkers in the early 1970s [107]. Quinone-containing compounds were among the first compounds to be explored as bioreductive prodrugs due to susceptibility of the quinone moiety to undergo reductive metabolism [108, 109]. The concept was based on the observation that human solid tumors contain cells that are remote from the vascular supply and most likely are deficient in oxygen. These cells possibly have a greater capacity for reductive metabolism and can potentially activate a latent alkylating group after reduction (Figure 7.27) [110].

7.3.2.1 Mitomycins
The quinone antibiotics mitomycins (Figure 7.28) were first discovered in 1950s, but it was in 1970 that they were approved for use as anticancer agents [111–113]. Most compounds in this class possess aziridine, quinone, and carbamate moieties arranged in a compact pyrrolo-[1,2-a] indole structure. Molecular pharmacology studies with mitomycin C revealed that this class of antitumor antibiotics was found to cross-link complementary strands of DNA [114–116]. Mitomycin C and its congener porfiromycin were shown to be selectively cytotoxic toward hypoxic cells [117]. Both these compounds are reductively activated, which converts the molecule to a short-lived and highly reactive quinone methide [111, 116, 118].

Reductive activation of mitomycin C involves a two-electron reduction of quinone moiety to the corresponding hydroquinone as the first step. The reduction disrupts the conjugation of the nitrogen lone pair electrons with the carbonyls, as speculated in the case of aziridinylquinones (see below), and substantially enhances the basicity of the aniline nitrogen [119]. This facilitates the elimination of the methoxy group (in the form of methanol). Subsequent tautomerism yields a highly reactive indole derivative called "mitosene" (Figure 7.29). Formation of the mitosene intermediate results in both the carbamate and the aziridine moieties to be "allylic" and is therefore capable of either mono- or dialkylating the DNA in a stepwise fashion [120, 121]. The first step involves opening of the aziridine functionality resulting in the exposure of the first electrophilic center (C1) (Figure 7.29).

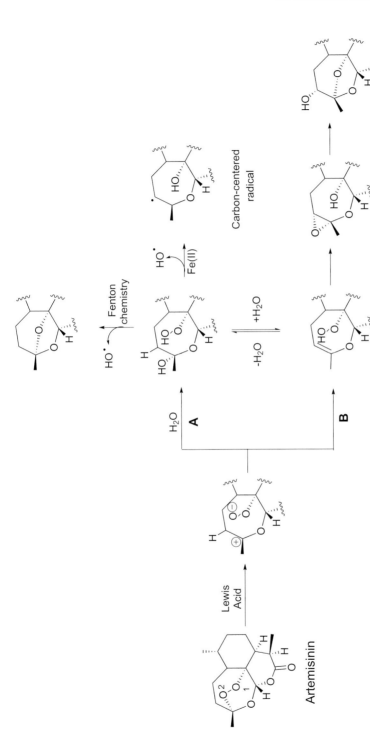

Figure 7.26 Bioactivation of artemisinin by heterolytic cleavage.

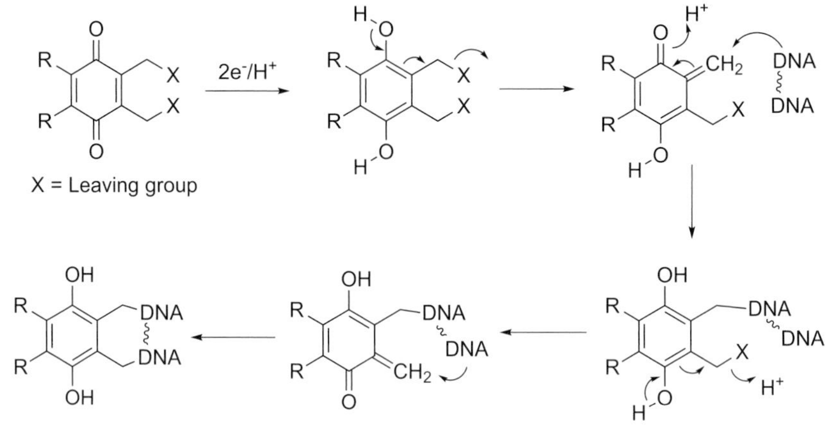

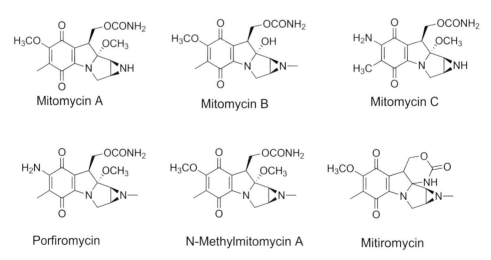

Figure 7.27 Reductive activation of substituted benzoquinones.

This is followed by elimination of the carbamate moiety to yield the second electrophilic carbon (C10). The alkylation appears to prefer the guanine bases in the GC-rich regions of the DNA with guanine alkylation at the 2-amino group.

7.3.2.2 Aziridinylbenzoquinones

The aziridinylbenzoquinones represent perhaps the simplest of the mitomycin C–like prodrugs (Figure 7.30) [24, 64, 122]. To date, only four benzoquinone-containing alkylating agents, diaziquone, carbazilquinone, triaziquone, and BZQ, have been used in the clinic, although other agents such as RH1 have received considerable attention.

Mitomycin A

Mitomycin B

Mitomycin C

Porfiromycin

N-Methylmitomycin A

Mitiromycin

Figure 7.28 Structures of mitomycin antibiotics.

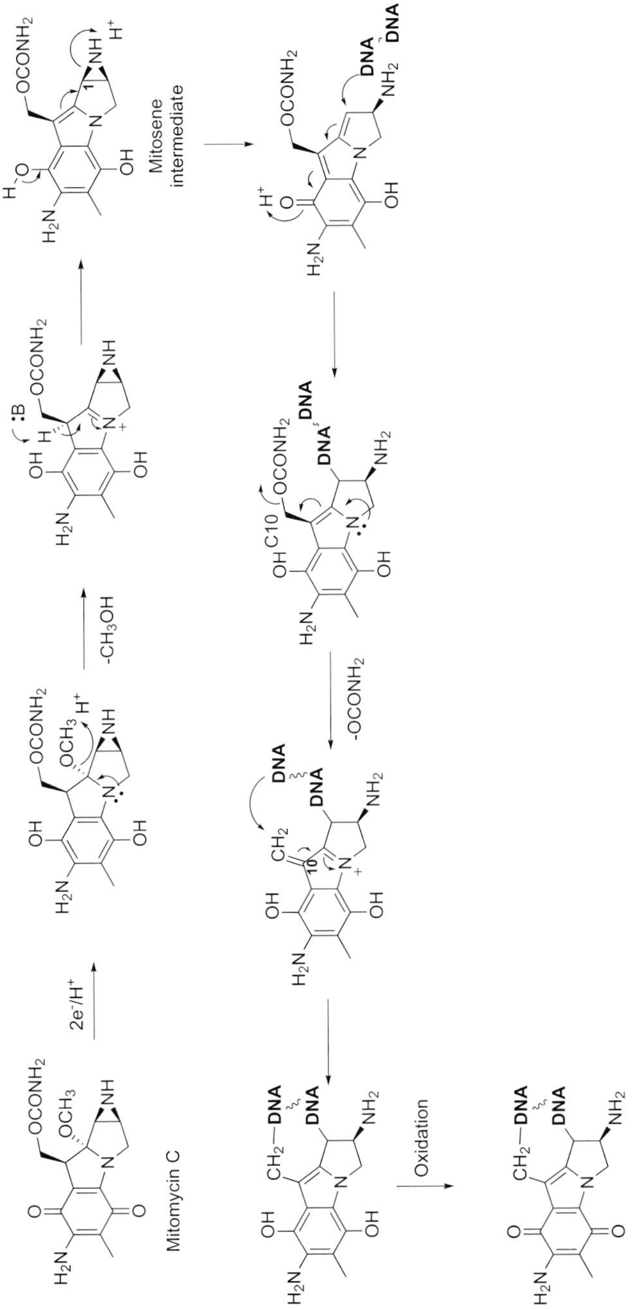

Figure 7.29 Reductive activation of mitomycin C.

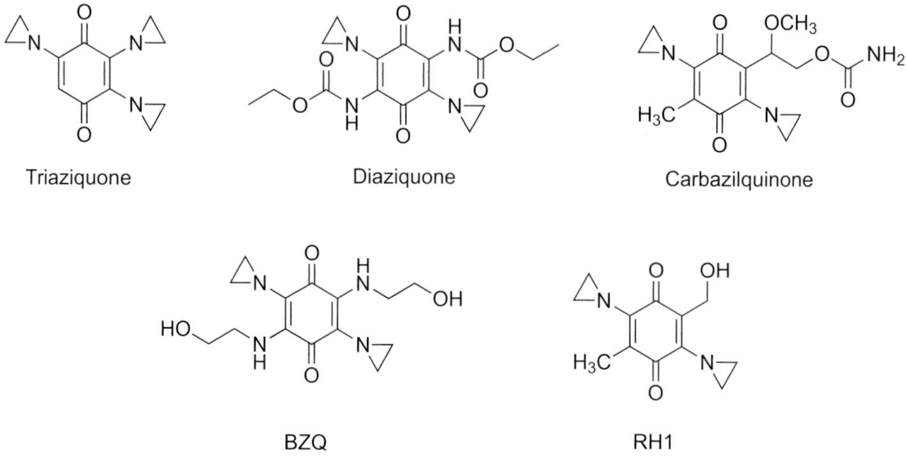

Figure 7.30 Structures of aziridinylbenzoquinones.

The activation of these compounds involves reduction of the quinone moiety from a nonaromatic quinone to the aromatic semiquinone or hydroquinone (one- and two-electron reductions, respectively) (Figure 7.31). The aziridine groups are quite unreactive when attached to quinones. However, as in the case of mitomycins, the reduction disrupts the conjugation between nitrogen lone pair of electrons and the carbonyl groups [119]. Consequently, there is an enhancement in the basicity of nitrogen atoms that results in their protonation and in the process vastly enhances the reactivity of the aziridine moieties and generates a species that is capable of cross-linking DNA (Figure 7.31). Following alkylation, autoxidation ensues, thus restoring the quinone moiety.

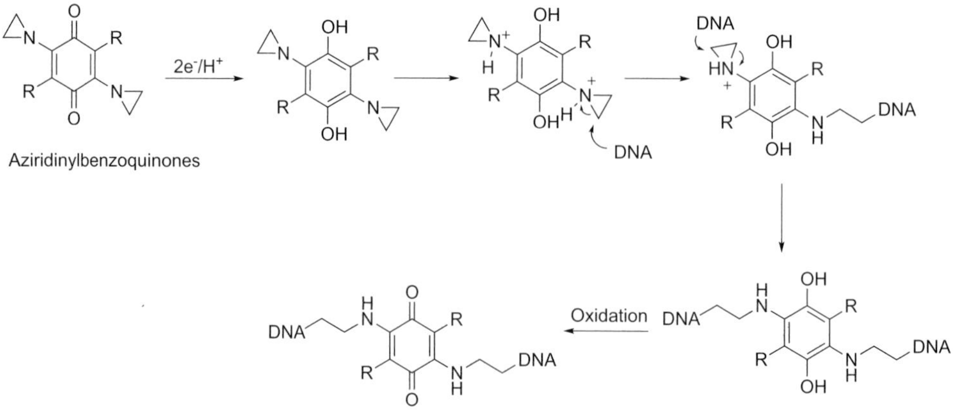

Figure 7.31 Metabolic activation of aziridinylbenzoquinones.

7.3.2.3 **Bioreductive Activation of Anthracyclines to Alkylating Species**

In addition to forming radicals, anthracyclines can also alkylate macromolecules via a reductive metabolic activation to electrophilic species. Figure 7.32 shows the proposed pathway for formation of a quinone methide by reductive activation of anthracyclines [108, 109]. The anthracycline hydroquinone formed by two-electron reduction of anthracycline can eliminate the sugar at the C7 position to form the corresponding quinone methide [123]. This intermediate can be efficiently trapped by thiolate nucleophiles such as *N*-acetylcysteine or glutathione [124] or the sulfydryl residues in proteins. Several groups have also revealed the formation of DNA adducts following reductive activation of anthracycline [125]. The ability of the hydroquinone to oxidize back to the quinone stabilizes the adduct formed following attack of the nucleophile [126].

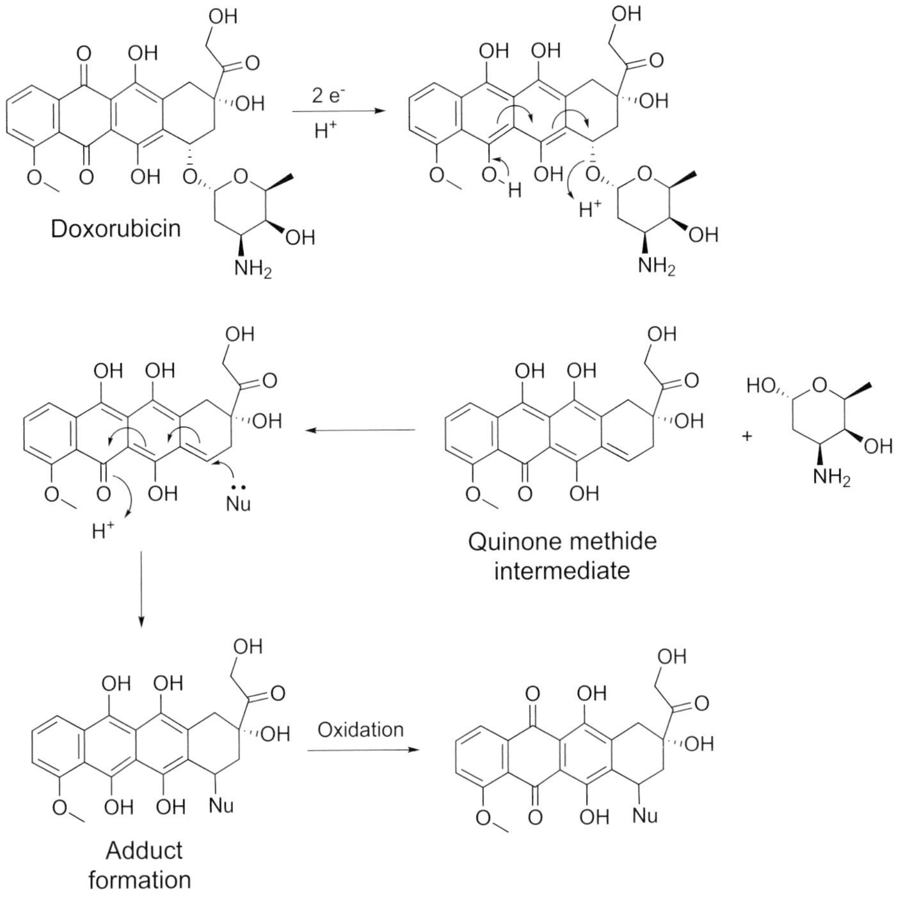

Figure 7.32 Bioreductive activation of doxorubicin to a reactive quinone methide intermediate.

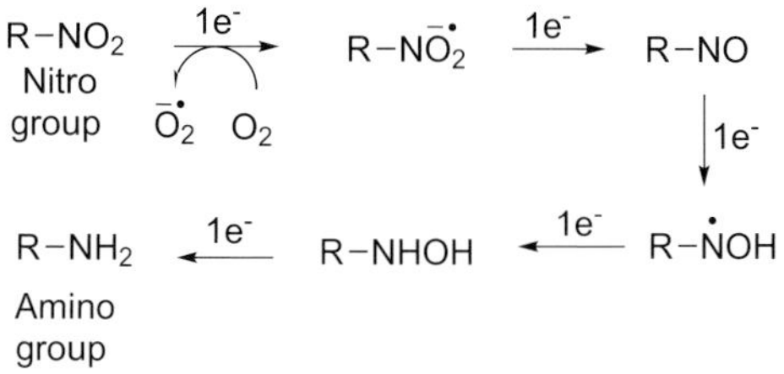

Figure 7.33 Six-electron reduction of nitro groups.

7.3.2.4 **Bioreductive Activation of Nitroaromatic Compounds**

The conversion of the electron-withdrawing nitro group to the electron-donating amine motif via a six-electron reduction (Figure 7.33) has been used as a means of reductively activating substituted nitroaromatic alkylating prodrugs. Nitrobenzyl compounds bearing leaving groups such as halides or carbamates at the benzylic position have shown hypoxic selectivities in cell culture and are proposed to behave as nucleic acid alkylating agents via generation of the iminoquinone methide intermediate (Figure 7.34) [127].

Many derivatives of nitro- and heteroaromatic chloromustards have been studies with respect to reduction of mustard reactivity (and therefore their toxicity) [24, 128]. Conjugation of the nitrogen mustard lone pair with the *para*-nitro group abrogates aziridinium ion formation. However, conversion of the nitro group to either the hydroxylamine or the fully reduced amine deconjugates this lone pair, thus facilitating the formation of the requisite reactive intermediate that can alkylate DNA (Figure 7.35).

Similarly, the nitroquinoline phosphoramide mustard is activated only after reduction of the nitro group to the corresponding aminoquinoline (Figure 7.36) [128]. The conversion of the electron-withdrawing nitro group to the electron-donating amine or intermediate hydroxylamine has also been used as a means of

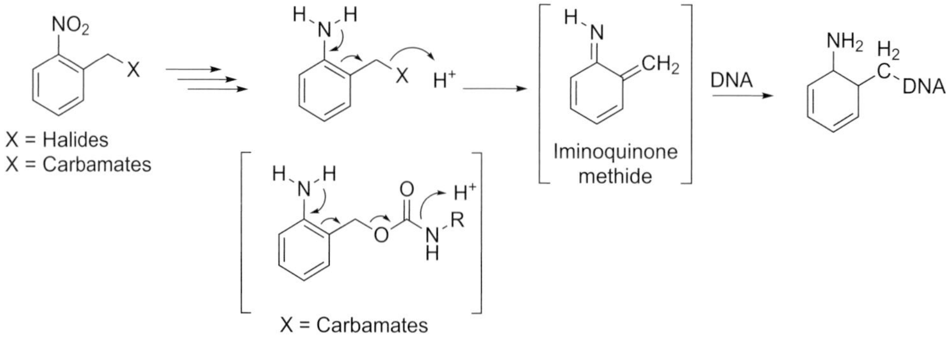

Figure 7.34 Bioreductive activation of nitroaromatic compounds.

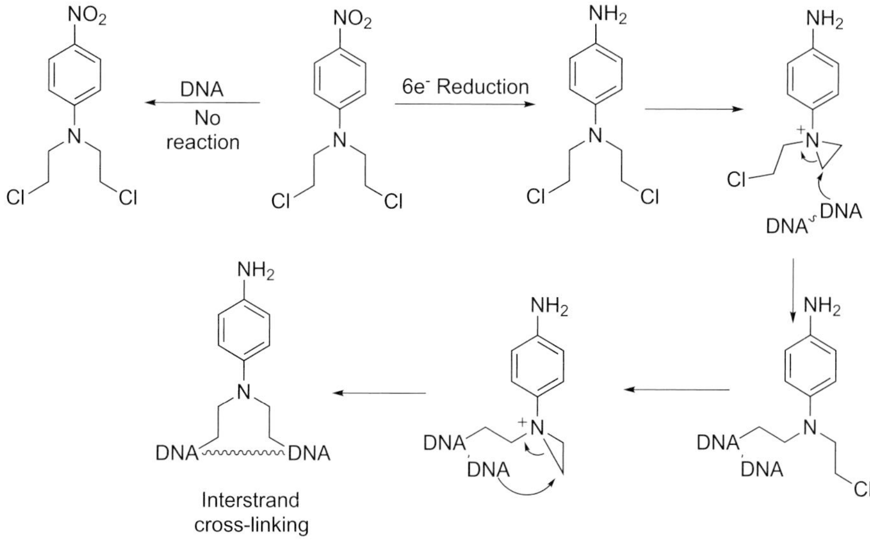

Figure 7.35 Bioactivation of nitroaromatic chloromustards.

reductively activating substituted nitroimidazoles toward mono- and bis-alkylation of DNA [129, 130].

7.4
Concluding Remarks

The examples presented in this chapter clearly show that bioactivation to yield a reactive intermediate is a perquisite for some drugs to exert their pharmacological

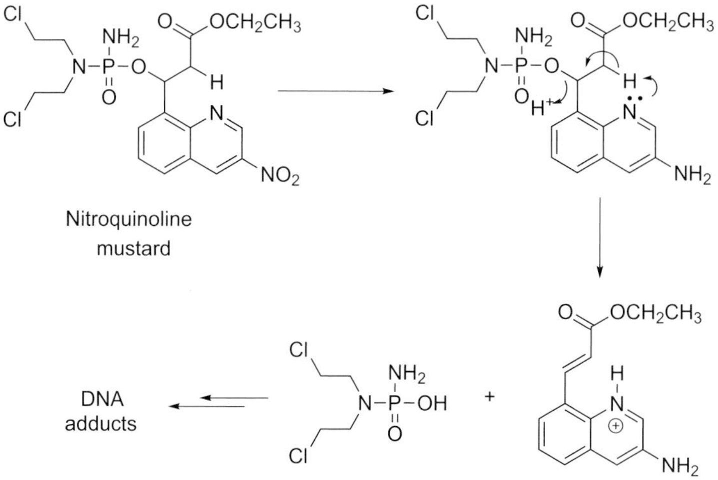

Figure 7.36 Reductive activation of nitroquinoline mustard.

effect. However, it is important to note that the reactive species formed in these cases can potentially act nonspecifically resulting in the irreversible binding to proteins. Thus, toxic effects observed following administration of these compounds could be due this nonspecific (and off-target) covalent binding of the reactive species to macromolecules.

References

1 Sachs, G., Shin, J.M., and Howden, C.W. (2006) Review article: the clinical pharmacology of proton pump inhibitors. *Alimentary Pharmacology and Therapeutics*, **23** (Suppl. 2), 2–8.

2 Lorentzon, P., Eklundh, B., Brandstrom, A., and Wallmark, B. (1985) The mechanism for inhibition of gastric (H++K+)-ATPase by omeprazole. *Biochimica Biophysica Acta*, **817** (1), 25–32.

3 Keeling, D.J., Fallowfield, C., Milliner, K.J., Tingley, S.K., Ife, R.J., and Underwood, A.H. (1985) Studies on the mechanism of action of omeprazole. *Biochemical Pharmacology*, **34** (16), 2967–2973.

4 Lindberg, P., Nordberg, P., Alminger, T., Brandstrom, A., and Wallmark, B. (1986) The mechanism of action of the gastric acid secretion inhibitor omeprazole. *Journal of Medicinal Chemistry*, **29** (8), 1327–1329.

5 Carter, S.K., Schabel, F.M. Jr., Broder, L.E., and Johnston, T.P. (1972) 1,3-Bis(2-chloroethyl)-1-nitrosourea (bcnu) and other nitrosoureas in cancer treatment: a review. *Advances in Cancer Research*, **16**, 273–332.

6 Schabel, F.M. Jr. (1976) Nitrosoureas: a review of experimental antitumor activity. *Cancer Treatment Reports*, **60** (6), 665–698.

7 Colvin, M., Brundrett, R.B., Cowens, W., Jardine, I., and Ludlum, D.B. (1976) A chemical basis for the antitumor activity of chloroethylnitrosoureas. *Biochemical Pharmacology*, **25** (6), 695–699.

8 Schabel, F.M. Jr., Johnston, T.P., Mc, C.G., Montgomery, J.A., Laster, W.R., and Skipper, H.E. (1963) Experimental evaluation of potential anticancer agents. VIII. Effects of certain nitrosoureas on

intracerebral L1210 leukemia. *Cancer Research*, **23**, 725–733.

9 Johnston, T.P., McCaleb, G.S., and Montgomery, J.A. (1963) The synthesis of antineoplastic agents. XXXII. *N*-Nitrosoureas. I. *Journal of Medicinal Chemistry*, **6**, 669–681.

10 Johnston, T.P., McCaleb, G.S., Opliger, P.S., and Montgomery, J.A. (1966) The synthesis of potential anticancer agents. XXXVI. *N*-Nitrosoureas. II. Haloalkyl derivatives. *Journal of Medicinal Chemistry*, **9**, 892–911.

11 Walker, M.D., Alexander, E. Jr., Hunt, W.E., MacCarty, C.S., Mahaley, M.S. Jr., Mealey, J. Jr., Norrell, H.A., Owens, G., Ransohoff, J., Wilson, C.B., Gehan, E.A., and Strike, T.A. (1978) Evaluation of BCNU and/or radiotherapy in the treatment of anaplastic gliomas. A cooperative clinical trial. *Journal of Neurosurgery*, **49** (3), 333–343.

12 Walker, M.D. (1978) The contemporary role of chemotherapy in the treatment of malignant brain tumor. *Clinical Neurosurgery*, **25**, 388–396.

13 Weiss, R.B. (1982) Streptozocin: a review of its pharmacology, efficacy, and toxicity. *Cancer Treatment Reports*, **66** (3), 427–438.

14 Weiss, R.B. and Issell, B.F. (1982) The nitrosoureas: carmustine (BCNU) and lomustine (CCNU). *Cancer Treatment Reviews*, **9** (4), 313–330.

15 Brundrett, R.B., Cowens, J.W., and Colvin, M. (1976) Chemistry of nitrosoureas. Decomposition of deuterated 1,3-bis(2-chloroethyl)-1-nitrosourea. *Journal of Medicinal Chemistry*, **19** (7), 958–961.

16 Lemoine, A., Lucas, C., and Ings, R.M. (1991) Metabolism of the

chloroethylnitrosoureas. *Xenobiotica*, **21** (6), 775–791.

17 Chen, F.X., Bodell, W.J., Liang, G., and Gold, B. (1996) Reaction of *N*-(2-chloroethyl)-*N*-nitrosoureas with DNA: effect of buffers on DNA adduction, cross-linking, and cytotoxicity. *Chemical Research in Toxicology*, **9** (1), 208–214.

18 Kohn, K.W. (1977) Interstrand cross-linking of DNA by 1,3-bis(2-chloroethyl)-1-nitrosourea and other 1-(2-haloethyl)-1-nitrosoureas. *Cancer Research*, **37** (5), 1450–1454.

19 Tong, W.P., Kirk, M.C., and Ludlum, D.B. (1982) Formation of the cross-link 1-[N3-deoxycytidyl],2-[N1-deoxyguanosinyl] ethane in DNA treated with *N,N'*-bis(2-chloroethyl)-*N*-nitrosourea. *Cancer Research*, **42** (8), 3102–3105.

20 Tong, W.P., Kohn, K.W., and Ludlum, D.B. (1982) Modifications of DNA by different haloethylnitrosoureas. *Cancer Research*, **42** (11), 4460–4464.

21 Ross, D., Langdon, S.P., Gescher, A., and Stevens, M.F. (1984) Studies of the mode of action of antitumour triazenes and triazines – V. The correlation of the in vitro cytotoxicity and in vivo antitumour activity of hexamethylmelamine analogues with their metabolism. *Biochemical Pharmacology*, **33** (7), 1131–1136.

22 Stevens, M.F., Hickman, J.A., Stone, R., Gibson, N.W., Baig, G.U., Lunt, E., and Newton, C.G. (1984) Antitumor imidazotetrazines. 1. Synthesis and chemistry of 8-carbamoyl-3-(2-chloroethyl)imidazo[5,1-d]-1,2,3,5-tetrazin-4(3 H)-one, a novel broad-spectrum antitumor agent. *Journal of Medicinal Chemistry*, **27** (2), 196–201.

23 Vaughan, K., Tang, Y., Llanos, G., Horton, J.K., Simmonds, R.J., Hickman, J.A., and Stevens, M.F. (1984) Studies of the mode of action of antitumor triazenes and triazines. 6. 1-Aryl-3-(hydroxymethyl)-3-methyltriazenes: synthesis, chemistry, and antitumor properties. *Journal of Medicinal Chemistry*, **27** (3), 357–363.

24 Rajski, S.R. and Williams, R.M. (1998) DNA cross-linking agents as antitumor drugs. *Chemical Reviews*, **98** (8), 2723–2796.

25 Agarwala, S.S., Kirkwood, J.M., Gore, M., Dreno, B., Thatcher, N., Czarnetski, B., Atkins, M., Buzaid, A., Skarlos, D., and Rankin, E.M. (2004) Temozolomide for the treatment of brain metastases associated with metastatic melanoma: a phase II study. *Journal of Clinical Oncology*, **22** (11), 2101–2107.

26 Eggermont, A.M. and Kirkwood, J.M. (2004) Re-evaluating the role of dacarbazine in metastatic melanoma: what have we learned in 30 years? *European Journal of Cancer*, **40** (12), 1825–1836.

27 Canellos, G.P. (2004) Lymphoma: present and future challenges. *Seminars in Hematology*, **41** (4 Suppl. 7), 26–31.

28 Legha, S.S. (1989) Current therapy for malignant melanoma. *Seminars in Oncology*, **16** (1 Suppl. 1), 34–44.

29 Legha, S.S., Ring, S., Papadopoulos, N., Plager, C., Chawla, S., and Benjamin, R. (1989) A prospective evaluation of a triple-drug regimen containing cisplatin, vinblastine, and dacarbazine (CVD) for metastatic melanoma. *Cancer*, **64** (10), 2024–2029.

30 Gibson, N.W., Erickson, L.C., and Hickman, J.A. (1984) Effects of the antitumor agent 8-carbamoyl-3-(2-chloroethyl)imidazo[5,1-d]-1,2,3,5-tetrazin-4(3 H)-one on the DNA of mouse L1210 cells. *Cancer Research*, **44** (5), 1767–1771.

31 Gibson, N.W., Hickman, J.A., and Erickson, L.C. (1984) DNA cross-linking and cytotoxicity in normal and transformed human cells treated in vitro with 8-carbamoyl-3-(2-chloroethyl)imidazo[5,1-d]-1,2,3,5-tetrazin-4(3H)-one. *Cancer Research*, **44** (5), 1772–1775.

32 Denny, B.J., Wheelhouse, R.T., Stevens, M.F., Tsang, L.L., and Slack, J.A. (1994) NMR and molecular modeling investigation of the mechanism of activation of the antitumor drug temozolomide and its interaction with DNA. *Biochemistry*, **33** (31), 9045–9051.

33 Danson, S.J. and Middleton, M.R. (2001) Temozolomide: a novel oral alkylating

agent. *Expert Review of Anticancer Therapy*, **1** (1), 13–19.

34 Hill, D.L. (1975) Microsomal metabolism of triazenylimidazoles. *Cancer Research*, **35** (11 Pt 1), 3106–3110.

35 Skibba, J.L., Beal, D.D., Ramirez, G., and Bryan, G.T. (1970) N-Demethylation the antineoplastic agent 4(5)-(3,3-dimethyl-1-triazeno)imidazole-5(4)-carboxamide by rats and man. *Cancer Research*, **30** (1), 147–150.

36 Skibba, J.L., Ramirez, G., Beal, D.D., and Bryan, G.T. (1970) Metabolism of 4(5)-(3,3-dimethyl-1-triazeno)-imidazole-5(4)-carboxamide to 4(5)-aminoimidazole-5(4)-carboxamide in man. *Biochemical Pharmacology*, **19** (6), 2043–2051.

37 Meer, L., Janzer, R.C., Kleihues, P., and Kolar, G.F. (1986) In vivo metabolism and reaction with DNA of the cytostatic agent, 5-(3,3-dimethyl-1-triazeno) imidazole-4-carboxamide (DTIC). *Biochemical Pharmacology*, **35** (19), 3243–3247.

38 Farid, N.A., Kurihara, A., and Wrighton, S.A. (2010) Metabolism and disposition of the thienopyridine antiplatelet drugs ticlopidine, clopidogrel, and prasugrel in humans. *Journal of Clinical Pharmacology*, **50** (2), 126–142.

39 Savi, P., Combalbert, J., Gaich, C., Rouchon, M.C., Maffrand, J.P., Berger, Y., and Herbert, J.M. (1994) The antiaggregating activity of clopidogrel is due to a metabolic activation by the hepatic cytochrome P450-1A. *Thrombosis and Haemostasis*, **72** (2), 313–317.

40 Savi, P., Herbert, J.M., Pflieger, A.M., Dol, F., Delebassee, D., Combalbert, J., Defreyn, G., and Maffrand, J.P. (1992) Importance of hepatic metabolism in the antiaggregating activity of the thienopyridine clopidogrel. *Biochemical Pharmacology*, **44** (3), 527–532.

41 Savi, P., Pereillo, J.M., Uzabiaga, M.F., Combalbert, J., Picard, C., Maffrand, J.P., Pascal, M., and Herbert, J.M. (2000) Identification and biological activity of the active metabolite of clopidogrel. *Thrombosis and Haemostasis*, **84** (5), 891–896.

42 Hagihara, K., Kazui, M., Kurihara, A., Iwabuchi, H., Ishikawa, M., Kobayashi,

H., Tanaka, N., Okazaki, O., Farid, N.A., and Ikeda, T. (2010) Biotransformation of prasugrel, a novel thienopyridine antiplatelet agent, to the pharmacologically active metabolite. *Drug Metabolism and Disposition*, **38** (6), 898–904.

43 Farid, N.A., Smith, R.L., Gillespie, T.A., Rash, T.J., Blair, P.E., Kurihara, A., and Goldberg, M.J. (2007) The disposition of prasugrel, a novel thienopyridine, in humans. *Drug Metabolism and Disposition*, **35** (7), 1096–1104.

44 Williams, E.T., Jones, K.O., Ponsler, G. D., Lowery, S.M., Perkins, E.J., Wrighton, S.A., Ruterbories, K.J., Kazui, M., and Farid, N.A. (2008) The biotransformation of prasugrel, a new thienopyridine prodrug, by the human carboxylesterases 1 and 2. *Drug Metabolism and Disposition*, **36** (7), 1227–1232.

45 Friedman, O.M., Wodinsky, I., and Myles, A. (1976) Cyclophosphamide (NSC-26271)-related phosphoramide mustards – recent advances and historical perspective. *Cancer Treatment Reports*, **60** (4), 337–346.

46 Sladek, N.E. (1988) Metabolism of oxazaphosphorines. *Pharmacology and Therapeutics*, **37** (3), 301–355.

47 Connors, T.A., Cox, P.J., Farmer, P.B., Foster, A.B., and Jarman, M. (1974) Some studies of the active intermediates formed in the microsomal metabolism of cyclophosphamide and isophosphamide. *Biochemical Pharmacology*, **23** (1), 115–129.

48 Schmidt, R., Baumann, F., Knupfer, H., Brauckhoff, M., Horn, L.C., Schonfelder, M., Kohler, U., and Preiss, R. (2004) CYP3A4, CYP2C9 and CYP2B6 expression and ifosfamide turnover in breast cancer tissue microsomes. *British Journal of Cancer*, **90** (4), 911–916.

49 Xie, H.J., Yasar, U., Lundgren, S., Griskevicius, L., Terelius, Y., Hassan, M., and Rane, A. (2003) Role of polymorphic human CYP2B6 in cyclophosphamide bioactivation. *Pharmacogenomics Journal*, **3** (1), 53–61.

50 Griskevicius, L., Yasar, U., Sandberg, M., Hidestrand, M., Eliasson, E., Tybring, G., Hassan, M., and Dahl, M.L. (2003)

Bioactivation of cyclophosphamide: the role of polymorphic CYP2C enzymes. *European Journal of Clinical Pharmacology*, **59** (2), 103–109.

51 Highley, M.S., Schrijvers, D., Van Oosterom, A.T., Harper, P.G., Momerency, G., Van Cauwenberghe, K., Maes, R.A., De Bruijn, E.A., and Edelstein, M.B. (1997) Activated oxazaphosphorines are transported predominantly by erythrocytes. *Annals of Oncology*, **8** (11), 1139–1144.

52 Draeger, U. and Hohorst, H.J. (1976) Permeation of cyclophosphamide (NSC-26271) metabolites into tumor cells. *Cancer Treatment Reports*, **60** (4), 423–427.

53 Alarcon, R.A. and Meienhofer, J. (1971) Formation of the cytotoxic aldehyde acrolein during in vitro degradation of cyclophosphamide. *Nature New Biology*, **233** (42), 250–252.

54 Blomgren, H. and Hallstrom, M. (1991) Possible role of acrolein in 4-hydroperoxycyclophosphamide-induced cell damage in vitro. *Methods and Findings in Experimental and Clinical Pharmacology*, **13** (1), 11–14.

55 Flowers, J.L., Ludeman, S.M., Gamcsik, M.P., Colvin, O.M., Shao, K.L., Boal, J.H., Springer, J.B., and Adams, D.J. (2000) Evidence for a role of chloroethylaziridine in the cytotoxicity of cyclophosphamide. *Cancer Chemotherapy and Pharmacology*, **45** (4), 335–344.

56 Colvin, M., Brundrett, R.B., Kan, M.N., Jardine, I., and Fenselau, C. (1976) Alkylating properties of phosphoramide mustard. *Cancer Research*, **36** (3), 1121–1126.

57 Legha, S.S., Slavik, M., and Carter, S.K. (1976) Hexamethylmelamine. An evaluation of its role in the therapy of cancer. *Cancer*, **38** (1), 27–35.

58 Jackson, C., Hartley, J.A., Jenkins, T.C., Godfrey, R., Saunders, R., and Thurston, D.E. (1991) *N2,N4,N6*-Tri (hydroxymethyl)-*N2,N4,N6*-trimethylmelamine (trimelamol) is an efficient DNA cross-linking agent in vitro. *Biochemical Pharmacology*, **42** (11), 2091–2097.

59 Patterson, A.V., Saunders, M.P., Chinje, E.C., Patterson, L.H., and Stratford, I.J. (1998) Enzymology of tirapazamine metabolism: a review. *Anticancer Drug Design*, **13** (6), 541–573.

60 Hwang, J.T., Greenberg, M.M., Fuchs, T., and Gates, K.S. (1999) Reaction of the hypoxia-selective antitumor agent tirapazamine with a C1′-radical in single-stranded and double-stranded DNA: the drug and its metabolites can serve as surrogates for molecular oxygen in radical-mediated DNA damage reactions. *Biochemistry*, **38** (43), 14248–14255.

61 Senan, S., Rampling, R., Graham, M.A., Wilson, P., Robin, H. Jr., Eckardt, N., Lawson, N., McDonald, A., von Roemeling, R., Workman, P., and Kaye, S.B. (1997) Phase I and pharmacokinetic study of tirapazamine (SR 4233) administered every three weeks. *Clinical Cancer Research*, **3** (1), 31–38.

62 Lee, D.J., Trotti, A., Spencer, S., Rostock, R., Fisher, C., von Roemeling, R., Harvey, E., and Groves, E. (1998) Concurrent tirapazamine and radiotherapy for advanced head and neck carcinomas: a phase II study. *International Journal of Radiation Oncology Biology Physics*, **42** (4), 811–815.

63 Minotti, G., Menna, P., Salvatorelli, E., Cairo, G., and Gianni, L. (2004) Anthracyclines: molecular advances and pharmacologic developments in antitumor activity and cardiotoxicity. *Pharmacological Reviews*, **56** (2), 185–229.

64 Powis, G. (1987) Metabolism and reactions of quinoid anticancer agents. *Pharmacology and Therapeutics*, **35** (1–2), 57–162.

65 Shao, R.G. (2008) Pharmacology and therapeutic applications of enediyne antitumor antibiotics. *Current Molecular Pharmacology*, **1** (1), 50–60.

66 Smith, A.L. and Nicolaou, K.C. (1996) The enediyne antibiotics. *Journal of Medicinal Chemistry*, **39** (11), 2103–2117.

67 Koide, Y., Ito, A., Edo, K., and Ishida, N. (1986) The biologically active site of neocarzinostatin-chromophore. *Chemical and Pharmaceutical Bulletin (Tokyo)*, **34** (10), 4425–4428.

68 Lam, K.S., Hesler, G.A., Gustavson, D.R., Crosswell, A.R., Veitch, J.M., Forenza, S., and Tomita, K. (1991) Kedarcidin, a new chromoprotein antitumor antibiotic. I. Taxonomy of producing organism, fermentation and biological activity. *Journal of Antibiotics (Tokyo)*, **44** (5), 472–478.

69 Shao, R.G. and Zhen, Y.S. (2008) Enediyne anticancer antibiotic lidamycin: chemistry, biology and pharmacology. *Anti-Cancer Agents in Medicinal Chemistry*, **8** (2), 123–131.

70 Thorson, J.S., Sievers, E.L., Ahlert, J., Shepard, E., Whitwam, R.E., Onwueme, K.C., and Ruppen, M. (2000) Understanding and exploiting nature's chemical arsenal: the past, present and future of calicheamicin research. *Current Pharmaceutical Design*, **6** (18), 1841–1879.

71 Long, B.H., Golik, J., Forenza, S., Ward, B., Rehfuss, R., Dabrowiak, J.C., Catino, J.J., Musial, S.T., Brookshire, K.W., and Doyle, T.W. (1989) Esperamicins, a class of potent antitumor antibiotics: mechanism of action. *Proceedings of the National Academy of Sciences of the United States of America*, **86** (1), 2–6.

72 Kamei, H., Nishiyama, Y., Takahashi, A., Obi, Y., and Oki, T. (1991) Dynemicins, new antibiotics with the 1,5-diyn-3-ene and anthraquinone subunit. II. Antitumor activity of dynemicin A and its triacetyl derivative. *Journal of Antibiotics (Tokyo)*, **44** (12), 1306–1311.

73 Bergman, R.G. (1973) Reactive 1,4-dehydroaromatics. *Accounts of Chemical Research*, **6**, 25–31.

74 Myers, A.G. (1987) Proposed structure of the neocarzinostatin chromophore–methyl thioglycolate adduct; A mechanism for the nucleophilic activation of neocarzinostatin. *Tetrahedron Letters*, **28**, 4493–4496.

75 Povirk, L.F. and Goldberg, I.H. (1984) Competition between anaerobic covalent linkage of neocarzinostatin chromophore to deoxyribose in DNA and oxygen-dependent strand breakage and base release. *Biochemistry*, **23** (26), 6304–6311.

76 Kappen, L.S. and Goldberg, I.H. (1978) Activation and inactivation of neocarzinostatin-induced cleavage of DNA. *Nucleic Acids Research*, **5** (8), 2959–2967.

77 Sugiura, Y., Shiraki, T., Konishi, M., and Oki, T. (1990) DNA intercalation and cleavage of an antitumor antibiotic dynemicin that contains anthracycline and enediyne cores. *Proceedings of the National Academy of Sciences of the United States of America*, **87** (10), 3831–3835.

78 Semmelhack, M.F., Gallagher, J., and Cohen, D. (1990) Bioreductive alkylations as a trigger for toxic effects of dynemicin. *Tetrahedron Letters*, **31**, 1521–1522.

79 Nicolaou, K.C., Dai, W.M., Wendeborn, S.V., Smith, A.L., Torisawa, Y., Maligres, P., and Hwang, C.-K. (1991) Enediyne compounds equipped with acid-, base-, and photo-sensitive triggering devices. Chemical simulation of the dynemicin A reaction cascade. *Angewandte Chemie International Edition in English*, **30**, 1032–1036.

80 Nicolaou, K.C. and Dai, W.-M.A. (1992) Molecular design and chemical synthesis of potent enediynes. 2. Dynemicin model systems equipped with C-3 triggering devices and evidence for quinone methide formation in the mechanism of action of dynemicin. *Journal of the American Chemical Society*, **114**, 8908–8921.

81 Abe, S. and Otsuki, M. (2002) Styrene maleic acid neocarzinostatin treatment for hepatocellular carcinoma. *Current Medicinal Chemistry – Anti-Cancer Agents*, **2**, 715–726.

82 Maeda, H. (1994) SMANCS/lipiodol. *Gan To Kagaku Ryoho*, **21**, 907–913.

83 Ikeda, K., Saitoh, S., Suzuki, Y., Tsubota, A., Koida, I., Kobayashi, M., Arase, Y., Chayama, K., Murashima, N., and Kumada, H. (1997) Effect of arterial administration of a high molecular weight anti-tumor agent, styrene maleic acid neocarzinostatin, for multiple small liver cancer – a pilot study. *Journal of Gastroenterology*, **32** (4), 513–520.

84 Hamann, P.R., Hinman, L.M., Beyer, C. F., Lindh, D., Upeslacis, J., Flowers, D. A., and Bernstein, I. (2002) An anti-CD33 antibody–calicheamicin conjugate for treatment of acute myeloid leukemia.

Choice of linker. *Bioconjugate Chemistry*, **13** (1), 40–46.

85 Hamann, P.R., Hinman, L.M., Hollander, I., Beyer, C.F., Lindh, D., Holcomb, R., Hallett, W., Tsou, H.R., Upeslacis, J., Shochat, D., Mountain, A., Flowers, D.A., and Bernstein, I. (2002) Gemtuzumab ozogamicin, a potent and selective anti-CD33 antibody–calicheamicin conjugate for treatment of acute myeloid leukemia. *Bioconjugate Chemistry*, **13** (1), 47–58.

86 Giles, F., Estey, E., and O'Brien, S. (2003) Gemtuzumab ozogamicin in the treatment of acute myeloid leukemia. *Cancer*, **98** (10), 2095–2104.

87 Alley, S.C., Okeley, N.M., and Senter, P.D. (2010) Antibody–drug conjugates: targeted drug delivery for cancer. *Current Opinion in Chemical Biology*, **14** (4), 529–537.

88 Senter, P.D. (2009) Potent antibody drug conjugates for cancer therapy. *Current Opinion in Chemical Biology*, **13** (3), 235–244.

89 Bross, P.F., Beitz, J., Chen, G., Chen, X. H., Duffy, E., Kieffer, L., Roy, S., Sridhara, R., Rahman, A., Williams, G., and Pazdur, R. (2001) Approval summary: gemtuzumab ozogamicin in relapsed acute myeloid leukemia. *Clinical Cancer Research*, **7** (6), 1490–1496.

90 Williams, J.P. and Handler, H.L. (2000) Antibody-targeted chemotherapy for the treatment of relapsed acute myeloid leukemia. *American Journal of Managed Care*, **6** (18 Suppl.), S975–S985.

91 DiJoseph, J.F., Armellino, D.C., Boghaert, E.R., Khandke, K., Dougher, M.M., Sridharan, L., Kunz, A., Hamann, P.R., Gorovits, B., Udata, C., Moran, J.K., Popplewell, A.G., Stephens, S., Frost, P., and Damle, N.K. (2004) Antibody-targeted chemotherapy with CMC-544: a CD22-targeted immunoconjugate of calicheamicin for the treatment of B-lymphoid malignancies. *Blood*, **103** (5), 1807–1814.

92 DiJoseph, J.F., Goad, M.E., Dougher, M. M., Boghaert, E.R., Kunz, A., Hamann, P.R., and Damle, N.K. (2004) Potent and specific antitumor efficacy of CMC-544, a CD22-targeted immunoconjugate of

calicheamicin, against systemically disseminated B-cell lymphoma. *Clinical Cancer Research*, **10** (24), 8620–8629.

93 O'Neill, P.M., Barton, V.E., and Ward, S. A. (2010) The molecular mechanism of action of artemisinin – the debate continues. *Molecules*, **15** (3), 1705–1721.

94 O'Neill, P.M. and Posner, G.H. (2004) A medicinal chemistry perspective on artemisinin and related endoperoxides. *Journal of Medicinal Chemistry*, **47** (12), 2945–2964.

95 Acton, N. and Klayman, D.L. (1985) Artemisitene, a new sesquiterpene lactone endoperoxide from *Artemisia annua*. *Planta Medica*, **51** (5), 441–442.

96 Klayman, D.L. (1985) In reply: antimalarial etymology. *Science*, **229** (4715), 706–708.

97 Klayman, D.L. (1985) Qinghaosu (artemisinin): an antimalarial drug from China. *Science*, **228** (4703), 1049–1055.

98 Meshnick, S.R., Jefford, C.W., Posner, G. H., Avery, M.A., and Peters, W. (1996) Second-generation antimalarial endoperoxides. *Parasitology Today*, **12** (2), 79–82.

99 Meshnick, S.R., Taylor, T.E., and Kamchonwongpaisan, S. (1996) Artemisinin and the antimalarial endoperoxides: from herbal remedy to targeted chemotherapy. *Microbiology Reviews*, **60** (2), 301–315.

100 Robert, A., Cazelles, J., and Meunier, B. (2001) Characterization of the alkylation product of heme by the antimalarial drug artemisinin. *Angewandte Chemie International Edition in English*, **40** (10), 1954–1957.

101 Olliaro, P.L., Haynes, R.K., Meunier, B., and Yuthavong, Y. (2001) Possible modes of action of the artemisinin-type compounds. *Trends in Parasitology*, **17** (3), 122–126.

102 Eckstein-Ludwig, U., Webb, R.J., Van Goethem, I.D., East, J.M., Lee, A.G., Kimura, M., O'Neill, P.M., Bray, P.G., Ward, S.A., and Krishna, S. (2003) Artemisinins target the SERCA of *Plasmodium falciparum*. *Nature*, **424** (6951), 957–961.

103 Berman, P.A. and Adams, P.A. (1997) Artemisinin enhances heme-catalysed

oxidation of lipid membranes. *Free Radicals in Biology and Medicine*, **22** (7), 1283–1288.

104 Haynes, R.K., Chan, H.W., Lung, C.M., Ng, N.C., Wong, H.N., Shek, L.Y., Williams, I.D., Cartwright, A., and Gomes, M.F. (2007) Artesunate and dihydroartemisinin (DHA): unusual decomposition products formed under mild conditions and comments on the fitness of DHA as an antimalarial drug. *ChemMedChem*, **2** (10), 1448–1463.

105 Haynes, R.K., Chan, W.C., Lung, C.M., Uhlemann, A.C., Eckstein, U., Taramelli, D., Parapini, S., Monti, D., and Krishna, S. (2007) The Fe2+-mediated decomposition, PfATP6 binding, and antimalarial activities of artemisone and other artemisinins: the unlikelihood of C-centered radicals as bioactive intermediates. *ChemMedChem*, **2** (10), 1480–1497.

106 Woerdenbag, H.J., Moskal, T.A., Pras, N., Malingre, T.M., el-Feraly, F.S., Kampinga, H.H., and Konings, A.W. (1993) Cytotoxicity of artemisinin-related endoperoxides to Ehrlich ascites tumor cells. *Journal of Natural Products*, **56** (6), 849–856.

107 Lin, A.J., Cosby, L.A., Shansky, C.W., and Sartorelli, A.C. (1972) Potential bioreductive alkylating agents. 1. Benzoquinone derivatives. *Journal of Medicinal Chemistry*, **15** (12), 1247–1252.

108 Moore, H.W. (1977) Bioactivation as a model for drug design bioreductive alkylation. *Science*, **197** (4303), 527–532.

109 Moore, H.W. and Czerniak, R. (1981) Naturally occurring quinones as potential bioreductive alkylating agents. *Medicinal Research Reviews*, **1** (3), 249–280.

110 Kennedy, K.A., Teicher, B.A., Rockwell, S., and Sartorelli, A.C. (1980) The hypoxic tumor cell: a target for selective cancer chemotherapy. *Biochemical Pharmacology*, **29** (1), 1–8.

111 Tomasz, M. and Palom, Y. (1997) The mitomycin bioreductive antitumor agents: cross-linking and alkylation of DNA as the molecular basis of their activity. *Pharmacology and Therapeutics*, **76** (1–3), 73–87.

112 Crooke, S.T. and Bradner, W.T. (1976) Mitomycin C: a review. *Cancer Treatment Reviews*, **3** (3), 121–139.

113 Crooke, S.T., Henderson, M., Samson, M., and Baker, L.H. (1976) Phase I study of oral mitomycin C. *Cancer Treatment Reports*, **60** (11), 1633–1636.

114 Iyer, V.N. and Szybalski, W. (1963) A molecular mechanism of mitomycin action: linking of complementary DNA strands. *Proceedings of the National Academy of Sciences of the United States of America*, **50**, 355–362.

115 Szybalski, W. and Iyer, V.N. (1964) Crosslinking of DNA by enzymatically or chemically activated mitomycins and porfiromycins, bifunctionally "alkylating" antibiotics. *Federation Proceedings*, **23**, 946–957.

116 Iyer, V.N. and Szybalski, W. (1964) Mitomycins and porfiromycin: chemical mechanism of activation and cross-linking of DNA. *Science*, **145**, 55–58.

117 Kennedy, K.A., Rockwell, S., and Sartorelli, A.C. (1980) Preferential activation of mitomycin C to cytotoxic metabolites by hypoxic tumor cells. *Cancer Research*, **40** (7), 2356–2360.

118 Suresh Kumar, G., Lipman, R., Cummings, J., and Tomasz, M. (1997) Mitomycin C–DNA adducts generated by DT-diaphorase. Revised mechanism of the enzymatic reductive activation of mitomycin C. *Biochemistry*, **36** (46), 14128–14136.

119 Mayalarp, S.P., Hargreaves, R.H., Butler, J., O'Hare, C.C., and Hartley, J.A. (1996) Cross-linking and sequence specific alkylation of DNA BY aziridinylquinones. 1. Quinone methides. *Journal of Medicinal Chemistry*, **39** (2), 531–537.

120 Maliepaard, M., de Mol, N.J., Tomasz, M., Gargiulo, D., Janssen, L.H., van Duynhoven, J.P., van Velzen, E.J., Verboom, W., and Reinhoudt, D.N. (1997) Mitosene–DNA adducts. Characterization of two major DNA monoadducts formed by 1,10-bis (acetoxy)-7-methoxymitosene upon reductive activation. *Biochemistry*, **36** (30), 9211–9220.

121 Tomasz, M. (1995) Mitomycin C: small, fast and deadly (but very selective). *Chemistry and Biology*, **2** (9), 575–579.

122 Begleiter, A. (2000) Clinical applications of quinone-containing alkylating agents. *Frontiers in Bioscience*, **5**, E153–E171.

123 Gaudiano, G., Resing, K., and Koch, T.H. (1994) Reaction of anthracycline antitumor drugs with reduced glutathione. Formation of aglycone conjugates. *Journal of the American Chemical Society*, **116**, 6537–6544.

124 Ramakrishnan, K. and Fisher, J. (1986) 7-Deoxydaunomycinone quinone methide reactivity with thiol nucleophiles. *Journal of Medicinal Chemistry*, **29** (7), 1215–1221.

125 Cullinane, C., Cutts, S.M., van Rosmalen, A., and Phillips, D.R. (1994) Formation of adriamycin–DNA adducts in vitro. *Nucleic Acids Research*, **22** (12), 2296–2303.

126 Abdella, B.R. and Fisher, J. (1985) A chemical perspective on the anthracycline antitumor antibiotics. *Environmental Health Perspectives*, **64**, 4–18.

127 Teicher, B.A. and Sartorelli, A.C. (1980) Nitrobenzyl halides and carbamates as prototype bioreductive alkylating agents. *Journal of Medicinal Chemistry*, **23** (8), 955–960.

128 Firestone, A., Mulcahy, R.T., and Borch, R.F. (1991) Nitroheterocycle reduction as a paradigm for intramolecular catalysis of drug delivery to hypoxic cells. *Journal of Medicinal Chemistry*, **34** (9), 2933–2935.

129 O'Neill, P., Jenkins, T.C., Stratford, I.J., Silver, A.R., Ahmed, I., McNeil, S.S., Fielden, E.M., and Adams, G.E. (1987) Mechanism of action of some bioreducible 2-nitroimidazoles: comparison of in vitro cytotoxicity and ability to induce DNA strand breakage. *Anti-Cancer Drug Design*, **1** (4), 271–280.

130 O'Neill, P., McNeil, S.S., and Jenkins, T.C. (1987) Induction of DNA crosslinks in vitro upon reduction of the nitroimidazole-aziridines RSU-1069 and RSU-1131. *Biochemical Pharmacology*, **36** (11), 1787–1792.

8
Retrospective Analysis of Structure–Toxicity Relationships of Drugs

Abbreviations

BSEP	Bile salt export pump
CYP	Cytochrome P450
COX-2	Cyclooxygenase-2
HEK	Human embryonic kidney
IADRs	Idiosyncratic adverse drug reactions
GSH	Glutathione
NSAIDs	Nonsteroidal anti-inflammatory drugs
UDPGA	UDP-glucuronic acid
UGT	UDP-glucuronosyltransferase

8.1
Introduction

In analyzing drug–structure human toxicity relationships, one of the most difficult aspects is that clinical data are often sparse and highly subjective. Many human toxicities, particularly the severe ones, are low-frequency idiosyncratic reactions to the drug. This is almost always the case since a high-frequency event would be rapidly observed in preclinical or early clinical development studies. It is arguable that preclinical toxicology is remarkably predictive of drug safety in the vast majority of human individuals, something that is not stated perhaps forcibly enough. With low-incidence events, normal statistical patterns are not observed until thousands of individuals have been observed. Much attention is focused on drugs withdrawn from the market and issued black box warnings. These certainly highlight major issues but bias any analysis, since all drugs cause adverse side effects and the issuing of black box warnings and even market withdrawals is not a precise science and does not fully take into account efficiency of side effect reporting, incorrect or correct usage of the drug, timing of adverse events relative to drug introduction, and so on. One factor in benefit/risk assessment is the availability of similar drugs, in many cases from the same pharmacological class, which show a real (or apparent)

Reactive Drug Metabolites, First Edition. Amit S. Kalgutkar, Deepak Dalvie, R. Scott Obach, and Dennis A. Smith.
© 2012 Wiley-VCH Verlag GmbH & Co. KGaA. Published 2012 by Wiley-VCH Verlag GmbH & Co. KGaA.

lower incidence of the effect and several classes have seen the more apparently hazardous drugs removed from the market, the most dominant class being the non-steroidal anti-inflammatory drugs (NSAIDs).

Many idiosyncratic adverse drug reactions (IADRs) occur at rates around 1 in 30 000 individuals. To show that a side effect has definitely a lower incidence than 1 in 30 000 treated individuals requires 90 000 treated patients. Similarly, there is a much greater than 50% chance that until 30 000 are treated the frequency of observations will exceed 1 in 30 000. When a new drug is launched, frequency of reporting side effects is heightened. Large-scale launches may contribute to the skewing of reported side effects so that a drug, which may be comparable to others, becomes seen as having more adverse effects than others, and the drug becomes subject to warnings and withdrawals. Drugs such as trovafloxacin and benoxaprofen had unprecedented rapid large-scale launches that may have contributed to their marketing withdrawals. These drugs are now labeled as "toxic" (hepatotoxic) and frequently compared to other less toxic drugs. Sometimes, in this labeling, multiple side effects are ignored. Benoxaprofen was a strong photosensitizer [1] in addition to any hepatic events. Although sketchy, most patients exhibiting side effects were elderly, for instance, the incidence of photosensitivity was 30% in this group [2]. The major clearance route of benoxaprofen was via acyl glucuronidation, which was cleared by renal and biliary excretion. Biliary excretion was followed by hydrolysis in the lower gut and reabsorption. Lowered renal function in the elderly and longer colonic transit (increased hydrolysis of acyl glucuronide) has been suggested as a reason for extensive accumulation of the drug [3]. In elderly patients, the drug half-life was 100 h compared to the half-life of 30–35 h in younger subjects.

Without correct prescribing guidance, benoxaprofen was given to all individuals as a standard dose size. Thus, in comparing the drug to others, the label of "hepatotoxic" may simply refer to incorrect dosage in a patient subgroup rather than an intrinsic property in the molecule.

It is useful to try to separate the most probable causes of the toxicity into those caused by the primary pharmacology of the drug and those caused due to secondary pharmacology effects. Terms such as "on target" and "off target" are also used to discriminate these. Different definitions such as A to D have been also used historically, in which type A is the toxic mechanism that has a pharmacological basis. There are two subtypes of type A, one based on the primary pharmacology (A1) of the drug (i.e., selective activity against the intended target of the drug) and the other based on other secondary pharmacology(s) (A2) of the drug (nonselective activity against non-intended receptors/enzymes/ion channels, etc.). The further categories are type B, which probably has an immunological base and is idiosyncratic (low frequency) and was not viewed as having a classic dose–response relationship; type C in which the effect of the drug is also due to a chemical reaction between drug or metabolite and tissue macromolecules, but there is a rapidly ensuing response with a more classical dose–response relationship; and type D toxicity that includes carcinogenesis and teratogenesis. Types B, C, and D cover the area of toxicity due to reactive metabolites. To cover these categories this chapter will review toxicity by primary and secondary pharmacology and subdivide the latter category into reversible and irreversible

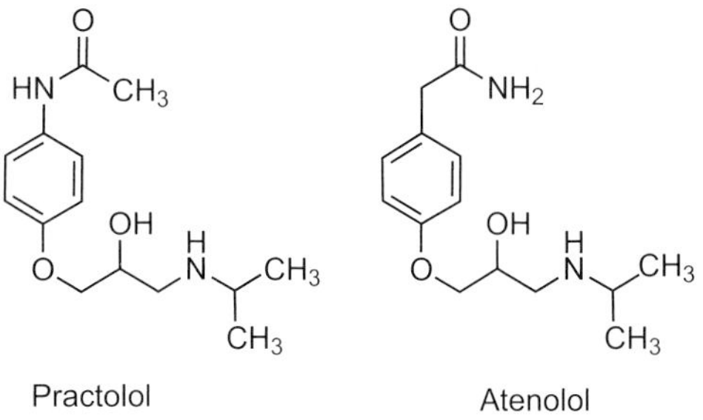

Figure 8.1 Structures of practolol and atenolol.

receptor effects. The term receptor is used to cover any macromolecule that the drug or metabolites interact with to trigger beneficial effects.

In certain cases the toxicity seen is of an unusual type and similar or follow-on compounds are devoid of the effects. This is comparatively rare but allows structural comparisons. As with most clinical toxicities, the actual mechanism is only partially understood. A prime example is practolol, a β-adrenoceptor antagonist with an acetylated aniline template (Figure 8.1), which was shown to be responsible for oculomucocutaneous syndrome. An antibody specific to a practolol reactive metabolite, most probably formed by oxidation of the aniline nitrogen, was found in the plasma of practolol-treated patients with or without a history of adverse reaction to the drug. No antibody was present in patients treated with other β-blocking drugs.

Atenolol (Figure 8.1) is structurally similar to practolol, but the amide has been reversed to remove the anilino function. The drug has been safely used for many years without any evidence of oculomucocutaneous syndrome. The aniline moiety has a long history of association with different drug toxicities. For instance, in 1955, Barnes and Barnes [4] observed the hypersensitivity reactions (reported as a syndrome similar to glandular fever) to *para*-aminosalicylic acid, diaminodiphenylsulfone, and procainamide and associated this with them all being primary aromatic amines.

Research on procainamide (Figure 8.2) showed that metabolism of the drug to a reactive hydroxylamine and nitroso metabolites could occur with human neutrophils and mononuclear leukocytes [5]. The metabolism only occurred if the cells had been stimulated to have a respiratory burst. The formation of reactive metabolites by these cells was deemed to be of great significance in the mechanism of procainamide-induced agranulocytosis (formation of a reactive metabolite by neutrophils) and procainamide-induced lupus (formation of a reactive metabolite by monocytes). Importantly, such metabolism was thought to be a possible general

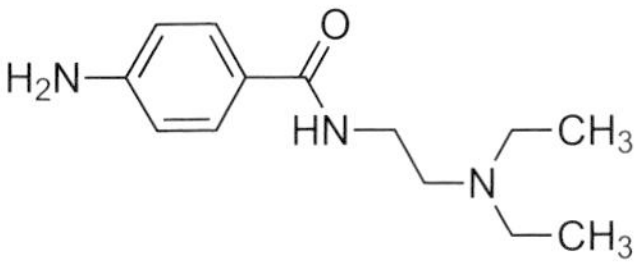

Figure 8.2 Structure of procainamide.

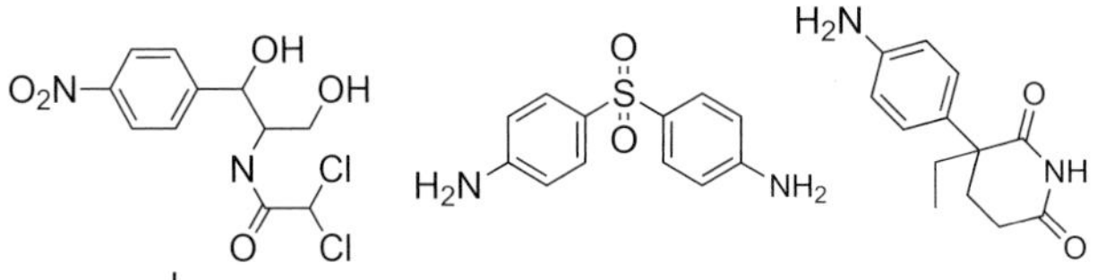

Figure 8.3 Structures of aniline or aniline precursor drugs chloramphenicol (I), dapsone (II), and aminoglutethimide (III).

mechanism for hypersensitivity reactions because of the role monocytes play in the processing of antigen and stimulation of antibody synthesis. Other aniline precursors or aniline-containing drugs causing aplastic anemia and agranulocytosis include the antibacterials chloramphenicol, aminoglutethimide, aminosalicilic acid, and dapsone (Figure 8.3) [6]. The aniline structure can be linked to mutagenicity, carcinogenicity, hepatic toxicity, skin toxicity, and blood toxicity (also including methemoglobinemia) (see Chapter 2). The facile formation of reactive hydroxylamine and nitroso metabolites that can react with macromolecules or undergo redox recycling is a compelling set of evidence for structure–toxicity relationships. Outside of this the work becomes less compelling, with fewer structural examples and more diverse toxicity.

In defining how structure–toxicity relationships can be best developed, it is useful to consider fairly recent drug side effect events. Table 8.1 lists drugs withdrawn

Table 8.1 Drug withdrawals from 1980 to date grouped into three categories of reason for withdrawal.

Primary Pharmacology		Reversible Secondary Pharmacology		Irreversible Secondary Pharmacology	
Generic Name	Daily Dose (mg)	Generic Name	Daily Dose (mg)	Generic Name	Daily Dose (mg)
Alosetron	1	Astemizole	10	Amineptine	300
Cerivastatin	0.3	Cisapride	40	Benoxaprofen	600
Encainide	150	Dexfenfluramine	15	Bromfenac	100
Flosequinan	100	Fenfluramine	15	Nomifensine	125
Rofecoxib	25	Grepafloxacin	400	Mibefradil	100
Valdecoxib	40	Rapacuronium	100	Remoxipride	300
		Terfenadine	120	Rofecoxib	25
		Troglitazone	400	Suprofen	800
				Temafloxacin	600
				Ticrynafen	400
				Tolcapone	300
				Troglitazone	400
				Trovafloxacin	200
				Valdecoxib	40
				Zomepirac	400

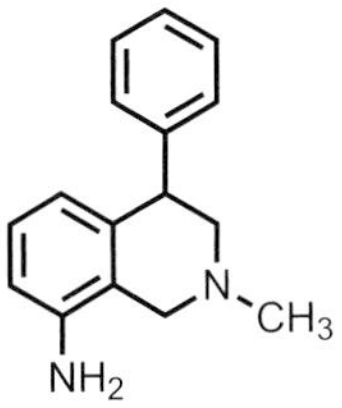

Figure 8.4 Structure of the aniline-containing antidepressant nomifensine.

since 1980 to date from the US and European markets. Below some of the drugs from this list will be examined in detail to understand the difficulties in defining the extent of the toxicity, the cause, and possible mechanisms and in doing so a basis for structure–toxicity relationships will be provided.

Although some of these drugs contain structural alerts, the only "validated" structure–toxicity relationship is with nomifensine (Figure 8.4). The drug was withdrawn for immunohemolytic (aplastic) anemia, in accord with the above aniline-containing drugs.

8.2
Irreversible Secondary Pharmacology

Amineptine, benoxaprofen, bromfenac, ticrynafen, troglitazone, tolcapone, and trovafloxacin were withdrawn from the market place due to hepatotoxicity. Temafloxacin, nomifensine, and remoxipride were withdrawn due to hemolytic and aplastic anemia. Suprofen was withdrawn due to flank pain syndrome, zomepirac due to anaphylaxis, rofecoxib due to cardiovascular toxicity, and valdecoxib due to skin and cardiovascular toxicity. The flank pain syndrome with suprofen is accompanied by renal dysfunction and associated changes in the excretion of uric acid. In many of the cases more than one toxicity finding also contributed to the withdrawal. For instance, temafloxacin was also associated with renal and liver toxicity and ticrynafen also exhibited flank pain syndrome [7].

8.2.1
Common Structural Features: Carboxylic Acids

Amineptine, benoxaprofen, bromfenac, suprofen, temafloxacin, ticrynafen, trovafloxacin, and zomepirac are all carboxylic acids. A major route of metabolism for carboxylic acids is the formation of acyl glucuronides and all but amineptine form this type of metabolite. To varying degrees acyl glucuronides are unstable and form positional isomers by acyl migration. The proposed pathway of protein covalent binding by acyl glucuronides involves condensation between the aldehyde group of a rearranged acyl glucuronide and a lysine residue or an amine group (of the N-terminus) leading to the formation of a glycated protein. Historically, much attention was focused on their possible role in toxicity since the isomers can bind covalently to proteins. Zomepirac is an α-unsubstituted acetic acid and as such has the highest reactivity and instability. This reactivity was initially linked, once the reactivity was revealed, to the hypersensitivity reactions that led to its withdrawal. This relationship looks scientifically robust, but studies have shown that NSAIDs are the second most important cause of drug anaphylaxis after penicillins in hospitalized patients, and the leading cause in ambulatory patients [8]. The finding is therefore general and while zomepirac may exhibit as the most pronounced case, anaphylaxic reactions have also been recorded for other NSAIDs including ibuprofen, indomethacin, sulindac, fenoprofen, meclofenamate, naproxen, piroxicam, tolmetin, acetaminophen, aspirin, diclofenac, ketorolac, valdecoxib, and celecoxib [7]. Many of these NSAIDs form acyl glucuronides, but compounds such as acetaminophen, piroxicam, valdecoxib, and celecoxib do not. With the suggestions of hypersensitivity being linked to acyl glucuronides, similar observations were made for other toxicities such as hepatic toxicity. While ibuprofen is considered to be one of the safest over-the-counter NSAIDs in the market, its close-in analogue ibufenac was withdrawn due to severe hepatotoxicity. Again, the α-unsubstituted carboxylic acid led to a much higher level of acyl glucuronide rearrangement and covalent binding suggestive of the role of highly unstable glucuronic acids in toxicity. Ibufenac caused raised liver function tests in a high number of patients with only a handful exhibiting actual frank hepatotoxicity.

Even with this distinction acyl glucuronides of α-substituted carboxylic acids have been implicated and investigated as possible causes of toxicity. Benoxaprofen was compared to flunoxaprofen, a structural analogue that appeared to be less toxic. When administered to rats, similar concentrations of plasma protein and liver protein adducts for benoxaprofen and flunoxaprofen were detected [9]. When this study was recreated in human hepatocytes, covalent binding was noted for both compounds and the proportion correlated to acyl glucuronide formation. 1,7-Phenanthroline increased the rate of glucuronidation but did not increase the rate of covalent binding. This is suggestive of other metabolites contributing to the covalent binding [10]. The fact that acyl glucuronides bind to protein in certain cases may have no link to toxicity. In studies [11] examining the cytotoxicity and genotoxicity of acyl glucuronides of NSAIDs, human embryonic kidney (HEK) 293 cells expressing UDP-glucuronosyltransferase (UGT) 1A3 (HEK/UGT1A3) and HEK/UGT1A4 cells were used. Acyl glucuronides are formed by (UGT) 1A3 and not (UGT) 1A4. Although HEK/UGT1A3 cells produced acyl glucuronides of ketoprofen, ibuprofen, diclofenac, and naproxen in a time-linear manner and HEK/UGT1A4 cells did not, there were no differences in the cytotoxicity profile of the drugs. (−)-Borneol, an inhibitor of acyl glucuronidation, increased the cytotoxicity strongly indicating that acyl glucuronidation in this test system was a detoxification process. Similarly, using COMET assays no evidence of genotoxicity could be found.

8.3
Primary Pharmacology and Irreversible Secondary Pharmacology

A confounding factor in structural comparison is the finding that covalent binding occurs in drugs that are deemed safe and can occur to an extent equal to or greater than the toxic drugs (see Chapter 14). Many of the withdrawn drugs in Table 8.1 including some of the NSAIDs were examined for reactive metabolite formation and covalent binding by acyl glucuronidation and oxidative mechanisms [12]. The *in vitro* comparison compared drugs labeled as hepatotoxic (acetaminophen, alpidem, bromfenac, carbamazepine, diclofenac, flutamide, imipramine, nefazodone, tacrine, ticlopidine, tienilic acid, and troglitazone) with those labeled as nonhepatotoxic (acetylsalicylic acid, caffeine, dexamethasone, losartan, ibuprofen, paroxetine, pioglitazone, rosiglitazone, sertraline, theophylline, venlafaxine, and zolpidem). There was considerable overlap between the toxic and nontoxic drugs in covalent binding after incubation with human liver microsomes in the presence of NADPH. On addition of UDP-glucuronic acid (UDPGA) as a cofactor for glucuronidation, the covalent binding levels of bromfenac and diclofenac were increased indicative of more than one mechanism. The greatest discriminator between the two groups was daily dose when the drugs were used clinically. This study does not discount the role of reactive metabolites, but implies that the total amount formed may be the most important factor. It also demonstrates that reactive metabolite formation is commonplace in many, perhaps the majority, of drug molecules. It also suggests that structure–toxicity relationships may reflect drug efficiency in many cases. Drug efficiency is the dose delivering the effective concentration to the target receptor and is defined by the affinity and potency of the drug against the target receptor, the fraction of the administered drug absorbed, and the intrinsic clearance of the drug. It can be seen as the partner to ligand efficiency, which calculates the real affinity against that expected by hydrophobic forces for the molecular weight of the compound.

The concept that the most efficient drugs in the class have the best safety record is illustrated by the glitazones. The PPARγ agonist troglitazone was withdrawn from the market due to hepatotoxicity. The drug had several follow-on compounds (rosiglitazone and pioglitazone) with similar structural template. The glitazones act as insulin sensitizers and improve insulin resistance. The acidic thiazolidinedione grouping present in this class gives the glitazones unique potency as PPARγ agonists. When troglitazone was withdrawn, the thiazolidinedione group was subject to detailed metabolism investigations [13]. Metabolism of this group leads to an ultimate reactive sulfonium ion. This can be formed from an initial sulfoxide, followed by a formal Pummerer rearrangement, or a C5 thiazolidinedione radical or a sulfur cation radical. Other reactive metabolites such as the quinone methide have also been identified. Rosiglitazone and pioglitazone can also form similar metabolites but are 100-fold more potent as PPARγ agonists [14]. These differences are reflected in clinical dose with rosiglitazone and pioglitazone dosed at 4–8 and 15–45 mg/day, respectively, in contrast to 400–600 mg/day of troglitazone. The outcome of this difference in potency and lower dose is a dramatic shift in hepatotoxicity. For instance, when increases in liver enzyme levels were compared, they were similar to placebo for rosiglitazone and pioglitazone, whereas troglitazone was associated with a threefold greater incidence of raised levels. Acute liver failure was seen in approximately 1 in 5000 patients receiving troglitazone, in contrast to negligible hepatotoxicity for rosiglitazone (with the few incidents having uncertain causality) and no hepatotoxicity reported with pioglitazone.

8.4
Primary or Secondary Pharmacology and Reactive Metabolites: the Possibility for False Structure–Toxicity Relationships

Rofecoxib and valdecoxib belong to the class of drugs termed cyclooxygenase-2 (COX-2)–selective inhibitors that include several other examples such as celecoxib, rofecoxib, and etoricoxib. These were compounds with advantages over conventional nonselective COX inhibitors (NSAIDs) since the anti-inflammatory effects are mediated through attenuation of COX-2-derived inflammatory prostaglandins while the gastrointestinal effects such as ulceration, which is mediated by COX-1, are reduced. Unfortunately, under some conditions of use these drugs may increase the risk of thrombotic cardiovascular events and this was first noted for rofecoxib and led to its subsequent withdrawal. Similar findings with valdecoxib contributed partly to its marketing withdrawal, but this drug had a higher incidence of serious skin toxicity. Investigations into the stability of rofecoxib in tissues suggested that the drug could bind to the elastin in the aorta. These investigations showed that rofecoxib reacts with the aldehyde group of allysine to give a condensation adduct (Figure 8.5). Allysine normally undergoes condensation with lysine residues to provide the cross-linking of elastin. The rofecoxib adduct would therefore inhibit cross-linking and could cause degradation of elastin fibers leading to aortic rupture. Other COX-2 inhibitors, including celecoxib, valdecoxib, and etoricoxib, did not undergo this adduct formation [15, 16].

These results would favor categorizing rofecoxib under irreversible secondary pharmacology and the furanone group as the heterocyclic core that is a key structural feature, which discriminated valdecoxib from other COX-2 inhibitors in causing the cardiovascular events.

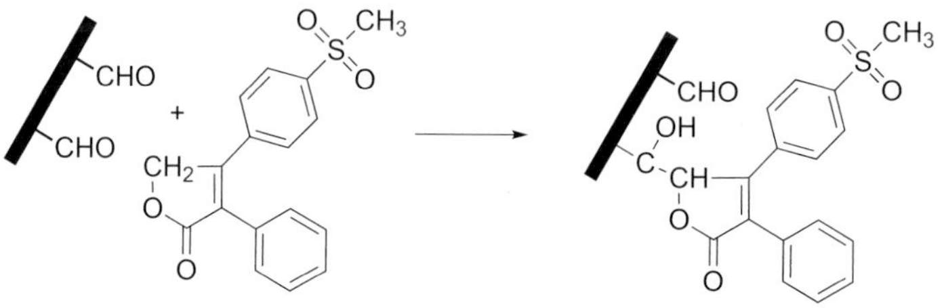

Figure 8.5 Proposed covalent binding mechanism for rofecoxib binding with elastin.

Considered alone, the above observations seem to present a plausible mechanism, but when the drugs are closely examined other differences arise in reversible secondary pharmacology. Celecoxib, but not rofecoxib or diclofenac, at therapeutically relevant concentrations, can act as a Kv7 potassium channel activator and an L-type calcium channel opener [17]. These vasorelaxant ion channel effects could account for different cardiovascular risk profiles for the compound. These findings would suggest that it is different, beneficial secondary pharmacology, which accounts for the difference in frequency of cardiovascular events. Pharmacological mechanisms, relating to primary pharmacology, advanced to explain the cardiovascular events include suppression of endothelial vascular prostaglandin I_2 while not inhibiting platelet-derived thromboxane A_2 production resulting in an imbalance of homeostatic mechanisms. The incidence of these effects with this rationale should show a relationship to dose and to the actual drug used (potency against COX-2).

Many subsequent studies [18] have been conducted to clarify the cardiovascular risks of remaining COX-2 inhibitors and the earlier nonselective compounds. A key finding has been that drugs showing <90% inhibition of COX-2 inhibition at the normal clinical doses (celecoxib, etoricoxib, ibuprofen, and meloxicam) have a relative risk of 1.18 for cardiovascular events, whereas for drugs giving >90% COX-2 inhibition the relative risk is 1.60 (rofecoxib and diclofenac). These studies show a common risk heightened by how far the clinical dose is placing the drug on the dose–response curve. They indicate that differentiation in terms of irreversible secondary pharmacology and adduct formation or beneficial secondary pharmacology are not major factors. The commonality of mechanism, via primary pharmacology, has led to a blanket black box warning on all NSAIDs with the wording "NSAIDs may cause an increased risk of serious cardiovascular thrombotic events, myocardial infarction, and stroke, which can be fatal." This risk may increase with duration of use. Patients with cardiovascular disease or risk factors for cardiovascular disease may be at a greater risk. All NSAIDs are contraindicated for the treatment of perioperative pain in the setting of coronary artery bypass graft surgery.

As described earlier, tienilic acid is a uricosuric/diuretic drug, which is activated by metabolism of its thiophene ring to a reactive metabolite that is likely to be involved in an autoimmune response. The metabolism of the thiophene to electrophilic sulfoxide or epoxide metabolites has been explored in a number of studies. Suprofen, a NSAID, is somewhat similar in structure with a thiophene ring system (Figure 8.6).

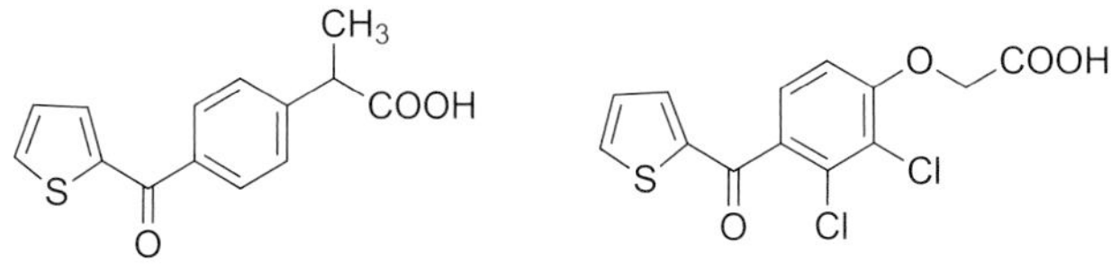

Figure 8.6 Structures of suprofen (I) and tienilic acid (II) illustrating the similarities in structure that may lead to speculation on common toxicity mechanisms involving reactive metabolites.

Suprofen was withdrawn due to acute flank pain syndrome and acute renal injury. Within the 700 000 persons who used the drug in the United States, 163 cases of acute flank pain syndrome were reported [19]. Possible risk factors included young age, concurrent use of other analgesic agents (especially ibuprofen), preexisting renal disease, a history of kidney stones, and a history of gout. It is tempting to link the presence of the thiophene and possible reactive metabolites to the syndrome and some reports have appeared to this effect showing suprofen, like ticrynafen, forms a reactive sulfoxide metabolite [20] that binds to cytochrome P450 (CYP) 2C9 and inactivates it. Both compounds cause kidney flank pain, but importantly both have uricosuric properties. Acute kidney injury is a common, but rare finding with all NSAIDs. NSAIDs inhibit prostaglandin synthesis in the kidney allowing vasoconstrictors such as angiotensin II and vasopressin to exert maximal effect. The risk of acute kidney injury varies among different NSAIDs with risk generally increasing with decrease in selectivity toward COX-2 [21]. The most selective COX inhibitors have the lowest risk. The adjusted odds ratios for various drugs for acute kidney injury are 0.95 (rofecoxib), 0.96 (celecoxib), 1.13 (meloxicam), 1.31 (), 1.11 (diclofenac), 1.53 (piroxicam), 1.61 (sulindac), 2.25 (ibuprofen), 1.72 (naproxen), 3.64 (high-dose aspirin), 1.94 (indomethacin), and 2.07 (ketorolac). Suprofen has a similar selectivity to ketorolac, being around 100-fold more potent for COX-1/COX-2. The acute renal failure may therefore be a symptom of selectivity and final clinical dose. The flank pain syndrome occurs rapidly and lasts for a period of several hours. Detailed clinical pharmacology studies [22] have shown that within 90 min after suprofen administration, the fractional excretion of uric acid increased from 8.8 to 35.5%. Urine became supersaturated with uric acid while glomerular filtration rate, renal plasma flow, and the excretion of Na^+ decreased. The findings are consistent with acute uric acid nephropathy, including crystallization of uric acid in the nephron as a mechanism of suprofen-induced renal dysfunction. Consideration of structure could indicate that suprofen is an inhibitor of URAT1, the apical surface reuptake urate transporter, as part of its secondary pharmacology.

Two COX-2 inhibitors initially had a labeling indicating warning on cutaneous reactions: celecoxib and valdecoxib. Valdecoxib was withdrawn due to a combination of this warning and excess cardiovascular mortality. Researchers from the FDA have used the Adverse Event Reporting System database to compare valdecoxib, celecoxib, rofecoxib, and meloxicam. They report no instances of Stevens–Johnson syndrome for meloxicam and an incidence of valdecoxib > celecoxib > rofecoxib. Valdecoxib and celecoxib were referred to as sulfonamide COX-2 inhibitors due to the presence of this function and a connection was made to sulfonamide antibacterials, a group of drugs widely associated with skin toxicity [23]. This finding would apparently implicate the sulfonamide group as a key determinant of toxicity. Sulfonamide antibacterials however are essential anilines with the sulfonamide being the surrogate for a carboxylic acid. Sulfonamide antibacterials are particularly associated with effects on the skin. Rashes are relatively common, but serious skin conditions also occur. The most serious skin reactions are severe forms of Stevens–Johnson syndrome and toxic epidermal necrolysis. Although the

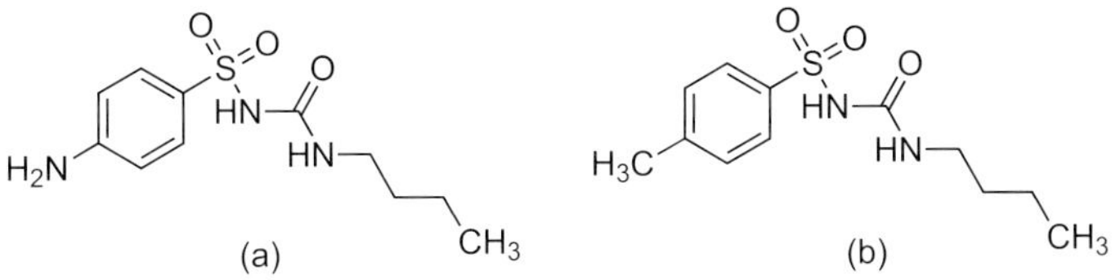

Figure 8.7 Structure of the aniline amino containing carbutamide (a), a drug associated with an array of toxicities including skin, which has been withdrawn, and its safer alternative tolbutamide (b).

mechanisms involved in these toxicities have not been fully elucidated, reactive metabolites appear to play a pivotal role. The N-4-hydroxylamine and N-4-nitroso metabolites, which are formed by oxidation of the aniline nitrogen, can bind covalently to proteins and are part of a cascade of events resulting in the induction of specific adverse immune responses.

The sulfonamide antibacterials, in some cases, had glucose-lowering activity. This activity was exploited in the development of the antidiabetic sulfonylureas [24]. These drugs bind and block an ATP-sensitive K^+ channel that stimulates insulin release from pancreatic β cells. The original drug, carbutamide, retained the N-4 aniline amine grouping. This drug had a variety of toxic effects on the blood and the skin including bone marrow depression, aplastic anemia, agranulocytosis, hypersensitivity, epidermal necrosis, and severe skin eruptions. Tolbutamide, its later derivative, in which the aniline nitrogen was replaced with a methyl function, proved much safer (Figure 8.7).

These major differences in allergic reactions implicate the N-4 aniline amine group as the functionality most responsible for these side effects of sulfonamide antibacterials and their antidiabetic sulfonylurea derivatives. The association of the sulfonamide functionality as important in the cutaneous reactions of antibacterials and the COX-2 inhibitors is false [24]. Other structural features, which differ between the COX-2 inhibitors, are the heterocyclic core with celecoxib having an imidazole, valdecoxib an oxazole, and rofecoxib a furanone (Figure 8.8).

NSAIDs, in general, have an association with erythema multiforme, Stevens–Johnson syndrome, and toxic epidermal necrolysis. The oxicam and butazone classes of NSAIDs have also been implicated. Isoxicam, in particular, was withdrawn

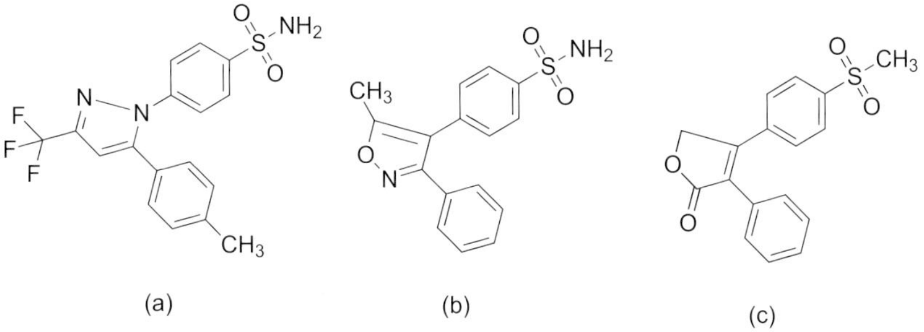

Figure 8.8 Structures of COX-2 inhibitors: celecoxib (a), valdecoxib (b), and rofecoxib (c).

from the market in France due to a high rate of dermal toxicity. It is tempting to correlate the methyl isoxazole group present in valdecoxib and isoxicam as being a common structural feature leading to similar outcomes. However, metabolism studies indicate no ring cleavage products and show hydroxylation of the methyl group as the sole metabolite of this functionality [25]. It is difficult to link such benign metabolism products to a toxicological outcome.

8.5
Multifactorial Mechanisms as Causes of Toxicity

The example of the cardiovascular toxicity of rofecoxib illustrates how a number of plausible scenarios can be constructed from different research areas leading to different implications on the structure. Amineptine is a tricyclic antidepressant (Figure 8.9) with the unusual structural feature of a carboxylic group attached to a six-carbon alkyl chain.

The major metabolic pathway is β-oxidation of the heptanoic side chain to pentanoic and propanoic side chain metabolites [26]. The dibenzocycloheptyl ring is also subject to oxidation on the unsubstituted benzylic position. Investigations into the hepatotoxicity initially focused on the generation of oxidative reactive metabolites. Irreversible binding was observed in microsomal systems and was mediated by CYP enzymes. Binding was attenuated by glutathione (GSH) and enhanced by the epoxide hydrolase inhibitor 1,1,1-trichloropropene-2,3-oxide suggesting an epoxide was the reactive metabolite [27]. These findings were felt by the authors as highly relevant to amineptine's hepatotoxicity. In further investigations the authors found that only when GSH was depleted *in vivo* using hamsters was covalent binding observed. To accomplish the GSH depletion hamsters were pretreated with phorone. At 300 mg/kg with or without this pretreatment no evidence of hepatic necrosis was observed [28]. Attention then focused on the possible implication of β-oxidation being inhibited or modified as a result of amineptine's metabolism. In rats, at 200 mg/kg the oxidation of ^{14}C-labeled palmitic acid was inhibited and was suggested as being related to the hepatotoxicity [29]. After administration to mice microvesicular steatosis was observed mimicking some observations of the human toxicity. A similar compound, tianeptine (Figure 8.10), was marketed in France, also undergoing β-oxidation as the main metabolic pathway [30]. Again, with this compound inhibition of β-oxidation of medium- and short-chain fatty acids and microvesicular steatosis was observed at high doses in mice [31]. The safety margin for this was 600-fold compared to 10-fold for amineptine. Metabolic activation [32] by CYP enzymes was also observed *in vitro* and *in vivo* in hamsters, similar to

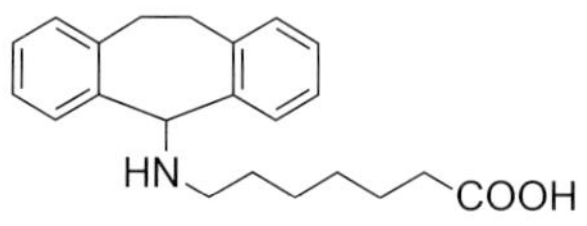

HN $\diagdown\diagup\diagdown\diagup\diagdown$ COOH

Figure 8.9 Structure of amineptine.

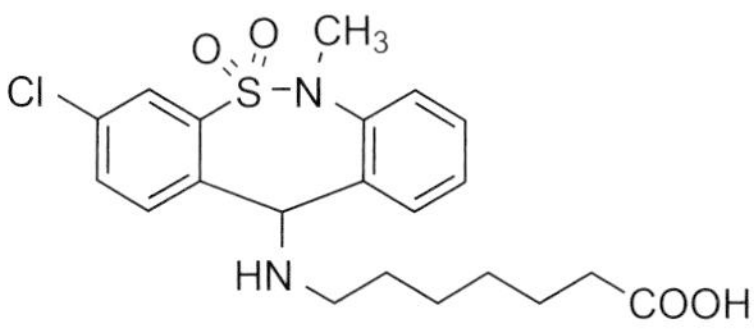

Figure 8.10 Structure of tianeptine.

amineptine. Hepatitis occurring in patients was described as hypersensitivity manifestations suggestive of an immunoallergic mechanism with histological examination revealing microvesicular steatosis [33].

The description of toxicity incorporates the types of finding one could associate partly with either mechanism. A possible and plausible outcome is that both contribute and are necessary. In other scenarios this can be described as a stress phenomenon, in that inhibition of function receives a stress of a different kind and is expressed as frank toxicity. Thus, while the heptanoic acid chain is a key structural feature, it by itself does not fully explain the toxicity.

Several of the drugs discussed have possible multifactorial mechanisms. For instance, bile salt export pump (BSEP) inhibition is suggested as a contributing mechanism to the idiosyncratic cholestasis caused by troglitazone [34]. BSEP is an ATP-binding cassette transporter critically involved in the secretion of bile salts into bile; its impairment leads to accumulation of cytotoxic bile salts in hepatocytes and, consequently, to hepatotoxicity. Both the parent drug and its sulfate metabolite are likely to be involved in the inhibition. Similar to the discussion above on the reactive metabolites of the glitazones, rosiglitazone and pioglitazone are equipotent inhibitors of BSEP [34]. The authors of this study incorrectly assume that the equipotency means that BSEP inhibition is not significant due to the different toxicological outcomes. The arguments for primary pharmacology apply equally here in terms of dose, and so on. Both rosiglitazone and pioglitazone are more selective in terms of this aspect of their reversible secondary pharmacology.

8.6
Clear Correlation between Protein Target and Reactive Metabolites

Certain compounds produce reactive metabolites that bind to the protein or heme component of P450 and inactivate the enzyme leading to potential and serious drug interactions.

Mibefradil (Figure 8.11) is a long-acting calcium channel antagonist, with particular activity against the T-type channel (transient, low-voltage-activated). The drug was effective in hypertension and chronic stable angina pectoris. At the clinical dose of 50–100 mg mibefradil was a potent inhibitor of CYP3A4, which resulted in multiple clinically relevant drug interactions. These included very important comedications such as simvastatin, which showed a large sevenfold elevation, sufficient to enhance potential adverse events, including rhabdomyolysis. Mibefradil was

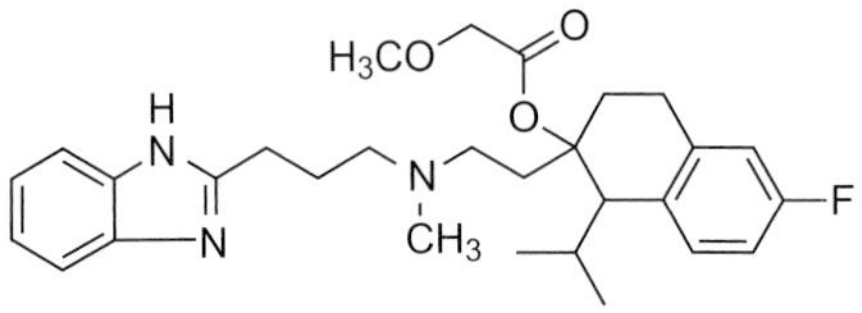

Figure 8.11 Structure of mibefradil.

shown to be a potent reversible ($IC_{50} = 0.3$–$2.0\,\mu M$) and subsequently and more importantly a "mechanism-based inhibitor" (see Chapter 3) of CYP3A4-catalyzed statin metabolism [35].

The mechanism of this inhibition is via formation of a reactive metabolite and the rate of CYP3A4 inactivation and the low partition ratio (moles mibefradil metabolized per mole enzyme inactivated) make mibefradil one of the most potent known "mechanism-based inhibitors" ($K_I = 2.3\,\mu M$ and $k_{inact} = 0.4\,min^{-1}$). This rate of inactivation is illustrated by the rapid and irreversible decrease in CYP3A4-catalyzed 1'-hydroxymidazolam formation with approximately 70% of CYP3A4 activity lost in the first minute of incubation with mibefradil. This decrease in CYP3A4 activity correlates with the time-dependent loss of CO binding, which, coupled with the lack of stable heme and/or apoprotein adducts, suggests heme destruction as the mechanism of inactivation of CYP3A4 rather than reaction with the protein.

8.7
Conclusion – Validation of Reactive Metabolites as Causes of Toxicity

Despite considerable research, the mechanistic pathways leading to idiosyncratic toxicity from reactive metabolites have not been established. With the aniline-containing compounds the evidence is overwhelming for the group to be implicated in many of the toxicities the drugs cause. Clearly, to include an aniline motif that either is present de novo or can be liberated by metabolism is a major risk. For other functional groups in drugs and their metabolites considerable extrapolation is needed. In this chapter emphasis has been placed on how some of these extrapolations may be misplaced. The gaps in the pathway are exemplified by remoxipride, which was withdrawn due to aplastic anemia. Like the aniline drugs, attention has focused on reactive metabolites present in blood. Remoxipride forms hydroquinone (NCQ-344) and catechol (NGQ-436) metabolites, which are capable of forming reactive *para*- and *ortho*-quinones (Figure 8.12). NCQ-344 is present in plasma and can be converted to GSH conjugates demonstrating its reactivity [36]. These conjugates could be formed by human neutrophils illustrating that the oxidation of the metabolites to *para*- and *ortho*-quinones can occur at or close to the site of toxicity.

Perturbation of apoptosis leads to a pathogenesis of various diseases such as aplastic anemia [37]. The hydroquinone, NCQ-344, causes apoptosis and necrosis

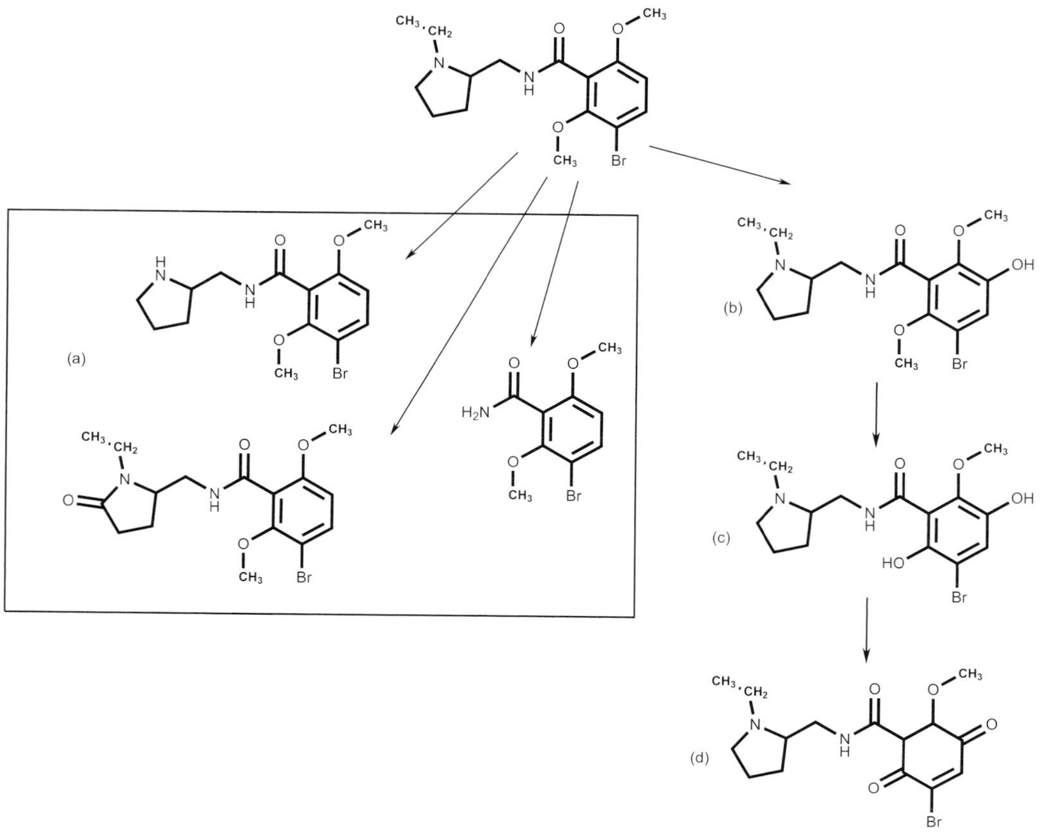

Figure 8.12 Metabolism of remoxipride to its predominant major metabolites involving oxidation of the pyrrolidone ring and hydrolysis (a); also shown is the very minor pathway of aromatic hydroxylation (b) leading to formation of the hydroquinone NCQ-344 (c) that can be activated to an *ortho*-quinone (d).

in human bone marrow progenitor cells and is accompanied by externalization of phosphatidylserine, activation of caspase-9/-3/-7, and fragmentation of DNA into nucleosomal fragments [38]. In this example the pathway from reactive metabolite looks clear until one examines the relative amounts and concentrations used in the various experiments. NCQ-344 is a small abundance metabolite in human. Quantification of the concentration present in patients [39] demonstrates circulating concentrations of between 0.1 and 1 nM; corresponding remoxipride concentrations were 5000–20 000 nM. These low circulating concentrations should be compared [37, 38] with those required to trigger apoptosis (35–75 μM) in the cell lines, which are approximately 35 000-fold higher.

In almost all cases examined these missing or broken links occur that attenuate the progress toward fully understanding and validating the role of reactive metabolites in toxicity. As outlined in this chapter the identification of a reactive metabolite may give false assumptions about the response for the toxicity. Certainly, reversible pharmacology in terms of primary and secondary needs to be further explored to help to determine the pivotal role of reactive metabolites.

References

1 Diffey, B.L. and Daymond, T.J. (1983) Photosensitivity studies and benoxaprofen. *Photobiochemistry and Photobiophysics*, **5** (3), 169–179.

2 Halsey, J.P. and Cardoe, N. (1982) Benoxaprofen: side-effect profile in 300 patients. *British Medical Journal (Clinical Research Edition)*, **284** (6326), 1365–1368.

3 Kamal, A. and Koch, I.M. (1982) Pharmacokinetic studies of benoxaprofen in geriatric patients. *European Journal of Rheumatology and Inflammation*, **5** (2), 76–81.

4 Barnes, J. and Barnes, E.J. (1955) Hypersensitivity to primary aromatic amines. *Lancet*, **268**, 455.

5 Uetrecht, J., Zahid, N., and Rubin, R. (1988) Metabolism of procainamide to a hydroxylamine by human neutrophils and mononuclear leukocytes. *Chemical Research in Toxicology*, **1** (1), 74–78.

6 Utrecht, J. (1989) Mechanism of hypersensitivity reactions: proposed involvement of reactive metabolites generated by activated leukocytes. *Trends in Pharmaceutical Sciences*, **10** (11), 463–467.

7 Smith, D. and Schmid, E.F. (2006) Drug withdrawals and the lessons within. *Current Opinion in Drug Discovery & Development*, **9** (1), 38–46.

8 Sánchez-Borges, M., Capriles-Hulett, A., and Caballero-Fonseca, F. (2004) The multiple faces of nonsteroidal antiinflammatory drug hypersensitivity. *Journal of Investigative Allergy and Immunology*, **14** (4), 329–334.

9 Dong, J.Q., Liu, J., and Smith, P.C. (2005) Role of benoxaprofen and flunoxaprofen acyl glucuronides in covalent binding to rat plasma and liver proteins in vivo. *Biochemical Pharmacology*, **70** (6), 937–948.

10 Dong, J.Q. and Smith, P.C. (2009) Glucuronidation and covalent binding of benoxaprofen in sandwich-cultured rat and human hepatocytes. *Drug Metabolism and Disposition*, **37** (12), 2314–2322.

11 Koga, T., Fujiwara, R., Nakajima, M., and Yokoi, T. (2011) Toxicological evaluation of acyl glucuronides of nonsteroidal anti-inflammatory drugs using human embryonic kidney 293 cells stably expressing human UDP-glucuronosyltransferase and human hepatocytes. *Drug Metabolism and Disposition*, **39** (1), 54–60.

12 Usui, T., Mise, M., Hashizume, T., Yabuki, M., and Komuro, S. (2009) Evaluation of

the potential for drug-induced liver injury based on in vitro covalent binding to human liver proteins. *Drug Metabolism and Disposition*, **37** (12), 2383–2392.

13 He, K., Talaat, R.E., Pool, W.F., Reily, M.D., Reed, J.E., Bridges, A.J., and Woolf, T.F. (2004) Metabolic activation of troglitazone: identification of a reactive metabolite and mechanisms involved. *Drug Metabolism and Disposition*, **32** (6), 639–646.

14 Smith, D.A., Harrison, A., and Morgan, P. (2011) Multiple factors govern the association between pharmacology and toxicity in a class of drugs: toward a unification of class effect terminology. *Chemical Research in Toxicology*, **24** (4), 463–474.

15 Oitata, M., Hirota, T., Murai, T., Miura, S., and Ikeeda, T. (2007) Covalent binding of rofecoxib, but not other cyclooxegenases-2 inhibitors, to allysine aldehyde in elastin of human aorta. *Drug Metabolism and Disposition*, **35** (10), 1846–1852.

16 Oitata, M., Hirota, T., Takahashi, M., Murai, T., Miura, S., Senoo, A., Hosokawa, T., Oonishi, T., and Ikeeda, T. (2007) Mechanism for covalent binding of rofecoxib to elastin of rat aorta. *Journal of Pharmacology and Experimental Therapeutics*, **320** (3), 1195–1203.

17 Brueggemann, L.I., Mani, B.K., Mackie, A.R., Cribbs, L.L., and Byron, K.L. (2010) Novel actions of nonsteroidal anti-inflammatory drugs on vascular ion channels: accounting for cardiovascular side effects and identifying new therapeutic applications. *Molecular and Cellular Pharmacology*, **2** (1), 15–19.

18 Meek, I.L., van de Laar, M., and Vonkeman, H.E. (2010) Non-steroidal anti-inflammatory drugs: an overview of cardiovascular risks. *Pharmaceuticals*, **3**, 2146–2162.

19 Strom, B.L., West, S.L., Sim, E., and Carson, J.L. (1989) The epidemiology of the acute flank pain syndrome from suprofen. *Clinical Pharmacology and Therapeutics*, **46**, 693–699.

20 O'Donnell, J.P., Dalvie, D.K., Kalgutkar, A.S., and Obach, R.S. (2003) Mechanism-based inactivation of human recombinant P450 2C9 by the nonsteroidal anti-inflammatory drug suprofen. *Drug Metabolism and Disposition*, **31** (11), 1369–1377.

21 Lafrance, J.-P. and Miller, D.R. (2009) Selective and non-selective non-steroidal anti-inflammatory drugs and the risk of acute kidney injury. *Pharmacoepidemiology and Drug Safety*, **18** (10), 923–931.

22 Abraham, P.A., Halstenson, C.E., Opsahl, J.A., Matzke, G.R., and Keane, W.F. (1988) Suprofen-induced uricosuria. A potential mechanism for acute nephropathy and flank pain. *American Journal of Nephrology*, **8** (2), 90–95.

23 La Grenade, L., Lee, L., Weaver, J., Bonnel, R., Karwoski, C., Governale, L., and Brinker, A. (2005) Comparison of reporting of Stevens–Johnson syndrome and toxic epidermal necrolysis in association with selective COX-2 inhibitors. *Drug Safety*, **28** (10), 917–924.

24 Smith, D.A. and Jones, R.M. (2008) The sulfonamide group as a structural alert: a distorted story? *Current Opinion in Drug Discovery & Development*, **11** (1), 72–79.

25 Osman, M., Chandrasekaran, A., Chan, K., Scatina, J., Erner, J., Cevallos, W., and Sisenwine, S. (1998) Metabolic disposition of 14-C bromfenac in healthy male volunteers. *Journal of Clinical Pharmacology*, **38**, 744–752.

26 Grislain, L., Gele, P., Bromet., N., Luijten, W., Volland, J.P., Mocaer, E., and Kamoun, A. (1990) Metabolism of amineptine in rat, dog and man. *European Journal of Drug Metabolism and Pharmacokinetics*, **15** (4), 339–345.

27 Geneve, J., Larrey, D., Amouyal, G., Belghiti, J., and Pessayre, J. (1987) Metabolic activation of the tricyclic antidepressant amineptine by human liver P-450. *Biochemical Pharmacology*, **36** (14), 2421–2424.

28 Geneve, J., Degott, C., Letteron, P., Tinel, M., Descatoire, V., Larrey, D., Amouyal, G., and Pessayre, D. (1987) Metabolic activation of the tricyclic antidepressant amineptine. II. Protective role of glutathione against in vitro and in vivo covalent binding. *Biochemical Pharmacology*, **36** (3), 331–337.

29 Ego, D., Gervais, P., and Strolin Benedetti, M. (1984) Amineptine hepatotoxicity and

inhibition of the β-oxidation of fatty acids. *Therapie*, **39** (1), 56–57.

30 Grislan, L., Gele, P., Bertrand, M., Luijten, W., Bromet, N., Salvadori, C., and Kamoun, A. (1990) The metabolic pathways of tianeptine, a new antidepressant, in healthy volunteers. *Drug Metabolism and Disposition*, **18** (5), 804–808.

31 Fromenty, B., Frenaux, E., Labbe, G., Deschamps, D., Larrey, D., Letteron, P., and Pessayre, D. (1989) Tianeptine, a new tricyclic antidepressant metabolized by β-oxidation of its heptanoic side chain, inhibits the mitochondrial oxidation of medium and short chain fatty acids in mice. *Biochemical Pharmacology*, **38** (21), 3743–3751.

32 Letteron, P., Labbe, G., Descatoire, V., Degott, C., Loeper, J., Tinel, M., Larrey, D., and Pessayre, D. (1989) Metabolic activation of the antidepressant tianeptine. II. In vivo covalent binding and toxicological studies at sublethal doses. *Biochemical Pharmacology*, **38** (19), 3247–3251.

33 Le Briquir, Y., Larrey, D., Blanc, P., Pageaux, G.P., and Michel, H. (1994) Tianeptine – an instance of drug induced hepatotoxicity predicted by prospective experimental studies. *Journal of Hepatology*, **21** (5), 771–773.

34 Snow, K.L. and Moseley, R.H. (2007) Effect of thiazolidinediones on bile acid transport in rat liver. *Life Sciences*, **80** (8), 732–740.

35 Foti, R.S., Rock, D.A., Pearson, J.T., Wahlstrom, J.L., and Wienkers, L.C.

(2011) Mechanism-based inactivation of cytochrome P450 3A4 by mibefradil through heme destruction. *Drug Metabolism and Disposition*, **39** (7), 1188–1195.

36 Erve, J.C.L., Svensson, M.A., von Euler-Chelpin, H., and Klasson-Wehler, E. (2004) Characterization of glutathione conjugates of the remoxipride hydroquinone metabolite NCQ-344 formed in vitro and detection following oxidation by human neutrophils. *Chemical Research in Toxicology*, **17** (4), 564–571.

37 Inayat-Hussain, S.H., McGuinness, S.M., Johansson, R., Lundstrom, J., and Ross, D. (2006) Caspase-dependent and-independent mechanisms in apoptosis induced by hydroquinone and catechol metabolites of remoxipride in HL-60 cells. *Chemico-Biological Interactions*, **128** (1), 51–63.

38 McGuinness, S.M., Johansson, R., Lundstrom, J., and Ross, D. (1999) Induction of apoptosis by remoxipride metabolites in HL60 and CD34+/CD19– human bone marrow progenitor cells: potential relevance to remoxipride-induced aplastic anemia. *Chemico-Biological Interactions*, **121** (3), 253–265.

39 Nilsson, L.B. (1998) High sensitivity determination of the remoxipride hydroquinone metabolite NCQ-344 in plasma by coupled column reversed-phase liquid chromatography and electrochemical detection. *Biomedical Chromatography*, **12** (2), 65–68.

9
Bioactivation and Natural Products

Abbreviations

COX Cyclooxygenase
CYP Cytochrome P450
GSH Glutathione
MeIQx 2-Amino-3,8-dimethylimidazo[4,5-f]quinoxaline
PhIP 2-Amino-1-methyl-6-phenylimidazo[4,5-b]pyridine

9.1
Introduction

Prior to the advent of modern pharmaceutical sciences, the use of naturally occurring materials in medicine was prevalent, and such practice remains a standard part of therapy in many parts of the world. Furthermore, many of the most widely used medications are either compounds purified from plants and fungi (e.g., opiates, *Cinchona* alkaloids, *Artemisia* terpenoids, etc.) or synthetic compounds based on such structures, or they originate from science derived from the study of the effects of natural products on mammalian systems. However, among many individuals who lack a thorough understanding of pharmacology and toxicology, there can be a misunderstanding that causes such individuals to equate "all natural" with "safe" [1]. Clearly, this is a position of ignorance, as many of the best known and most potent human toxins are derived from natural sources, such as saxitoxin, tetrodotoxin, maitotoxin, ricin, botulinum toxin, strychnine, nicotine, coniine, and tubocurarine, among many others (Figure 9.1). Thus, while the synthetic chemist can certainly produce a vast array of potentially toxic chemicals, this is not an exclusive license as Mother Nature has offered many herself. It can be rationalized that species of plants and fungi possessing an ability to protect themselves from ingestion by

Reactive Drug Metabolites, First Edition. Amit S. Kalgutkar, Deepak Dalvie, R. Scott Obach, and Dennis A. Smith.
© 2012 Wiley-VCH Verlag GmbH & Co. KGaA. Published 2012 by Wiley-VCH Verlag GmbH & Co. KGaA.

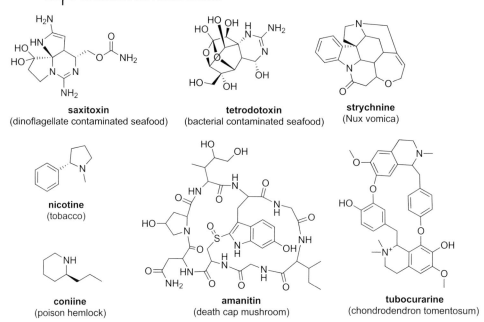

Figure 9.1 Chemical structures of known toxins saxitoxin, tetrodotoxin, strychnine, nicotine, coniine, tubocurarine, and amanitin. These are not known to be bioactivated, but rather act by specific interactions with various ion channels and proteins.

animals would possess a selective advantage. This has been termed "plant–animal warfare," which states that animals must develop means by which to either develop resistance to the plant-derived toxins or develop an ability to detoxify them, such as xenobiotic metabolizing enzymes, for example, cytochrome P450 (CYP) [2]. Most toxins of natural origin target ion channels causing toxicity at neuromuscular junctions, leading to paralysis and death. However, there are other mechanisms of toxicity of natural agents such as the hepatotoxicity caused by α-amanitin via inhibition of RNA polymerase.

Since this is a book on the bioactivation of compounds to chemically reactive intermediates, this chapter will focus only on those naturally derived agents that are poisonous via this type of mechanism. The toxic outcomes for this group of natural compounds typically include hepatic injury, immunoallergy, and carcinogenesis. The natural compounds described below are present either as plant secondary metabolites in herbal remedies or as accidental contaminants in foods. The types of chemical mechanisms of bioactivation fall within those described in Chapter 5 – there is nothing new among the bioactivation chemistries offered by these naturally occurring compounds. However, because these are derived from plants, they are generally devoid of many of the substituents present in synthetic drugs and the compounds are mostly restricted to carbon, hydrogen, nitrogen, and oxygen.

9.2
Well-Known Examples of Bioactivation of Compounds Present in Herbal Remedies

9.2.1
Germander and Teucrin A

Germander has been a plant used in various folk remedies. Several cases of hepato-toxicity were observed in the late 1980s when it was introduced in France as a weight control agent. In almost all cases, patients presenting with hepatotoxicity recovered on discontinuation of the use of the herb. Also it was shown that toxicity returned when the herb was reintroduced [3]. Germander possesses several plant secondary metabolites, among them diterpenoids (Figure 9.2). Considerable study has been done with the diterpenoid teucrin A, which possesses a pendant 3-furan substituent. In Chapter 5, the bioactivation of furan rings was described and teucrin A serves as a good example of this. The necessity of CYP activation in toxicity was demonstrated by showing that inhibition of protein adduct formation occurred with tritiated teucrin A when hepatocytes were treated with an inhibitor of CYP3A4 (troleandomycin) and increased adduct formation when CYP enzyme activities were induced with dexamethasone [4]. This same trend was observed *in vivo* [5]. An analogue wherein the furan was replaced with a tetrahydrofuran showed no toxic-ity, offering evidence of the importance of the furan substituent.

The mechanism of teucrin A bioactivation is proposed to begin with epoxidation of the furan ring followed by opening of the ring to the enedial, as with other furans (Figure 9.3) [6]. The enedial is the reactive entity to which nucleophiles, such as amines and thiols, can form adducts. The study of teucrin A has even extended to attempts to identify the proteins to which the reactive enedial interme-diate can form adducts [7]. Using immunochemical methods to help isolate adducts followed by mass spectrometric analysis yielded multiple proteins identi-fied in rat liver as targets for adduction by teucrin A. Interestingly, in earlier efforts, patients who had taken germander showed evidence of anti-epoxide hydrolase anti-bodies [8]. *In vitro* work showed that in the presence of CYP activity, teucrin A was shown to inactivate epoxide hydrolase, suggesting the possible formation of adducts to this specific protein.

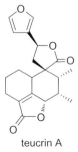

teucrin A

Figure 9.2   Teucrin A.

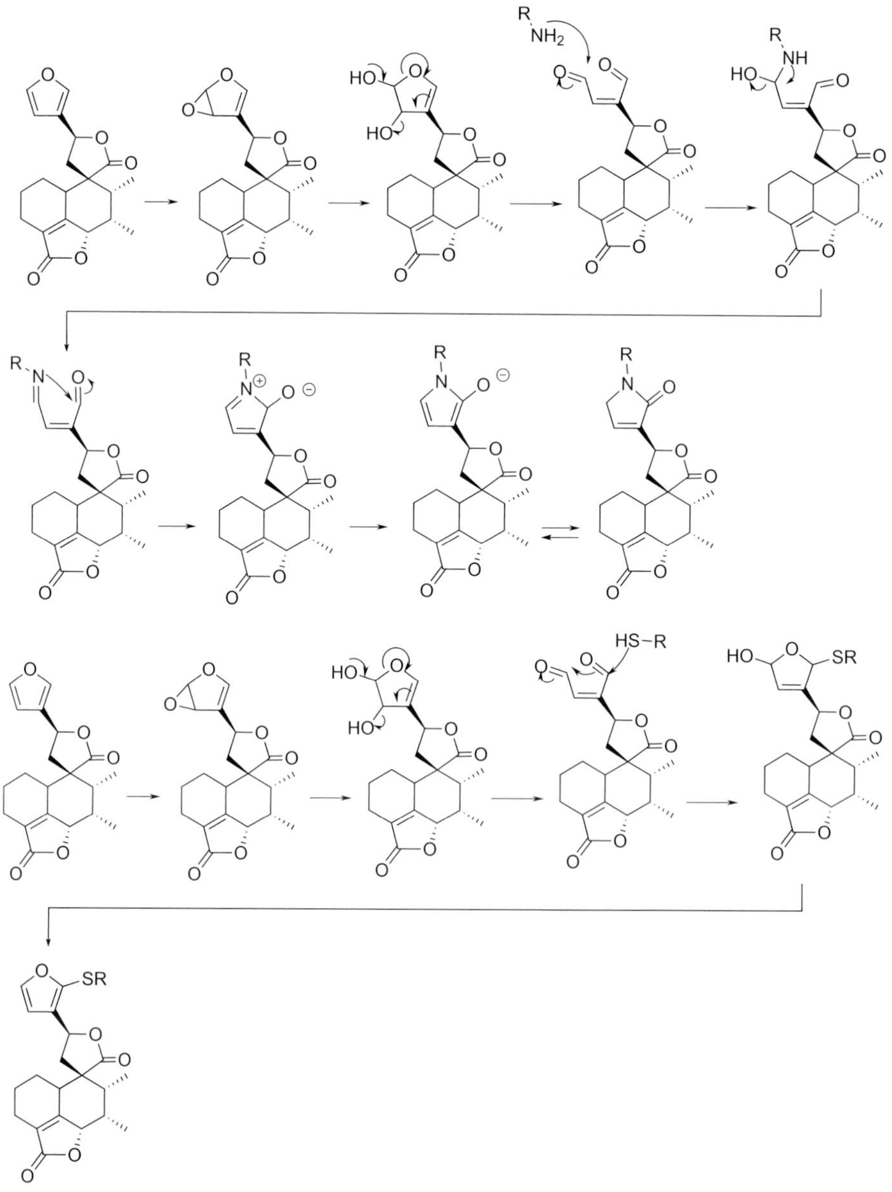

Figure 9.3 Mechanism of adduct formation to teucrin A by amines and thiols.

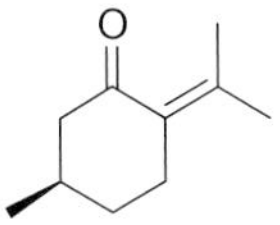

pulegone

Figure 9.4 Structure of pulegone.

9.2.2
Pennyroyal Oil and Menthofuran

Pennyroyal (Figure 9.4) is a plant in the mint genus and is used to make teas. The concentrated oil contains high quantities of pulegone (several hundred mg/mL) and the oil has been used as an agent to induce abortion [9]. While the herb in small amounts is used as a flavorant, the oil is dangerous and has caused several cases of hepatic and multiorgan failure resulting in death [10, 11]. Pulegone is a terpenoid structure (Figure 9.4) and is first metabolized to menthofuran [12], which is the compound that is bioactivated via an epoxide mechanism to yield a conjugated enedial structure (Figure 9.5) [13, 14]. Subsequently, adducts are formed to macromolecules [15] and glutathione (GSH), and in mice adducts have been shown with amines and sulfite anion [16]. Pulegone is also metabolized to *para*-cresol, a known hepatotoxicant [17]; however, in an *in vitro* model of hepatotoxicity evidence was obtained to show that it is the menthofuran bioactivation pathway(s) that generates reactive metabolites that is responsible for toxicity, not *para*-cresol [18].

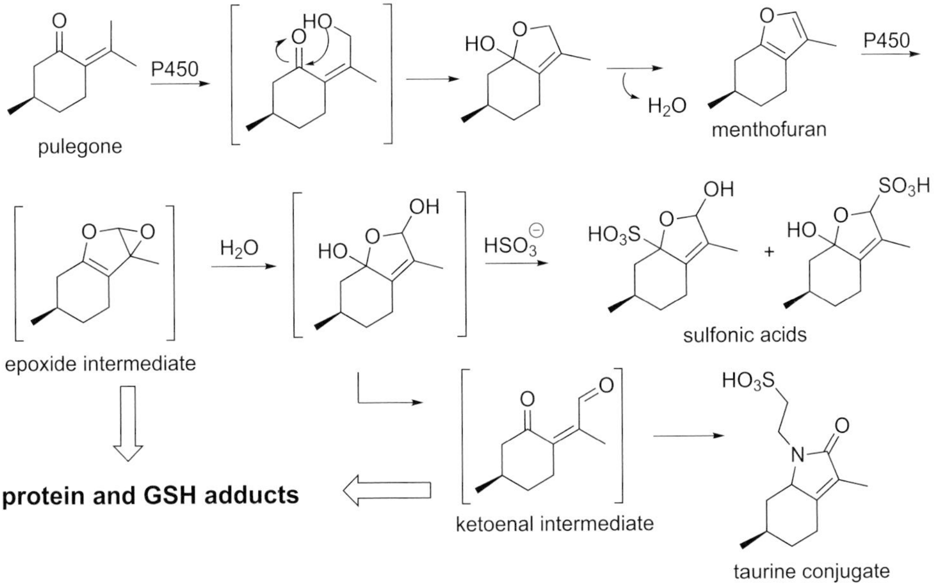

Figure 9.5 Conversion of pulegone to menthofuran and bioactivation of menthofuran.

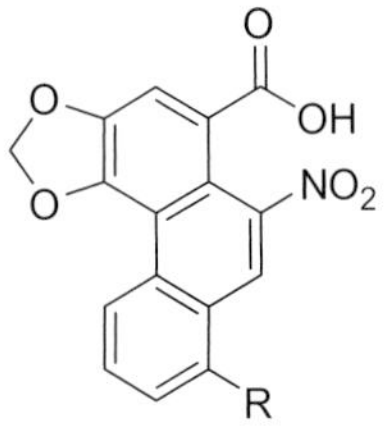

aristolochic acid
I: R=OMe
II: R=H

Figure 9.6 Aristolochic acid.

9.2.3
Aristolochia **and Aristolochic Acid**

In the early 1990s, an increased incidence of renal fibrosis was observed in Belgium and was associated with use of a herbal weight loss agent [19]. It was determined that the agent was contaminated with *Aristolochia fangchi*, and that the toxicity could be associated with aristolochic acids (Figure 9.6). *Aristolochia* herb has been used in traditional Chinese medicine as a treatment in obstetrics (to aid in ejection of the placenta), and is currently used as a treatment for arthritis and gout. Investigation of purified aristolochic acid as a potential pharmaceutical led to its identification as a mutagen and rodent carcinogen. Patients treated with *Aristolochia* show an incidence of urothelial cancer. Furthermore, the incidence of renal fibrosis in several Balkan countries has been linked to ingestion of *Aristolochia* seeds.

Aristolochic acid is bioactivated by reduction of the nitro group and spontaneous ring closure to form an aryl *N*-hydroxamic acid (Figure 9.7) [20, 21]. The reduction has been shown to be catalyzed by several enzymes such as CYP1A1, CYP1A2, CYP oxidoreductase (OR), cyclooxygenase-1 (COX-1), and NAD(P)H:quinone oxidoreductase (NQO1) [22–24]. As the target organ for toxicity is the kidney, greater focus is placed on the last two enzymes as these are highly expressed in kidney. The *N*-aryl hydroxamic acid can spontaneously lose water to yield a nitrenium ion, or it is possible that this group is conjugated (e.g., sulfated, acetylated) and that the conjugate eliminates to form the nitrenium species. The nitrenium ion charge is delocalized and the carbon center can react with hard nucleophiles such as water (to form the hydroxyl metabolite) or the amino nitrogen of purine rings. Examination of the structures of adducts to DNA has yielded the site of addition to be with the exocyclic nitrogens of deoxyadenosine and deoxyguanosine (Figure 9.7) [22]. DNA adducts of aristolochic acid have been observed *in vivo* in both animals and patients suffering from nephropathy [25, 26]. Recently, a second possible pathway of adduct formation has been proposed, based on the observation of aristoxazole (Figure 9.7) [27].

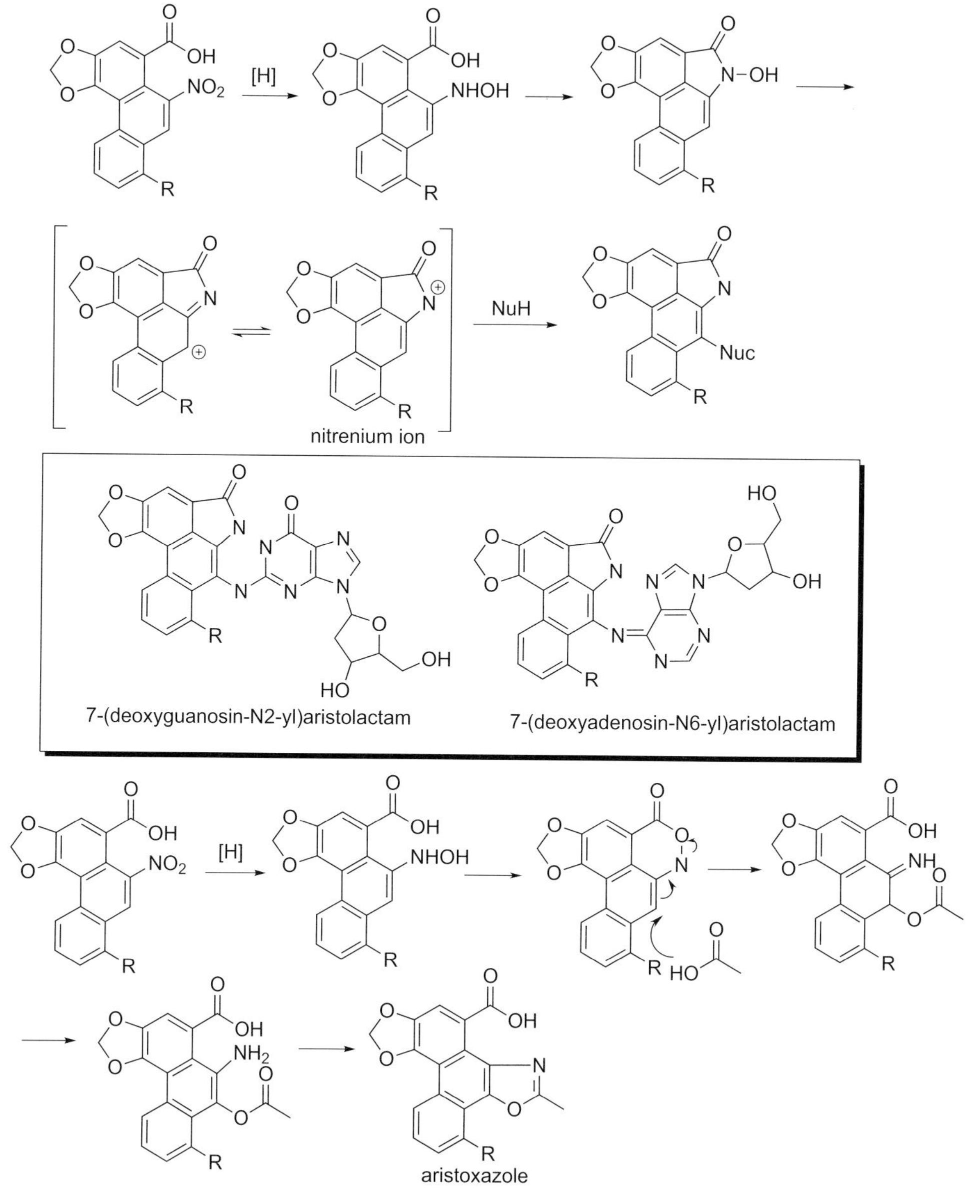
[H]
NuH
nitrenium ion
Nuc
7-(deoxyguanosin-N2-yl)aristolactam
7-(deoxyadenosin-N6-yl)aristolactam
[H]
aristoxazole

Figure 9.7 Metabolism and bioactivation of aristolochic acids.

9.2.4
Comfrey, Coltsfoot, and Pyrrolizidine Alkaloids

Pyrrolizidine alkaloids are constituents of a wide number of plants, and there are several hundred known compounds within the pyrrolizidine family. Plants of the families Boraginaceae and Asteraceae are most commonly associated with pyrrolizidine alkaloids. Exposure to pyrrolizidines can be through purposeful ingestion of herbal remedies containing these agents as well as through accidental ingestion of contaminated foodstuffs (e.g., honey obtained from bees harvesting nectar from pyrrolizidine-containing plants). The common core structure is the fused pyrrolizine structure with substituents at the 1- and 7-positions. Several of the pyrrolizidine alkaloids are hepatotoxic, mutagenic, and carcinogenic, and several are associated with reports of veno-occlusive disease [28, 29]. Comfrey leaves are frequently used in poultices to aid in wound healing and the roots are used to make teas. It is this latter usage that is most associated with toxicity since the roots also have considerably greater quantities of these toxins, and several nations have restricted the sale of comfrey for external uses only. Comfrey contains 14 pyrrolizidines including lycopsamine, echimidine, and lasiocarpine [28, 30]. It is not believed that the pyrrolizidines are pharmacologically active, and there are efforts to make comfrey preparations that retain their putative wound healing properties without the pyrrolizidines [31]. Coltsfoot (*Tussilago farfara*) has been used to relieve

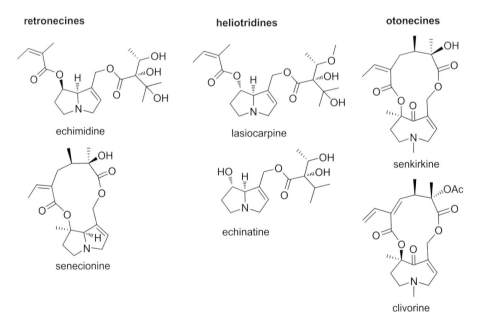

Figure 9.8 Structures of pyrrolizidine alkaloids.

cough and other lung ailments. It contains the pyrrolizidine senecionine and also the related compound senkirkine, both of which are mutagenic [32].

The pyrrolizidine alkaloids can be categorized into three family types that when undergoing bioactivation can all give rise to a common type of pyrrolic ester intermediate [33]. N-Oxidation and ester hydrolysis biotransformations serve to detoxify this class of compounds. Activation begins with CYP-catalyzed hydroxylation at the α-position to the nitrogen of the pyrroline side of the ring (Figure 9.9). On rearrangement, a pyrrolic ester is formed that can spontaneously eliminate the acyl moiety to yield a reactive carbocation. The carbocation can react with various macromolecular nucleophiles or water. For example, the metabolism of riddelliine, a component of ragwort that can be eaten by grazing ranch animals and result in

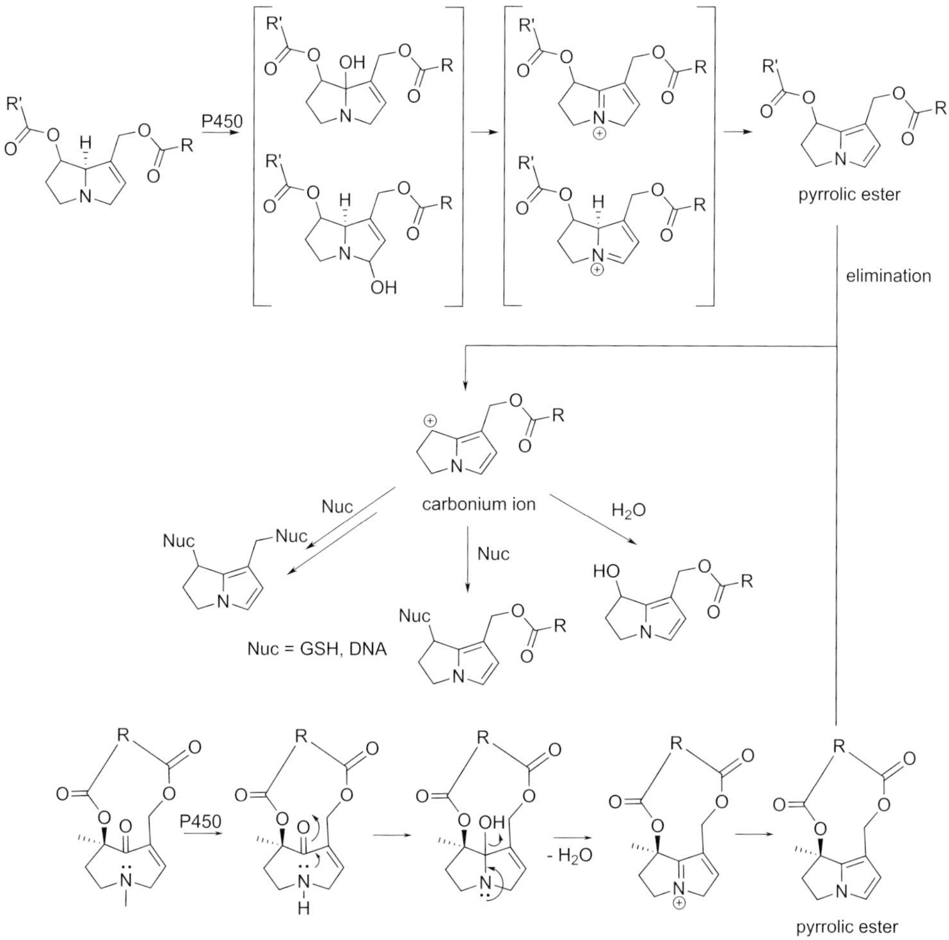

Figure 9.9 Bioactivation mechanisms of pyrrolizidine alkaloids.

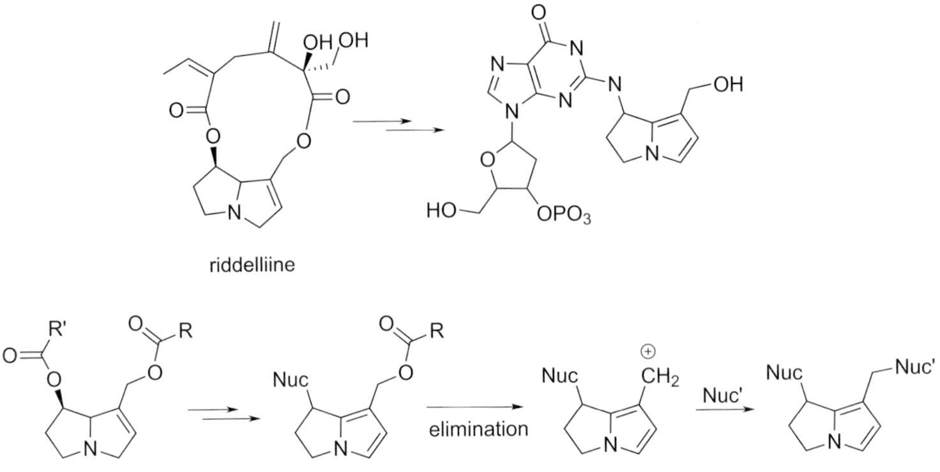

riddelliine

Figure 9.10 Adduct formed by riddelliine and mechanism of DNA cross-link formation by pyrrolizidine alkaloids.

toxicity, was shown to form adducts with the 2-amino position of guanidine in DNA (Figure 9.10) [34, 35].

Pyrrolizidine alkaloids may be particularly mutagenic because they can form cross-linked nucleic acids, due to the presence of two ester groups that are allylic to the intermediate pyrrole [36]. If an adduct to a nucleic acid forms before the second ester is hydrolyzed, then a second elimination reaction of that ester can yield a reactive carbocation adjacent to other nucleophiles on the nucleic acid. Formation of cross-linked adducts to nucleic acids and protein has also been demonstrated [37].

9.3
Well-Known Examples of Bioactivation of Compounds Present in Foods

9.3.1
Cycasin

Cycasin is an azoxy glycoside produced by cycad plants (Figure 9.11). The relevance of human exposure to cycasin is via ingestion of starches prepared from cycad plant and seeds. Improper soaking of the plant material fails to adequately remove the toxic glycoside. Reported toxic effects include hepatotoxicity, carcinogenicity, and interestingly a neurodegenerative disease of extraordinarily high prevalence among natives of Guam referred to as *lytico-bodig* that resembles a combination of amyotrophic lateral sclerosis, Parkinson's disease, and Alzheimer's disease. The Alzheimer's disease has been proposed to arise from neurotoxicity caused by cycasin or by β-methylamino-L-alanine, a neurotoxin that is generated by bacteria that commonly inhabit the cycad roots [38].

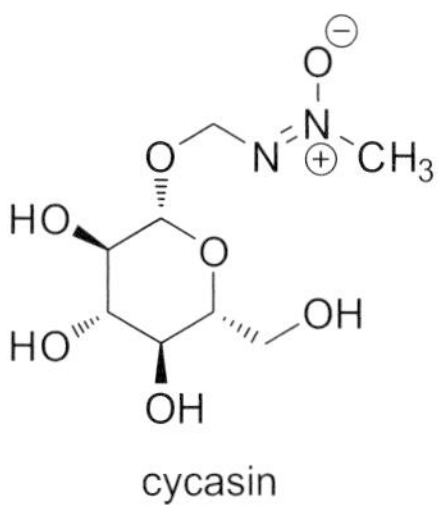

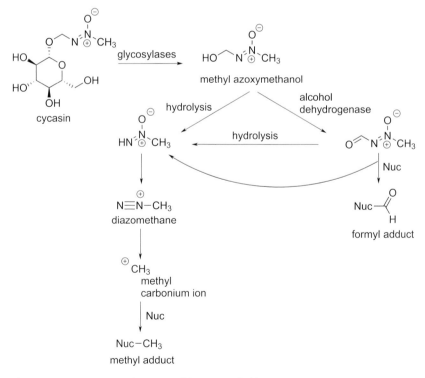

cycasin

Figure 9.11 Structure of cycasin.

The metabolism and activation of cycasin is shown in Figure 9.12. Cycasin is initially metabolized by glycosylases in intestinal microflora to yield the aglycone methylazoxymethanol [39]. The role of gut microflora is supported by metabolism studies in germ-free rats wherein the substantial portion of a dose of cycasin is excreted unchanged in contrast to normal rats in which unchanged cycasin is a minor component of excreted cycasin-derived material. Following deglycosylation, methylazoxymethanol can undergo spontaneous hydrolysis to an intermediate that will lose water to yield methyl diazonium ion. This is a well-established progenitor of methyl carbonium ion, which can methylate biological nucleophiles, such as

Figure 9.12 Bioactivation of cycasin and formation of adducts.

nucleic acids, and cause genetic mutation. Alternately, methylazoxymethanol has been shown to undergo oxidation catalyzed by alcohol dehydrogenases. This is even more sensitive to hydrolysis, and thus more readily able to enter the reaction cascade that yields the methyl carbonium ion. The role of methylazoxymethanol in the mutagenic activity of cycasin is supported by the observation that *in vitro* mutagenicity is reduced in the presence of methylpyrazole, an inhibitor of alcohol dehydrogenase.

9.3.2
Aflatoxin

Aflatoxins are a family of related compounds that are produced by strains of *Aspergillus*, and the threat to human health derives from ingestion of foodstuffs contaminated with *Aspergillus*, including peanuts, corn, rice, and others (Figure 9.13) [40]. It is more frequently a public health concern in developing areas of the world. Chronic exposure can result in hepatocellular carcinoma, and ingestion of high quantities (e.g., ~1 mg) can result in acute hepatotoxicity and death. Characteristics of aflatoxin toxicity are well represented in animals (and, in fact, the first established observation of aflatoxin-induced toxicity was observed in farm poultry).

There are four main aflatoxins termed aflatoxin B_1, B_2, G_1, and G_2, with most studies conducted with aflatoxin B_1 (the designations derive from the fluorescent characteristics of the molecules, i.e., blue or green fluorescent emission). Aflatoxin B_1 is a furanocoumarin, which is bioactivated by epoxidation at the 8,9-double bond to yield a very highly reactive epoxide (Figure 9.14) [41]. The epoxidation is catalyzed by human CYP3A4 and the resulting epoxide has a half-life in aqueous solution of seconds. The flat structure of the remaining part of the molecule intercalates into the base pair structure of DNA and aligns the reactive epoxide such that it can react with nucleophilic groups in DNA such as the N7 position on

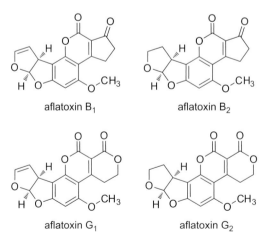

Figure 9.13 Structures of aflatoxins.

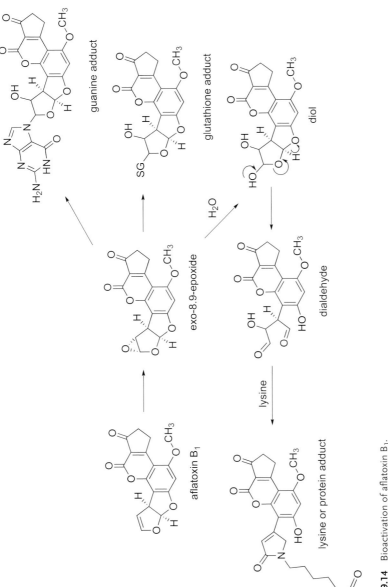

Figure 9.14 Bioactivation of aflatoxin B_1.

guanine. Hydrolysis of the epoxide to the dihydrodiol occurs spontaneously (as opposed to being catalyzed by epoxide hydrolase) and is followed by rearrangement to a dialdehyde that can react with lysine to form protein adducts (e.g., with albumin). Finally, the reactive epoxide can also be conjugated with GSH by glutathione transferases (especially glutathione transferase M1-1 in human).

9.3.3
3-Methylindole

3-Methylindole represents an unusual example of a natural product (tryptophan) being ingested and converted by endogenous microflora to the proximate toxicant, 3-methylindole, which is subsequently bioactivated by CYP enzymes in lung tissue to a reactive iminium species (Figure 9.15) that covalently binds to nucleophiles and results in pulmonary disease (reviewed in [42]). Investigation of this phenomenon had its origins in the observation of pulmonary toxicity observed in ruminant livestock. What has been learned about the bioactivation mechanism of 3-methylindole has been able to be applied to bioactivation mechanisms of 3-alkylindole-containing drugs such as zafirlukast [43, 44]. Human exposure to 3-methylindole can be traced to reductive metabolism of dietary tryptophan as well as in tobacco smoke.

3-Methylindole metabolism has been examined in detail with much focus on the initial CYP-catalyzed hydroxylation of the 3-methyl position as the step that begins the bioactivation and generation of the intermediate 3-methyleneindolene and subsequent nucleophile adducts and covalent binding (pathway a in Figure 9.15). This is observed in lung microsomes and is cited as an explanation for the pneumotoxicity. Further detailed investigations using GSH as a nucleophile trapping agent revealed multiple oxidation reactions that can occur on 3-methylindole to yield several adducts (pathways b–e in Figure 9.15) [45]. These can proceed via epoxidation reactions and hydroxylation to phenols that can give rise to reactive electrophilic quinone imines.

9.3.4
Polycyclic Azaheterocyclic Compounds in Cooked Meats

Cooking of meat leads to the formation of numerous polycyclic aromatic amines derived from oxidative condensations of amino acids and creatinine, many of which have been shown to be mutagenic and carcinogenic [46]. These compounds require bioactivation by CYP enzymes and can also be bioactivated by COX. Two of the most studied are 2-amino-3,8-dimethylimidazo[4,5-f]quinoxaline (MeIQx) and 2-amino-1-methyl-6-phenylimidazo[4,5-b]pyridine (PhIP) (Figure 9.16).

The bioactivation of MeIQx and PhIP commences with the hydroxylations of the exocyclic amino groups that are catalyzed by CYP1A1, 1A2, and 1B1 (Figure 9.16). Conjugation of the N-hydroxy with acetate or sulfate via N-acetyltransferase and sulfotransferases yields a highly unstable ester that undergoes elimination to yield a highly reactive nitrenium ion. This can form adducts with tissue nucleophiles,

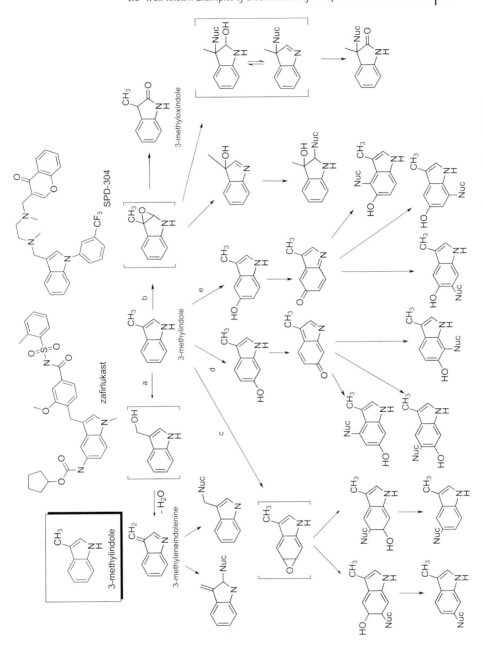

Figure 9.15 Structures of 3-methylindole and 3-alkylindole-containing drugs, and bioactivation mechanism of 3-methylindole.

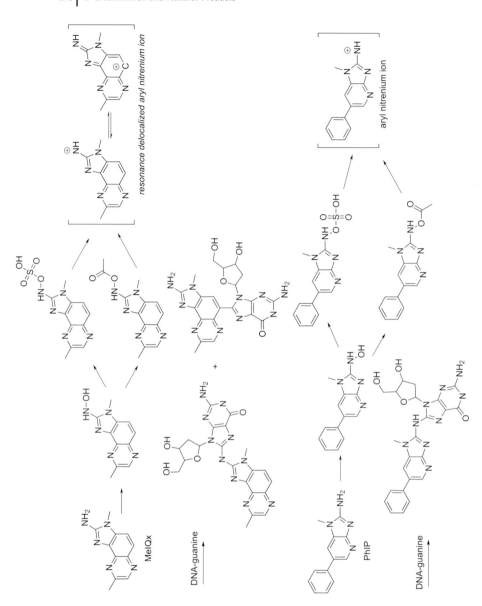

Figure 9.16 Bioactivation of the dietary polycyclic aromatic amines MeIQx and PhIP.

such as DNA bases, and structures of adducts have been determined [47, 48]. For MeIQx, rearrangement to a carbonium ion occurs based on the structure of an alternate adducts. Detoxification of these compounds occurs via alternate oxidation and glucuronidation pathways that occur prior to N-hydroxylation, or via glucuronidation of the hydroxylamine. While it could be expected that there would be an effect of N-acetyltransferase genetics in DNA adduct formation and possibly carcinogenesis caused by polycyclic aromatic amines, results have been mixed in this regard [49–51].

9.3.5
Nitrosamines

As explained in Chapter 2, exposure to N-nitrosamines can occur via either direct exposure to such compounds (e.g., 4-(methylnitrosamino)-1-(3-pyridyl)-1-butanone and N-nitrosonornicotine from smokeless tobacco products) or nitrosation of secondary amine xenobiotics ingested along with nitrite and nitrate (the latter is reduced to nitrite in the saliva and stomach). Nitrosation of secondary amines occurs at low pH, such as that encountered in the stomach, and for tobacco this can occur during curing and storage (Figure 9.17). For nitrosation of secondary

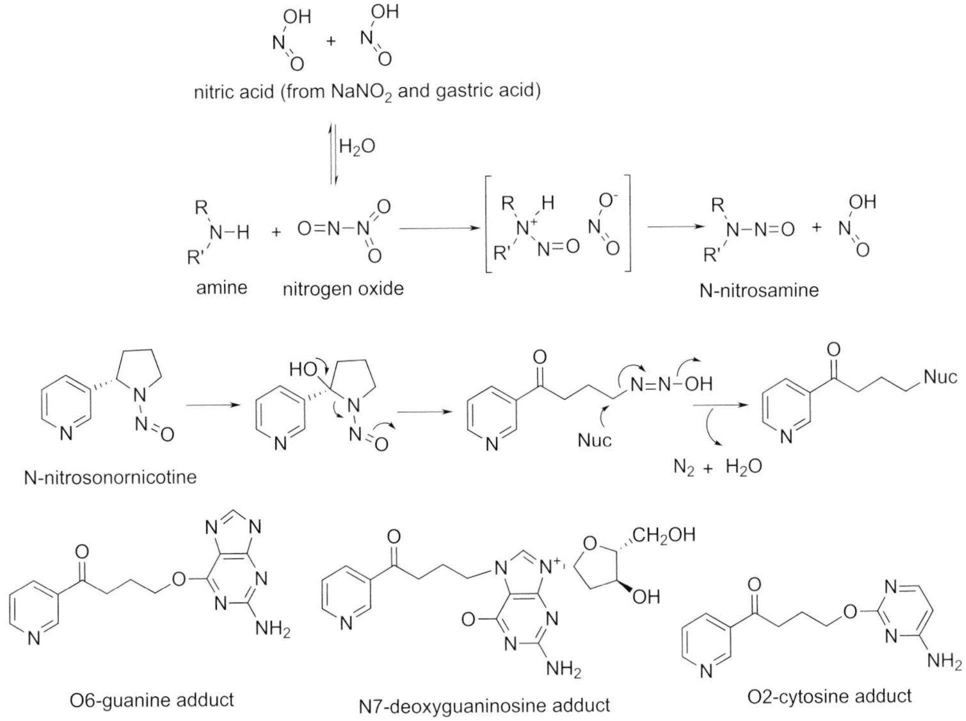

Figure 9.17 Formation and activation of nitrosamines, and structures of adducts with nucleic acid bases.

amines *in vivo*, gastric nitrite levels can be as high as 0.3 mM following a meal rich in nitrate. Nitrite and nitrate are used as preservatives in meat to help prevent bacterial contamination; thus, a balance must be met between risk of carcinogenicity and risk of bacterial infection. The nitrosation of amine-containing drugs and potential toxic effects is a controversial and perhaps somewhat overlooked topic [52]. Tobacco products have been a frequently cited source of direct exposure to nitrosamines, particularly cured materials used in chewing tobacco, and incidence of oral cancers is higher in users of these products. The nitrosamine content of chewing tobaccos has been measured to be about 0.1% of that of nicotine itself, with some unique preparations containing considerably greater levels [53].

The mechanism of bioactivation of *N*-nitrosamines begins with hydroxylation of the α-carbon by CYP enzymes [54]. Conversion to the carbonyl tautomer yields a reactive hydroxyl diazine, which on reaction with a nucleophile yields an adduct while releasing nitrogen and water. Adducts of nitroso-substituted tobacco alkaloids have been identified following chemical reaction with model acetoxy derivatives of the nitrosamines [55, 56]. Treatment of animals with nitroso tobacco alkaloids and extraction of the nucleic acids showed adducts containing the pyridylbutyl group.

9.4
Summary

From the examples described, it should be readily appreciated that bioactivation to reactive metabolites is not restricted to drugs and other man-made chemicals. Natural products are also subject to biotransformation by xenobiotic metabolizing enzymes and in some instances a reactive electrophile can be generated. Each herbal product is a complex mixture of hundreds of unique chemical constituents generated by plant secondary metabolism and any subsequent processing that the plant matter is subjected to postharvest. It can be expected that as the use of herbal remedies increases, instances of toxicity will also unfortunately increase. Investigation of the underlying mechanisms of these occurrences and identification of the constituents responsible poses a massive task for toxicologists and drug metabolism scientists.

References

1 Smith, A. (2002) It's natural so it must be safe. *Australian Prescriber*, **25** (3), 50–51.

2 Gonzalez, F.J. and Nebert, D.W. (1990) Evolution of the P450 gene superfamily: animal–plant 'warfare', molecular drive and human genetic differences in drug oxidation. *Trends in Genetics*, **6** (6), 182–186.

3 Stedman, C. (2002) Herbal hepatotoxicity. *Seminars in Liver Disease*, **22** (2), 195–206.

4 Lekehal, M., Passayre, D., Lereau, J.M., Moulis, C., Fouraste, I., and Fau, D. (1996) Hepatotoxicity of the herbal medicine germander: metabolic activation of its furano diterpenoids by cytochrome P450 3A depletes cytoskeleton-associated

protein thiols and forms plasma membrane blebs in rat hepatocytes. *Hepatology*, **24** (1), 212–218.

5 Kouzi, S.A., McMurtry, R.J., and Nelson, S.D. (1994) Hepatotoxicity of germander (*Teucrium chamaedrys* L.) and one of its constituent neoclerodane diterpenes teucrin A in the mouse. *Chemical Research in Toxicology*, **7** (6), 850–856.

6 Druckova, A. and Marnett, L.J. (2006) Characterization of the amino acid adducts of the enedial derivative of teucrin A. *Chemical Research in Toxicology*, **19** (10), 1330–1340.

7 Druckova, A., Mernaugh, R.L., Ham, A.L., and Marnett, L.J. (2007) Identification of the protein targets of the reactive metabolite of teucrin A in vivo in the rat. *Chemical Research in Toxicology*, **20** (10), 1393–1408.

8 De Berardinis, V., Moulis, C., Maurice, M., Beaune, P., Pessayre, D., Pompon, D., and Loeper, J. (2000) Human microsomal epoxide hydrolase is the target of germander-induced autoantibodies on the surface of human hepatocytes. *Molecular Pharmacology*, **58** (3), 542–551.

9 Petrakis, E.A., Kimbaris, A.C., Pappas, C.S., Tarantilis, P.A., and Polissiou, M.G. (2009) Quantitative determination of pulegone in pennyroyal oil by FT-IR spectroscopy. *Journal of Agricultural and Food Chemistry*, **57** (21), 10044–10048.

10 Seeff, L.B. (2007) Herbal hepatotoxicity. *Clinics in Liver Disease*, **11** (3), 577–596.

11 Chen, X.W., Serag, E.S., Sneed, K.B., and Zhou, S.F. (2011) Herbal bioactivation, molecular targets and the toxicity relevance. *Chemico-Biological Interactions*, **192** (3), 161–176.

12 Gordon, W.P., Huitric, A.C., Seth, C.L., McClanahan, R.H., and Nelson, S.D. (1987) The metabolism of the abortifacient terpene, (*R*)-(+)-pulegone, to a proximate toxin, menthofuran. *Drug Metabolism and Disposition*, **15** (5), 589–594.

13 Thomassen, D., Knebel, N., Slattery, J.T., McClanahan, R.H., and Nelson, S.D. (1992) Reactive intermediates in the oxidation of menthofuran by cytochromes P-450. *Chemical Research in Toxicology*, **5** (1), 123–130.

14 Khojasteh-Bakht, S.C., Chen, W., Koenigs, L.L., Peter, R.M., and Nelson, S.D. (1999) Metabolism of (*R*)-(+)-pulegone and (*R*)-(+)-menthofuran by human liver cytochrome P-450s: evidence for formation of a furan epoxide. *Drug Metabolism and Disposition*, **27** (5), 574–580.

15 Anderson, I.B., Mullen, W.H., Meeker, J.E., Khojasteh-Bakht, S.C., Oishi, S., Nelson, S.D., and Blanc, P.D. (1996) Pennyroyal toxicity: measurement of toxic metabolite levels in two cases and review of the literature. *Annals of Internal Medicine*, **124** (8), 726–734.

16 Chen, L.-J., Lebetkin, E.H., and Burka, L.T. (2003) Metabolism of (*R*)-(+)-menthofuran in Fischer-344 rats: identification of sulfonic acid metabolites. *Drug Metabolism and Disposition*, **31** (10), 1208–1213.

17 Madyastha, K.M. and Raj, C.P. (1991) Evidence for the formation of a known toxin, *p*-cresol, from menthofuran. *Biochemistry Biophysics Research Communications*, **177** (1), 440–446.

18 Khojasteh, S.C., Oishi, S., and Nelson, S.D. (2010) Metabolism and toxicity of menthofuran in rat liver slices and in rats. *Chemical Research in Toxicology*, **23** (11), 1824–1832.

19 Stiborova, M., Frei, E., Arlt, V.M., and Schmeiser, H.H. (2008) Metabolic activation of carcinogenic aristolochic acid, a risk factor for Balkan endemic nephropathy. *Mutation Research*, **658** (1–2), 55–67.

20 Chan, W., Cui, L., Xu, G., and Cai, Z. (2006) Study of the phase I and phase II metabolism of nephrotoxin aristolochic acid by liquid chromatography/tandem mass spectrometry. *Rapid Communications in Mass Spectrometry*, **20** (11), 1755–1760.

21 Chan, W., Luo, H.B., Zheng, Y., Cheng, Y.K., and Cai, Z. (2007) Investigation of the metabolism and reductive activation of carcinogenic aristolochic acids in rats. *Drug Metabolism and Disposition*, **35** (6), 866–874.

22 Stiborova, M., Frei, E., Sopko, B., Wiessler, M., and Schmeiser, H.H. (2002) Carcinogenic aristolochic acids upon activation by DT-diaphorase form adducts

found in DNA of patients with Chinese herbs nephropathy. *Carcinogenesis*, **23** (4), 617–625.

23 Stiborova, M., Frei, E., Sopko, B., Sopkova, K., Markova, V., Lankova, M., Kumstyrova, T., Wiessler, M., and Schmeiser, H.H. (2003) Human cytosolic enzymes involved in the metabolic activation of carcinogenic aristolochic acid: evidence for reductive activation by human NAD(P)H:quinone oxidoreductase. *Carcinogenesis*, **24** (10), 1695–1703.

24 Stiborova, M., Frei, E., Hodek, P., Wiessler, M., and Schmeiser, H.H. (2005) Human hepatic and renal microsomes, cytochromes P450 1A1/2, NADPH: cytochrome P450 reductase and prostaglandin H synthase mediate the formation of aristolochic acid–DNA adducts found in patients with urothelial cancer. *International Journal of Cancer*, **113** (2), 189–197.

25 Schmeiser, H.H., Bieler, C.A., Wiessler, M., van Ypersele de Strihou, C., and Cosyns, J.P. (1996) Detection of DNA adducts formed by aristolochic acid in renal tissue from patients with Chinese herbs nephropathy. *Cancer Research*, **56** (9), 2025–2028.

26 Nortier, J.L., Martinez, M.C., Schmeiser, H.H., Arlt, V.M., Bieler, C.A., Petein, M., Depierreux, M.F., De Pauw, L., Abramowicz, D., Vereerstraeten, P., and Vanherweghen, J.L. (2000) Urothelial carcinoma associated with the use of a Chinese herb (*Aristolochia fangchi*). *New England Journal of Medicine*, **342** (23), 1686–1692.

27 Priestap, H.A., de los Santos, C., and Quirke, J.M. (2010) Identification of a reduction product of aristolochic acid: implications for the metabolic activation of carcinogenic aristolochic acid. *Journal of Natural Products*, **73** (12), 1979–1986.

28 Mei, N., Guo, L., Fu, P.P., Fuscoe, J.C., Luan, Y., and Chen, T. (2010) Metabolism, genotoxicity, and carcinogenicity of comfrey. *Journal of Toxicology and Environmental Health, Part B*, **13** (7–8), 509–526.

29 Chen, Z. and Huo, J.R. (2010) Hepatic veno-occlusive disease associated with toxicity of pyrrolizidine alkaloids in herbal preparations. *The Netherlands Journal of Medicine*, **68** (6), 252–260.

30 Liu, F., Wan, S.Y., Jiang, Z., Li, S.F.Y., Ong, E.S., Castano, O., and Osorio, J.C.C. (2009) Determination of pyrrolizidine alkaloids in comfrey by liquid chromatography–electrospray ionization mass spectrometry. *Talanta*, **80** (2), 916–923.

31 Barbakadze, V., Mulkijanyan, K., Gogilashvili, L., Amiranashvili, L., Merlani, M., Novikova, Z., and Sulakvelidze, M. (2009) Allantoin- and pyrrolizidine alkaloids-free wound healing compositions from *Symphytum asperum*. *Bulletin of the Georgian National Academy of Sciences*, **3** (1), 159–164.

32 Candrian, U., Luethy, J., Graf, U., and Schlatter, C. (1984) Mutagenic activity of the pyrrolizidine alkaloids seneciphylline and senkirkine in *Drosophila* and their transfer into rat milk. *Food and Chemical Toxicology*, **22** (3), 223–225.

33 Fu, P.P., Xia, Q., Lin, G., and Chou, M.W. (2004) Pyrrolizidine alkaloids –genotoxicity, metabolism enzymes, metabolic activation, and mechanisms. *Drug Metabolism Reviews*, **36** (1), 1–55.

34 Yang, Y., Yan, J., Churchwell, M., Beger, R., Chan, P., Doerge, D.R., Fu, P.P., and Chou, M.W. (2001) Development of a (32) P-postlabeling/HPLC method for detection of dehydroretronecine-derived DNA adducts in vivo and in vitro. *Chemical Research in Toxicology*, **14** (1), 91–100.

35 Chou, M.W., Jian, Y., Williams, L.D., Xia, Q., Churchwell, M., Doerge, D.R., and Fu, P.P. (2003) Identification of DNA adducts derived from riddelliine, a carcinogenic pyrrolizidine alkaloid. *Chemical Research in Toxicology*, **16** (9), 1130–1137.

36 Petry, T.W., Bowden, G.T., Huxtable, R.J., and Sipes, I.G. (1984) Characterization of hepatic DNA damage induced in rats by the pyrrolizidine alkaloid monocrotaline. *Cancer Research*, **44** (4), 1505–1509.

37 Coulombe, R.A., Drew, G.L., and Stermitz, F.R. (1999) Highlight: pyrrolizidine alkaloids crosslink DNA with actin. *Toxicology and Applied Pharmacology*, **154** (2), 198–202.

38 Kirby, G.E., Kabel, H., Higon, J., and Spencer, P. (1999) Damage and repair of

nerve cell DNA in toxic stress. *Drug Metabolism Reviews*, **31** (3), 589–618.

39 Morgan, R.W. and Hoffmann, G.R. (1983) Cycasin and its mutagenic metabolites. *Mutation Research*, **114** (1), 19–58.

40 Kensler, T.W., Roebuck, B.D., Wogan, G.N., and Groopman, J.D. (2011) Aflatoxin: a 50-year odyssey of mechanistic and translational toxicology. *Toxicological Sciences*, **120** (Suppl. 1), s28–s38.

41 Guengerich, F.P., Johnson, W.W., Shimada, T., Ueng, Y.F., Yamazaki, H., and Langouet, S. (1998) Activation and detoxication of aflatoxin B1. *Mutation Research*, **402** (1–2), 121–128.

42 Yost, G.S. (1989) Mechanisms of 3-methylindole pneumotoxicity. *Chemical Research in Toxicology*, **2** (5), 273–279.

43 Kassahun, K., Skordos, K., McIntosh, I., Slaughter, D., Doss, G.A., Baillie, T.A., and Yost, G.S. (2005) Zafirlukast metabolism by cytochrome P450 3A4 produces an electrophilic alpha,beta-unsaturated iminium species that results in the selective mechanism-based inactivation of the enzyme. *Chemical Research in Toxicology*, **18** (9), 1427–1437.

44 Sun, H. and Yost, G.S. (2008) Metabolic activation of a novel 3-substituted indole-containing TNF-alpha inhibitor: dehydrogenation and inactivation of CYP3A4. *Chemical Research in Toxicology*, **21** (2), 374–385.

45 Yan, Z., Easterwood, L.M., Maher, N., Torres, R., Huebert, N., and Yost, G.S. (2007) Metabolism and bioactivation of 3-methylindole by human liver microsomes. *Chemical Research in Toxicology*, **20** (1), 140–148.

46 Schut, H.A.J. and Snyderwine, E.G. (1999) DNA adducts of heterocyclic amine food mutagens: implications for mutagenesis and carcinogenesis. *Carcinogenesis*, **20** (3), 353–368.

47 Turesky, R.J., Rossi, S.C., Welti, D.H., Lay, J.O. Jr., and Kadlubar, F.F. (1992) Characterization of DNA adducts formed in vitro by reaction of N-hydroxy-2-amino-3-methylimidazo[4,5-f]quinoline and N-hydroxy-2-amino-3,8-dimethylimidazo [4,5-f]quinoxaline at the C-8 and N2 atoms of guanine. *Chemical Research in Toxicology*, **5** (4), 479–490.

48 Lin, D., Kaderlik, K.R., Turesky, R.J., Miller, D.W., Lay, J.O. Jr., and Kadlubar, F.F. (1992) Identification of N-(deoxyguanosin-8-yl)-2-amino-1-methyl-6-phenylimidazo[4,5-b]pyridine as the major adduct formed by the food-borne carcinogen, 2-amino-1-methyl-6-phenylimidazo[4,5-b]pyridine, with DNA. *Chemical Research in Toxicology*, **5** (5), 691–697.

49 Minchin, R.F., Kadlubar, F.F., and Ilett, K.F. (1993) Role of acetylation in colorectal cancer. *Mutation Research/Fundamental and Molecular Mechanisms of Mutagenesis*, **290** (1), 35–42.

50 Butler, L.M., Millikan, R.C., Sinha, R., Keku, T.O., Winkel, S., Harlan, B., Eaton, A., Gammon, M.D., and Sandler, R.S. (2008) Modification by N-acetyltransferase 1 genotype on the association between dietary heterocyclic amines and colon cancer in a multiethnic study. *Mutation Research/Fundamental and Molecular Mechanisms of Mutagenesis*, **638** (1–2), 162–174.

51 Metry, K.J., Neale, J.R., Doll, M.A., Howarth, A.L., States, J.C., McGregor, W.G., Pierce, W.M. Jr., and Hein, D.W. (2010) Effect of rapid human N-acetyltransferase 2 haplotype on DNA damage and mutagenesis induced by 2-amino-3-methylimidazo-[4,5-f]quinoline (IQ) and 2-amino-3,8-dimethylimidazo-[4,5-f]quinoxaline (MeIQx). *Mutation Research/Fundamental and Molecular Mechanisms of Mutagenesis*, **684** (1–2), 66–73.

52 Brambilla, G. and Martelli, A. (2007) Genotoxic and carcinogenic risk to humans of drug–nitrite interaction products. *Mutation Research*, **635** (1), 17–52.

53 Brunnemann, K.D., Prokopczyk, B., Djordjevic, M.V., and Hoffmann, D. (1996) Formation and analysis of tobacco-specific N-nitrosamines. *Critical Reviews in Toxicology*, **26** (2), 121–137.

54 Hecht, S.S., Upadhyaya, P., and Wang, M. (2011) Evolution of research on the DNA adduct chemistry of N-nitrosopyrrolidine and related aldehydes. *Chemical Research in Toxicology*, **24** (6), 781–790.

55 Wang, L., Spratt, T.E., Liu, X.K., Hecht, S.S., Pegg, A.E., and Peterson, L.A. (1997) Pyridyloxobutyl adduct *O*6-[4-oxo-4-(3-pyridyl)butyl]guanine is present in 4-(acetoxymethylnitrosamino)-1-(3-pyridyl)-1-butanone-treated DNA and is a substrate for *O*6-alkylguanine-DNA alkyltransferase. *Chemical Research in Toxicology*, **10** (5), 562–567.

56 Upadhyaya, P., Sturla, S.J., Tretyakova, N., Ziegel, R., Villalta, P.W., Wang, M., and Hecht, S.S. (2003) Identification of adducts produced by the reaction of 4-(acetoxymethylnitrosamino)-1-(3-pyridyl)-1-butanol with deoxyguanosine and DNA. *Chemical Research in Toxicology*, **16** (2), 180–190.

10
Experimental Approaches to Reactive Metabolite Detection

Abbreviations

GSH   Glutathione
LC–MS/MS   Liquid chromatography–tandem mass spectrometry
qWBA   Quantitative whole-body autoradiography
TDI   Time-dependent inhibition
TOF   Time-of-flight
TQMS   Tandem-quadrupole mass spectrometry

10.1
Introduction

In other chapters in this book, the theoretical considerations of bioactivation and reactive metabolites have been discussed. All of this knowledge required the application of experimental approaches to gather data in support for various hypotheses of bioactivation of individual compounds and structural elements contained within them. In this chapter, experimental approaches that yield insight into reactive metabolite formation are described. These can be categorized into two main types: (a) experiments that are specifically designed to explore reactive metabolite generation and (b) experiments that are done with other objectives in mind but from which data can emerge to suggest the presence of reactive metabolites.

10.2
Identification of Structural Alerts and Avoiding them in Drug Design

Modern medicinal chemistry and drug design employ *in silico* methods, wherein virtual compounds are designed to optimize target potency (using custom-built models based on pharmacophore and/or target protein structure data) and physicochemical properties (for which commercially available computational programs exist). Knowledge-based *in silico* strategies can also be employed to avoid the

Reactive Drug Metabolites, First Edition. Amit S. Kalgutkar, Deepak Dalvie, R. Scott Obach, and Dennis A. Smith.
© 2012 Wiley-VCH Verlag GmbH & Co. KGaA. Published 2012 by Wiley-VCH Verlag GmbH & Co. KGaA.

inclusion of substituents known to generate chemically reactive intermediates. In any new structure if a substituent is included that could possibly be metabolized to a reactive entity, there is no guarantee that it will in fact be metabolized. Computational methods to predict metabolism of a new chemical from its structure alone have been described but have not yet fulfilled an acceptable level of reliability. Thus, *in silico* methods to address reactive metabolites are restricted to library-based approaches whereby the presence of a substituent that has been associated with reactive metabolites is noted. For example, the DEREK program employs this type of approach in alerting to the potential for mutagenicity [1]. Because the link between reactive metabolite generation and toxicity is not well defined in all cases, an approach that can be taken early in research programs is one whereby potentially offending substituents are purposefully avoided in the design of new drugs. Thus, there are specific substituents that are not permitted to be included in newly designed molecules, irrespective of whether such substituents would offer other advantages in drug performance (e.g., intrinsic potency, good biopharmaceutical properties, low clearance, etc.). These substituents are frequently referred to as "structure alerts" and lists of such alerts have been described [2, 3]. A brief list is included in Table 10.1. Lists of structural alerts are derived from experiences reported in the scientific literature in which mechanisms of bioactivation have been delineated for specific drugs that had been shown to cause toxicity believed to be associated with reactive metabolites. It is important to note that there are a vast number of substituents that have been shown to yield a reactive metabolite in at least one example. If structure alert lists were that comprehensive, a substituent as simple as a phenyl ring could be removed from consideration because it is possible to oxidize a phenyl to an epoxide or a quinone. Thus, structure alert lists must be constrained to those examples for which there is a high prevalence of examples that yield reactive metabolites.

There are two major shortcomings of the use of structure alerts in drug design. First, since the lists are based on knowledge, it is not possible to avoid as yet

Table 10.1 A list of common structural alerts associated with reactive metabolite formation and toxicity.

Precursor	Reactive Metabolite
Alkene	Epoxide
Alkyne	Ketene
Polycyclic arene	Epoxide
Aniline	Quinone imine
o- or *p*-dialkoxyarene; phenol	Quinone
Furan	α,β-Unsaturated aldehyde
Thiophene	*S*-Oxide
Methylenedioxyphenyl	*o*-Quinone
2-Aminothiazole	Thiourea *S*-oxide
3-Alkylindole	α,β-Unsaturated imine
Haloalkane	Acyl halide

unknown structures that can be bioactivated. Thus, lists of structure alerts will probably always be growing, as new structures are discovered to be subject to bioactivation. Second, and more importantly, the functional groups in structure alert lists are categorized into a simple binary categorization, that is, those known to be bioactivated versus everything else. Unfortunately, the above classification is arbitrary and there is no clear distinction as to when a particular group is classified as a structural alert. Additional context is needed when attempting to make design decisions when a structure alert is involved, since not all molecules possessing a structure alert have toxicity problems in the clinic, and there are molecules that lack known structure alerts that do cause toxicity. For example, the highly successful antidepressant agent paroxetine contains a methylenedioxyphenyl substituent, a well-established structural alert that can undergo metabolic bioactivation to reactive carbene and quinoid structures. Furthermore, it is known that paroxetine is metabolized on this substituent and nucleophilic adducts of paroxetine have been demonstrated *in vitro* [4]. However, paroxetine has been administered safely to millions of patients and it has not been shown to cause safety problems due to reactive metabolites. Thus, structural alert lists must be used with caution in early drug design. If the target pharmacophore lacks constraint such that a structure alerting substituent can be replaced with other substituents without loss of other desired attributes, then it is advisable to exclude the structure alert from the design. However, if the structure alert appears to be critical to the pharmacological properties of the new compound, other information is needed to aid in decision making. This can include the experimental approaches described in this chapter as well as knowledge of the total daily dose needed for efficacy, whether the drug will be used chronically, and the severity of the unmet medical need being targeted.

10.3
Assays for the Detection of Reactive Metabolites

There are a variety of methods to determine whether a new compound can generate reactive metabolites. These vary with regard to the thoroughness of the experiment and the confidence one can have in the conclusions. They range from resource-intensive approaches that can quantitate covalent adducts to macromolecules to approaches whereby the potential for bioactivation can be screened across thousands of compounds. All have limitations when attempting to use the results for predicting the potential for toxicity and comparing compounds.

10.3.1
Qualitative Electrophile Trapping Assays

The most widely used methodology for detecting the potential for bioactivation of new compounds to reactive electrophilic intermediates is mass spectrometry–based assays using glutathione (GSH) or a related thiol as a nucleophilic trapping agent

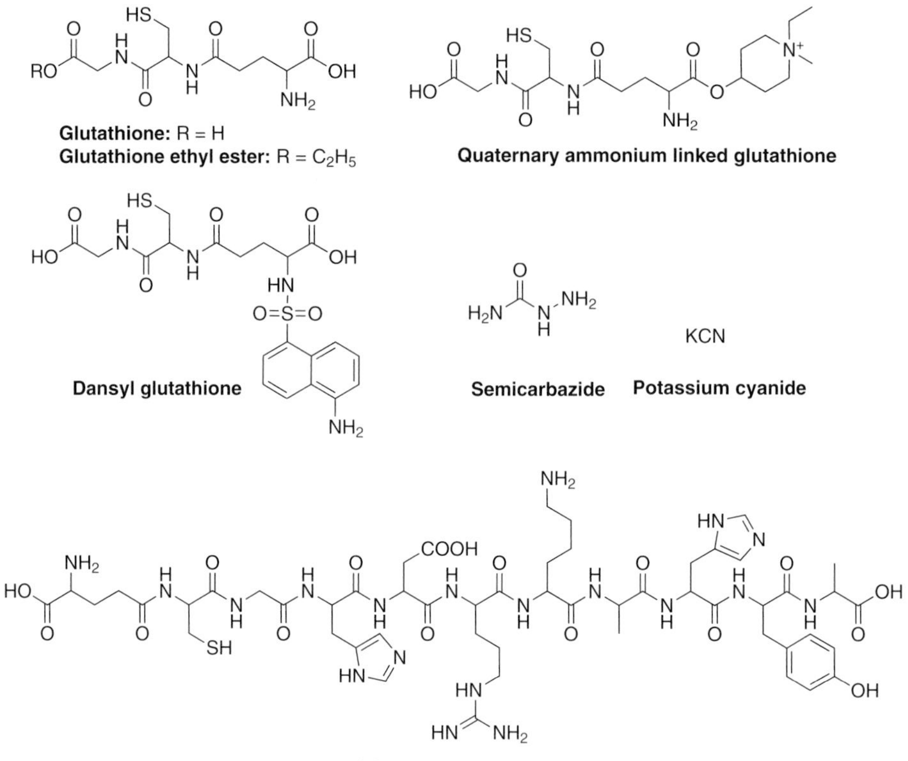

Glutathione: R = H
Glutathione ethyl ester: R = C₂H₅

Quaternary ammonium linked glutathione

Dansyl glutathione

Semicarbazide   **Potassium cyanide**

KCN

ECGHDRKAHYK peptide

Figure 10.1 Structures of nucleophiles used in trapping reactive metabolites.

(Figure 10.1) [5, 6]. Test compounds are incubated with liver microsomes (preferably human) supplemented with NADPH or an NADPH generation system to support cytochrome P450 activity, and nucleophilic thiol. After termination, the incubations mixtures are analyzed by HPLC with tandem-quadrupole mass spectrometry (TQMS) detection. The neutral loss scanning technique that can be done using TQMS is well suited to finding GSH adducts because in positive ion mode these adducts almost always fragment in the collision cell of TQMS instruments by the loss of the pyroglutamic acid moiety (from GSH), which is 129 mass units. Demonstration of a parent molecular ion that yields a neutral loss of 129 units in an incubation mixture is taken as proof that the compound forms a reactive electrophile capable of reacting with GSH. Additionally, other TQMS scanning algorithms can be employed to find GSH adducts (e.g., product scanning of ion currents corresponding to molecular ions of expected GSH adducts such as molecular ion +307, +323, etc.). A major shortcoming of this approach is that it is not quantitative – it only offers a yes/no answer to the question of whether a test compound can be detectably bioactivated to an electrophile that can react with GSH. MS response varies from compound to compound, so peak intensities cannot be quantitatively compared across compounds and their corresponding GSH adducts. Detection capability varies with the ionization properties of the GSH adduct and the rate at which such an adduct is formed. Furthermore, the use of liver microsomes and NADPH favors the generation of reactive metabolites and does not account for alternate, non-450 metabolic routes that may divert test compounds to other non-bioactivation pathways as well as missing metabolic pathways that can detoxify the reactive metabolite. Finally, since only a soft nucleophile is used to trap electrophiles, bioactivation can be missed if a test compound is metabolized to a hard electrophile. However, this assay approach has shown utility because it can be automated and carried out in high throughput. The data permit a medicinal chemist to prefer the pursuit of new compounds that do not show bioactivation over those that do.

Advances have been made in GSH trapping assays to enhance sensitivity and degree of quantitation. GSH ethyl ester is used as an alternative trapping agent to enhance the ionization in MS [7]. When an adduct is formed, GSH adds one amino and two carboxylic acid groups to a molecule. These two acid groups can cause a decrease in detection of ions when scanning in the positive ion mode. Esterifying one acid group enhances the detectability. Precursor ion scanning of m/z 272 in negative ionization mode can demonstrate GSH adducts that may not yield a neutral loss of 129 units [8]. Isotopically labeled mixtures of GSH have also been employed to enhance the selectivity and throughput of GSH trapping assays [9]. A 1:1 mixture of GSH and $[^{15}N^{13}C_2]$-GSH used in microsomal incubations leads to adducts that will show a characteristic mass spectral pattern of peaks 3 mass units apart. Solid-phase extraction of incubation mixtures permits samples to be analyzed by mass spectrometry without needing HPLC. Using stable-labeled GSH and gathering data on a linear ion trap permits the simultaneous detection of GSH adducts and daughter scanning of the adduct molecular ions to offer structural information [10]. High-resolution mass spectrometers can also be used in which the GSH adduct can be detected and fragmentation data can also be gathered to aid in the structural assignment of the adduct [11]. This has also been described using Q-trap mass spectrometry and time-of-flight (TOF) accurate mass with mass defect filtering of the data [12, 13]. Finally, the use of a cysteine-containing peptide in place of GSH, coupled with TOF–MS, and an ion exchange chip yields an assay that could be done without requiring HPLC [14]. These instruments and approaches make the detection of GSH adducts less dependent on neutral loss scanning of 129, and those adducts that do not yield this fragmentation can be detected. Ma and Zhu have recently reviewed recent advances in the detection and characterization of reactive metabolites by liquid chromatography–tandem mass spectrometry (LC–MS/MS) in drug discovery and development [15].

Hard electrophiles cannot be detected in microsomal incubations using thiol nucleophiles. Rather, the use of cyanide has been described to accomplish this [16]. By using a mixture of stable isotope-labeled $K^{13}C^{15}N$ with nonlabeled KCN, and mass spectrometric detection of the isotope pattern of cyanide adducts, the bioactivation of several alicyclic amine drugs could be detected (e.g., nicotine, nefazodone, etc.), whereas GSH adducts were not detected. Semicarbazide can be used to detect potentially reactive aldehydes as illustrated with reactive metabolites generated from heterocyclic ring scission [17].

10.3.2
Quantitative Electrophile Trapping Assays

A major shortcoming of nucleophile trapping assays described in Section 10.3.1 is that the assays yield binary outputs, that is, is an adduct detected or not? In the event that a particular chemical series demonstrates the formation of adducts, it is important to quantitatively compare across compounds and develop structure–activity relationships. While it is acknowledged that adduct detection assays are not necessarily predictive of toxicity, in the absence of other information during the early phase of drug research, selection of compounds with lower amounts of adduct formed is preferred. Thus, it can be desirable to be able to quantitate adducts in *in vitro* assays. Approaches include the use of radiometric methods, fluorescence detection, and mass spectrometric methods.

Use of a GSH analogue containing a quaternary ammonium group for semiquantitatively trapping reactive metabolites was demonstrated (see Figure 10.1) [18]. Ionization efficiency in mass spectrometers is greater for quaternary ammonium GSH adducts and response factors among adducts are more similar to each other, as compared to adducts using GSH. Thus, this approach can be considered semiquantitative. Dansylated GSH (see Figure 10.1), in which a fluorescent dansyl substituent is linked to the glycine amino group on GSH, has been used as a nucleophile trap [19]. Dansyl-GSH is incubated in place of GSH with test compounds and liver microsomes, and the mixture is analyzed by HPLC with in-line fluorescence and mass spectrometric detectors. Thus, the identity of the adduct and its quantity can be simultaneously determined, since the fluorescence response of the dansyl group is unchanged when the adduct is formed. This assay was used to demonstrate that compounds forming reactive metabolites could be associated with toxicity only after the quantitative adduct data were normalized with the daily dose of these drugs [20].

Radiometric measurement using radiolabeled nucleophiles is the other approach that can be used to gather quantitative data for reactive metabolites *in vitro*. ^{35}S-GSH has been used to quantify the adducts that are formed after the trapping of electrophiles [21]. The ready availability of [^{14}C]-KCN permits the quantitative measurement of hard electrophiles. Separation of unreacted cyanide from cyanide that is covalently bound to the test compound can be easily accomplished [22, 23]. Also, both [^{14}C]-NaCN and [^{35}S]-cysteine can be simultaneously used in liver microsomal incubations with incubation mixtures analyzed by HPLC–MS with in-line radiometric flow detection [24]. Results with this method correlated with covalent binding data gathered for the same compounds. Radiolabeled semicarbazide can be used to quantitatively assess the bioactivation of alicyclic amines to aldehydes. In this method, an amine is first incubated alone in a typical liver microsome system, and then postincubated to optimally trap reactive aldehyde intermediates with radiolabeled semicarbazide. The amount of adduct formed is then determined by using HPLC with in-line radiometric detection or collection of fractions and analysis in a liquid scintillation counter. The method has been applied to various compounds and has proven to be useful for the screening of covalent binding generated by newly synthesized compounds with alicyclic amine moieties [25].

10.3.3
Covalent Binding Assays

The determination of metabolism-dependent covalent binding of xenobiotics has been carried out for years to better understand mechanisms of toxicity. Application of covalent binding approaches in drug research was recently described in an article by Evans *et al.* [26]. These authors outlined an approach to utilizing covalent binding data in drug research in the selection of new drug candidates for clinical development. In an *in vitro* covalent binding study, radiolabeled test compound, a source of enzyme (e.g., liver microsomes), and cofactors required for enzyme activity are incubated. The incubations are terminated by precipitating the protein, and the precipitate is extensively washed to remove radioactivity that is not covalently bound. The results are compared to control incubations in which the precipitation and washing is done at time zero and in which incubation is carried out in the absence of cofactors (Figure 10.2).

Evans *et al.* [26] did not suggest that *in vitro* covalent binding data alone serve as a criterion for the acceptability of new compounds into clinical development, but that such data, along with *in vivo* covalent binding data gathered in rats, are used in combination with several other factors (e.g., attractive biopharmaceutical and pharmacokinetic properties, pharmacodynamics, daily dosing regimen, clinical indication). However, while at that time much was known about the metabolism-dependent covalent binding of several agents already shown to demonstrate toxicity likely related to this phenomenon, information on covalent binding capabilities among drugs not associated with toxicity was not known. Subsequent investigations showed that many drugs can demonstrate NADPH-dependent covalent binding *in vitro*, and that toxic ones cannot be distinguished from nontoxic ones based on covalent binding alone [27–29]. However, when covalent binding data are considered with the total daily dose, agents associated with hepatotoxicity can be distinguished from those not showing hepatotoxicity (Figure 10.3). The use of human hepatocytes, which possess a greater complement of xenobiotic metabolizing enzymes than liver microsomes, in covalent binding studies appears to provide a better capability to distinguish toxic from nontoxic. This could be due to the activities of enzymes that can detoxify reactive intermediates, such as glucuronyl transferases, methyltransferases, glutathione transferases, and others.

Because of the need for radiolabeled test compounds, covalent binding studies are not routinely conducted in early stages of drug discovery. Custom radiosynthesis of new agents is very resource intensive, especially due to the

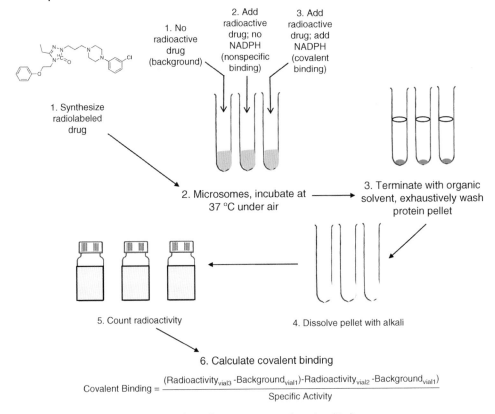

Figure 10.2 Experimental scheme for measurement of covalent binding.

need to place the radioactive atom at a position that is resistant to metabolism. Thus, simple radiosynthetic approaches, such as methylation of a heteroatom with readily available [^{14}C]-labeled methylating reagents, are not an option. Tritiation can sometimes serve as a valuable approach in the generation of radiolabeled test compounds for *in vitro* covalent binding experiments, but careful attention must be paid to the site(s) of incorporation of the tritium atom(s) to assure that the material will give an acceptable result in covalent binding experiments. As a specific compound gets closer to being the one nominated for clinical development, and certainly within the clinical development phase, the resource investment in preparing a radiolabeled compound becomes more worthwhile. However, the strategy of whether to conduct *in vitro* covalent binding experiments for a compound in clinical development remains controversial, due to ambiguity around the interpretation of data that show covalent binding [30].

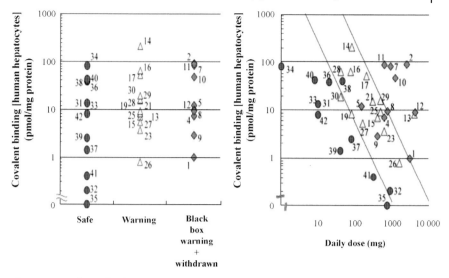

Figure 10.3 Relationship between *in vitro* covalent binding, dose, and toxicity (adapted from [29]).

10.3.4
Detecting and Characterizing Bioactivation by Enzymes Other than Cytochrome P450

There are other special instances that arise for particular compounds in which the electrophile trapping or covalent binding assays described in the preceding sections are not suitable. Acyl glucuronide metabolites have been proposed to be an underlying mechanism responsible for toxicity exhibited by many carboxylic acid–containing drugs [31, 32]. The challenge has been in distinguishing those agents that will generate acyl glucuronides that will be a problem from others that will not. Many drugs for which acyl glucuronides are quantitatively important metabolites in humans do not show toxicity associated with these metabolites (e.g., the nonsteroidal anti-inflammatory drug ibuprofen). But a few anti-inflammatory drugs, such as benoxaprofen and zomepirac, have been discontinued due to clinical toxicity for which reactive acyl glucuronides have been blamed as the underlying cause. To address the possibility that a new agent forms a reactive acyl glucuronide, an NMR-based approach has been disclosed in which the chemical kinetics of acyl glucuronide rearrangement are measured, which is reflection of its chemical reactivity [33].

For other drugs, bioactivation pathways catalyzed by enzymes other than cytochrome P450 may need to be considered, and the *in vitro* experiment adjusted to accommodate this. The initial judgment needs to be based on the structure of the new molecule that dictates the types of reactive metabolites that can arise. Drugs can be bioactivated by sulfotransferases (e.g., benzylic alcohols), acetyltransferases (e.g., aryl hydroxamic acids), myeloperoxidase (e.g., azaheterocyclics and phenols), cysteine conjugate β-lyase (e.g., alkyl halides), and acetyl coenzyme A transferase (e.g., carboxylic acids) [34–38]. As with the previously described assays designed to measure bioactivation, placing overall context to the findings generated in such specialized mechanistic studies can also be difficult.

10.4
Other Studies that can Show the Existence of Reactive Metabolites

Many standard drug metabolism studies can uncover the presence of reactive metabolites without specifically seeking this information out. These include *in vitro* metabolite identification studies, radiolabeled metabolism and excretion studies in animals and humans, whole-body autoradiography studies, and cytochrome P450 inhibition assays.

10.4.1
Metabolite Identification Studies

The identification of metabolites generated using *in vitro* systems is an activity that occurs at various stages throughout the drug discovery and development phases. The identification of sites of metabolism on a new molecule or chemical scaffold during early research can aid in predicting important routes of clearance in humans, drug design to reduce high rates of metabolic intrinsic clearance, and the identification of pharmacologically active metabolites. Reactive metabolites are generally not stable enough to be observed intact. However, during metabolite identification experiments, metabolites can be identified that can only arise via a reactive intermediate metabolite. A list of these is given in Table 10.2.

Table 10.2 Downstream metabolites that indicate the generation of a reactive intermediate.

Observed Metabolite	Precursor Structures	Possible Reactive Intermediate
Dihydrodiol	Alkene, arene	Epoxide
GSH adduct or mercapturic acid	Arene, alkene, aniline, phenol, thiophene, furan	Quinone, quinone methide, quinone imine, epoxide, thiophene-S-oxide, α,β-unsaturated carbonyl
2-, 3-, or 4-acyl glucuronide	Carboxylic acid	1-Acyl glucuronide
Acetic acid	Terminal acetylene	Ketene
Guaiacol	Arene, phenol, phenyl ether, methylenedioxy-phenyl	o-Quinone
Carboxylic acid	Amine, alcohol, ether, furan	Aldehyde, imine

If GSH is included in the *in vitro* incubations, then the presence of GSH adducts will indicate the presence of a reactive intermediate. Using spectroscopic tools (MS and NMR), the structure of the adduct can be elucidated and permit the proposal of the structure of the reactive intermediate. This information can be used in the design of alternate structures that cannot undergo the bioactivation reaction. The observation of dihydrodiols generated from arenes or alkenes indicates the formation of reactive epoxides. Observation of acetic acid metabolites from terminal alkynes indicates the presence of reactive ketenes. If a carboxylic acid is shown to be glucuronidated, the observation of rearranged glucuronides on the 2-, 3-, and 4-positions suggests that the acyl glucuronide is reactive.

10.4.2
Radiolabeled Metabolism and Excretion *In Vivo*

Radiolabeled excretion studies carried out in laboratory animals and humans are a standard part of drug development. The purpose of these studies is to provide an accounting of the total fate of drug-related material, and the use of drugs containing a radionuclide offers the best method whereby this accounting can occur. These data are used for several purposes:

1) to permit making quantitative comparisons of total circulating metabolite profiles in humans versus laboratory animal species used in safety assessments to assure that animals were exposed to the metabolites to which humans are exposed;
2) to define the time course of total excretion of drug-related material and the routes (i.e., urinary, fecal);
3) to define the clearance pathways for the new drug in humans, by reconstructing the total metabolism pathway tree (such knowledge can also be used to better understand sources of interpatient variability in pharmacokinetics and possibly drug response).

During these studies, the structures of metabolites are determined using spectroscopic and chemical techniques. The quantity of each metabolite in excreta is calculated, and the plasma exposure to each metabolite is estimated from the plasma radioactivity profile on HPLC. The metabolites observed in excreta could be indicative of the existence of a chemically reactive intermediate metabolite (Table 10.2). Thus, the drug metabolism scientist must be diligent in seeking out the presence of metabolites downstream of a reactive intermediate.

When processing plasma samples for metabolite profiling by HPLC–MS, plasma proteins must be removed prior to injection of the sample on HPLC. In most cases, adding miscible organic solvent, such as acetonitrile or methanol to plasma samples to precipitate the protein, does this. Prior to processing a plasma sample the total radioactivity present in that sample is determined as an important measurement used in the calculation of recovery of drug-related material through the extraction procedure to provide confidence that the subsequent radiometric HPLC data are adequately representative of the metabolite profile. In rare instances, the recovery of total drug-related radioactivity is low (e.g., <85%), which can be due to the covalent binding of drug-related material to plasma proteins. Such a finding can be of concern, as unrecoverable drug-related radioactivity that is present in the plasma protein can be indicative of covalent binding. It should be kept in mind that the actual plasma proteins to which the material is bound may not have anything to do with toxicity, but that the observation of covalently bound drug to plasma proteins indicates the existence of a reactive metabolite and may be a marker for other covalent binding occurring in tissues.

Finally, radiolabel studies are used to determine the total recovery of drug-related material in excreta along with a measurement of how long this takes. The overall mean mass balance obtained from an examination of radiolabel excretion data is determined. It is tempting to conclude that when mass balance is low (i.e., below 80% in humans), the drug-related material may be trapped in a tissue, very possibly by covalent incorporation into proteins. However, this is not necessarily the case and there is no association between low mass balance and covalent binding [39]. Low recovery can be due to a variety of technical challenges in collecting and measuring drug-related material in all excreta, and not due to covalent binding *in vivo*. Thus, mass balance data should not be used to conclude that a new compound may be undergoing bioactivation to a reactive intermediate.

10.4.3
Whole-Body Autoradiography and Tissue Binding

During the course of drug development, a tissue distribution study is done, usually in the rat. Quantitative whole-body autoradiography (qWBA) is currently the most commonly used modern method of determining tissue distribution of total drug-related material, while in the past such data were gathered by dissection of tissues from rats dosed with radiolabeled drug and radiometric analysis of the tissues. In qWBA studies, animals are administered a radioactive dose of test compound, they are sacrificed at various time points, the carcasses are frozen, thin slices of the whole bodies are prepared, and the radioactivity in the slices are quantitatively imaged on film. This yields a time course of total drug-related material in all tissues.

The long-term presence of drug-related material in a specific tissue(s) can serve as an alert to the possibility of covalently bound material arising from reactive metabolites. qWBA data have been described as delineating drugs known to cause toxicity via reactive metabolites from those that do not [40, 41]. The presence of unextractable drug-related material in the liver of the rat has been used, in conjunction with *in vitro* observations of metabolism-dependent covalent binding in a decision tree aimed to reduce the progression of compounds possessing bioactivation liabilities into clinical development [26]. The obvious shortcoming of the use of animal tissue retention is that the data may not be relevant to humans. Furthermore, as with *in vitro* covalent binding studies and ADME studies, these experiments require the synthesis of radiolabeled drug, with the isotope at a position not amenable to removal by metabolism. This requires considerable investment in each compound and is not readily amenable to use in early drug research when the study of large numbers of compounds is needed.

10.4.4
Inactivation of Cytochrome P450 Enzymes

In Chapter 3, the generation of reactive metabolites as it pertains to the inactivation of cytochrome P450 enzymes was discussed. In addition to the drug metabolism experiments described in Sections 10.4.1–10.4.3, detection of the time-dependent inhibition (TDI) of P450 enzymes can be indicative of the formation of reactive metabolites. The primary objective of such experiments is to address the possibility of drug–drug interactions, but one must be aware that TDI can be a harbinger of a reactive metabolite. If inactivation is due to formation of a protein or heme adduct, it is possible that the reactive metabolite that inactivates the P450 enzyme is also capable of diffusing from the enzyme active site and covalently binding to other proteins. For example, tienilic acid and its regioisomer wherein the thiophene is substituted on the 3-position demonstrate an interesting behavior in this regard [42]. The thiophene ring is bioactivated to a reactive S-oxide (or possibly an epoxide). For tienilic acid, the reactive metabolite binds to cytochrome P4502C9 that generates it, causing inactivation. For the regioisomer, the reactive intermediate is capable of diffusing from the enzyme and reacting with other proteins present in liver microsomes. The demonstration of P450 TDI is not proof of the generation of a reactive metabolite, but it can serve as a trigger point for further investigation of bioactivation potential.

10.5
Conclusion

In drug discovery/development, considerable effort has been made to develop methods whereby those compounds that have an ability to be metabolized to reactive intermediates can be identified and better characterized for potential risk. These various assays were described in this chapter, along with descriptions of how other data that are routinely gathered for other reasons can be used in gaining insight into reactive metabolites. While these assays can accomplish their objectives from a technical standpoint, the interpretation of the data for each individual compound in decision making remains a challenge [30]. Nucleophile trapping and covalent binding assays are used as methods to reduce the number of drug candidates that show toxicity later in clinical development, by removing compounds that can be metabolized to reactive entities from the development process. However, these assays must be interpreted in concert with other considerations in order to be successfully employed in drug research.

References

1 Richard, A.M. (1998) Structure-based methods for predicting mutagenicity and carcinogenicity: are we there yet? *Mutation Research*, **400**, 493–507.

2 Kalgutkar, A.S., Gardner, I., Obach, R.S., Shaffer, C.L., Callegari, E., Henne, K.R., Mutlib, A.E., Dalvie, D.K., Lee, J.S., Nakai, Y., O'Donnell, J.P., Boer, J., and Harriman, S.P. (2005) A comprehensive listing of bioactivation pathways of organic functional groups. *Current Drug Metabolism*, **6** (3), 161–225.

3 Kalgutkar, A.S. and Soglia, J.R. (2005) Minimising the potential for metabolic activation in drug discovery. *Expert Opinion in Drug Metabolism and Toxicology*, **1** (1), 91–142.

4 Zhao, S.X., Dalvie, D.K., Kelly, J.M., Soglia, J.R., Frederick, K.S., Smith, E.B., Obach, R.S., and Kalgutkar, A.S. (2007) NADPH-dependent covalent binding of [3H]paroxetine to human liver microsomes and S-9 fractions: identification of an electrophilic quinone metabolite of paroxetine. *Chemical Research in Toxicology*, **20** (11), 1649–1657.

5 Chen, W.G., Zhang, C., Avery, M.J., and Fouda, H.G. (2001) Reactive metabolite screen for reducing candidate attrition in drug discovery. *Advances in Experimental Medicine and Biology*, **500**, 521–524.

6 Samuel, K., Yin, W., Stearns, R.A., Tang, Y.S., Chaudhary, A.G., Jewell, J.P., Lanza, T., Lin, L.S., Hagmann, W.K., Evans, D.C., and Kumar, S. (2003) Addressing the metabolic activation potential of new leads in drug discovery: a case study using ion trap mass spectrometry and tritium labeling techniques. *Journal of Mass Spectrometry*, **38** (2), 211–221.

7 Soglia, J.R., Harriman, S.P., Zhao, S., Barberia, J., Cole, M.J., Boyd, J.G., and Contillo, L.G. (2004) The development of a higher throughput reactive intermediate screening assay incorporating micro-bore liquid chromatography–micro-electrospray ionization–tandem mass spectrometry and glutathione ethyl ester as an in vitro conjugating agent. *Journal of Pharmaceutical and Biomedical Analysis*, **36** (1), 105–116.

8 Dieckhaus, C.M., Fernandez-Metzler, C.L., King, R., Krolikowski, P.H., and Baillie, T.A. (2005) Negative ion tandem mass spectrometry for the detection of glutathione conjugates. *Chemical Research in Toxicology*, **18** (4), 630–638.

9 Yan, Z. and Caldwell, G.W. (2004) Stable-isotope trapping and high-throughput screenings of reactive metabolites using the isotope MS signature. *Analytical Chemistry*, **76** (23), 6835–6847.

10 Daniels, S., Espina, R., Kao, K., Yuan, H., Lin, J., Diamond, S., Johnson, B., Rodgers, J., Prakash, S., Unger, S., Christ, D., Miwa, G., Gan, L.S., and Mutlib, A.E. (2008) Application of stable isotope-labeled compounds in metabolism and in metabolism-mediated toxicity studies. *Chemical Research in Toxicology*, **21** (9), 1672–1689.

11 Castro-Perez, J., Plumb, R., Liang, L., and Yang, E. (2005) A high-throughput liquid chromatography/tandem mass spectrometry method for screening glutathione conjugates using exact mass neutral loss acquisition. *Rapid Communications in Mass Spectrometry*, **19** (6), 798–804.

12 Rousu, T., Pelkonen, O., and Tolonen, A. (2009) Rapid detection and characterization of reactive drug metabolites in vitro using several isotope-labeled trapping agents and ultra-performance liquid chromatography/time-of-flight mass spectrometry. *Rapid Communications in Mass Spectrometry*, **23** (6), 843–855.

13 Wen, B. and Fitch, W.L. (2009) Screening and characterization of reactive metabolites using glutathione ethyl ester in combination with Q-trap mass spectrometry. *Journal of Mass Spectrometry*, **44** (1), 90–100.

14 Mitchell, M.D., Elrick, M.M., Walgren, J.L., Mueller, R.A., Morris, D.L., and Thompson, D.C. (2008) Peptide-based in vitro assay for the detection of reactive metabolites. *Chemical Research in Toxicology*, **21** (4), 859–868.

15 Ma, S. and Zhu, M. (2009) Recent advances in applications of liquid

chromatography–tandem mass spectrometry to the analysis of reactive drug metabolites. *Chemico-Biological Interactions*, **179** (1), 25–37.

16 Argoti, D., Liang, L., Conteh, A., Chen, L., Bershas, D., Yu, C.P., Vouros, P., and Yang, E. (2005) Cyanide trapping of iminium ion reactive intermediates followed by detection and structure identification using liquid chromatography–tandem mass spectrometry (LC–MS/MS). *Chemical Research in Toxicology*, **18** (10), 1537–1544.

17 O'Donnell, J.P., Dalvie, D.K., Kalgutkar, A.S., and Obach, R.S. (2003) Mechanism-based inactivation of human recombinant P4502C9 by the nonsteroidal anti-inflammatory drug suprofen. *Drug Metabolism and Disposition*, **31** (11), 1369–1377.

18 Soglia, J.R., Contillo, L.G., Kalgutkar, A.S., Zhao, S., Hop, C.E.C.A., Boyd, J.G., and Cole, M.J. (2006) A semiquantitative method for the determination of reactive metabolite conjugate levels in vitro utilizing liquid chromatography–tandem mass spectrometry and novel quaternary ammonium glutathione analogs. *Chemical Research in Toxicology*, **19** (3), 480–490.

19 Gan, J., Harper, T.W., Hsueh, M.M., Qu, Q., and Humphreys, W.G. (2005) Dansyl glutathione as a trapping agent for the quantitative estimation and identification of reactive metabolites. *Chemical Research in Toxicology*, **18** (5), 896–903.

20 Gan, J., Ruan, Q., He, B., Zhu, M., Shyu, W.C., and Humphreys, G.W. (2009) In vitro screening of 50 highly prescribed drugs for thiol adduct formation – comparison of potential for drug-induced toxicity and extent of adduct formation. *Chemical Research in Toxicology*, **22** (4), 690–698.

21 Takakusa, H., Masumoto, H., Makino, C., Okazaki, O., and Sudo, K. (2009) Quantitative assessment of reactive metabolite formation using 35S-labeled glutathione. *Drug Metabolism and Pharmacokinetics*, **24** (1), 100–107.

22 Gorrod, J.W., Whittlesea, C.M.C., and Lam, S.P. (1991) Trapping of reactive intermediates by incorporation of 14C-sodium cyanide during microsomal

oxidation. *Advances in Experimental Medicine and Biology*, **283**, 657–664.

23 Meneses-Lorente, G., Sakatis, M.Z., Schulz-Utermoehl, T., De Nardi, C., and Watt, A.P. (2006) A quantitative high-throughput trapping assay as a measurement of potential for bioactivation. *Analytical Biochemistry*, **351** (2), 266–272.

24 Inoue, K., Shibata, Y., Takahashi, H., Ohe, T., Chiba, M., and Ishii, Y. (2009) A trapping method for semi-quantitative assessment of reactive metabolite formation using [35S]cysteine and [14C] cyanide. *Drug Metabolism and Pharmacokinetics*, **24** (3), 245–254.

25 Miura, M., Hori, W., Kasahara, Y., and Nakagawa, I. (2010) Quantitative assessment of the metabolic activation of alicyclic amines via aldehyde. *Journal of Pharmacological and Toxicological Methods*, **61** (1), 44–51.

26 Evans, D.C., Watt, A.P., Nicoll-Griffith, D.A., and Baillie, T.A. (2004) Drug–protein adducts: an industry perspective on minimizing the potential for drug bioactivation in drug discovery and development. *Chemical Research in Toxicology*, **17** (1), 3–16.

27 Obach, R.S., Kalgutkar, A.S., Soglia, J.R., and Zhao, S.X. (2008) Can in vitro metabolism-dependent covalent binding data in liver microsomes distinguish hepatotoxic from nonhepatotoxic drugs? An analysis of 18 drugs with consideration of intrinsic clearance and daily dose. *Chemical Research in Toxicology*, **21** (9), 1814–1822.

28 Bauman, J.N., Kelly, J.M., Tripathy, S., Zhao, S.X., Lam, W.W., Kalgutkar, A.S., and Obach, R.S. (2009) Can in vitro metabolism-dependent covalent binding data distinguish hepatotoxic from nonhepatotoxic drugs? An analysis using human hepatocytes and liver S-9 fraction. *Chemical Research in Toxicology*, **22** (2), 332–340.

29 Nakayama, S., Atsumi, R., Takakusa, H., Kobayashi, Y., Kurihara, A., Nagai, Y., Nakai, D., and Okazaki, O. (2009) A zone classification system for risk assessment of idiosyncratic drug toxicity using daily dose and covalent binding.

Drug Metabolism and Disposition, **37** (9), 1970–1977.

30 Park, B.K., Boobis, A., Clarke, S., Goldring, C.E., Jones, D., Kenna, J.G., Lambert, C., Laverty, H.G., Naisbitt, D.J., Nelson, S., Nicoll-Griffith, D.A., Obach, R.S., Routledge, P., Smith, D.A., Tweedle, D.J., Vermeulen, N., Williams, D.P., Wilson, I.D., and Baillie, T.A. (2011) Managing the challenge of chemically reactive metabolites in drug development. *Nature Reviews in Drug Discovery*, **10** (4), 292–306.

31 Stachulski, A.V. (2007) The chemistry and biological activity of acyl glucuronides. *Current Opinion in Drug Discovery and Development*, **10** (1), 58–66.

32 Shipkova, M., Armstrong, V.W., Oellerich, M., and Wieland, E. (2003) Acyl glucuronide drug metabolites: toxicological and analytical implications. *Therapeutic Drug Monitoring*, **25** (1), 1–16.

33 Walker, G.S., Atherton, J., Bauman, J., Kohl, C., Lam, W., Reily, M., Lou, Z., and Mutlib, A. (2007) Determination of degradation pathways and kinetics of acyl glucuronides by NMR spectroscopy. *Chemical Research in Toxicology*, **20** (6), 876–886.

34 Glatt, H. (1997) Bioactivation of mutagens via sulfation. *FASEB Journal*, **11** (5), 314–321.

35 Yeh, H.M. and Hanna, P.E. (1982) Arylhydroxamic acid bioactivation via acyl group transfer. Structural requirements for transacylating and electrophile-generating activity of N-(2-fluorenyl) hydroxamic acids and related compounds. *Journal of Medicinal Chemistry*, **25** (7), 842–846.

36 Tafazoli, S. and O'Brien, P.J. (2005) Peroxidases: a role in the metabolism and side effects of drugs. *Drug Discovery Today*, **10** (9), 617–625.

37 Anders, M.W. (2004) Glutathione-dependent bioactivation of haloalkanes and haloalkenes. *Drug Metabolism Reviews*, **36** (3–4), 583–594.

38 Skonberg, C., Olsen, J., Madsen, K.G., Hansen, S.H., and Grillo, M.P. (2008) Metabolic activation of carboxylic acids. *Expert Opinion in Drug Metabolism and Toxicology*, **4** (4), 425–438.

39 Roffey, S.J., Obach, R.S., Gedge, J.I., and Smith, D.A. (2007) What is the objective of the mass balance study? A retrospective analysis of data in animal and human excretion studies employing radiolabeled drugs. *Drug Metabolism Reviews*, **39** (1), 17–43.

40 Takakusa, H., Masumoto, H., Yukinaga, H., Makino, C., Nakayama, S., Okazaki, O., and Sudo, K. (2008) Covalent binding and tissue distribution/retention assessment of drugs associated with idiosyncratic drug toxicity. *Drug Metabolism and Disposition*, **36** (9), 1770–1779.

41 Masubuchi, N., Makino, C., and Murayama, N. (2007) Prediction of in vivo potential for metabolic activation of drugs into chemically reactive intermediate: correlation of in vitro and in vivo generation of reactive intermediates and in vitro glutathione conjugate formation in rats and humans. *Chemical Research in Toxicology*, **20** (3), 455–464.

42 Bonierbale, E., Valadon, P., Pons, C., Desfosses, B., Dansette, P.M., and Mansuy, D. (1999) Opposite behaviors of reactive metabolites of tienilic acid and its isomer toward liver proteins: use of specific anti-tienilic acid–protein adduct antibodies and the possible relationship with different hepatotoxic effects of the two compounds. *Chemical Research in Toxicology*, **12** (3), 286–296.

11
Case Studies on Eliminating/Reducing Reactive Metabolite Formation in Drug Discovery

Abbreviations

AKT	Protein kinase B
CL_p	Plasma clearance
c-Met	Mesenchymal–epithelial transition factor
COX-2	Cyclooxygenase-2
CRF_1	Corticotropin-releasing factor-1
CYP	Cytochrome P450
F	Oral bioavailability
FMS	A type III receptor tyrosine kinase
GSH	Glutathione
HLM	Human liver microsomes
IADRs	Idiosyncratic adverse drug reactions
PYK2	Proline-rich tyrosine kinase 2
$T_{1/2}$	Half-life
Tpo	Thrombopoietin
V_{dss}	Steady-state distribution volume

11.1
Medicinal Chemistry Tactics to Eliminate Reactive Metabolite Formation

Considering that a detailed understanding of the biochemical mechanisms of idiosyncratic adverse drug reactions (IADRs) remains poorly understood, it is currently impossible to accurately predict which new drugs will be associated with a significant incidence of IADRs and this poses a significant challenge in drug discovery/development. Because it is now widely appreciated that reactive metabolites, as opposed to the parent molecules from which they are derived, are responsible for the pathogenesis of immune-mediated IADRs, most pharmaceutical companies have implemented procedures to evaluate reactive metabolite formation potential of new chemical entities with the goal of eliminating or minimizing the liability by rational structural modification of the lead chemical series.

Reactive Drug Metabolites, First Edition. Amit S. Kalgutkar, Deepak Dalvie, R. Scott Obach, and Dennis A. Smith.
© 2012 Wiley-VCH Verlag GmbH & Co. KGaA. Published 2012 by Wiley-VCH Verlag GmbH & Co. KGaA.

Qualitative assessment of *in vitro* cytochrome P450 (CYP)–catalyzed reactive metabolite formation involves trapping studies conducted in NADPH-supplemented human liver microsomes (HLM) in the presence of exogenously added nucleophiles such as reduced glutathione (GSH), amines (e.g., semicarbazide and methoxylamine), or potassium cyanide. Liver microsomes can be replaced by alternate metabolism vectors (e.g., liver cytosol, liver S9 fractions, hepatocytes, neutrophils, etc.), to evaluate the participation of non-CYP enzymes in reactive metabolite formation. In case of reactive metabolite positives, characterization of the adduct structure provides insight into the reactive metabolite structure and the mechanism for its formation. The information is then used, as appropriate, to modify the structure of the reactive metabolite positives in order to eliminate the liability. In practice, however, this exercise is not trivial; medicinal chemistry tactics to eliminate reactive metabolite formation could confer a detrimental effect on primary pharmacology (e.g., changes in agonist/antagonist behavior, subtype selectivity for target receptor or enzyme) and/or pharmacokinetic attributes. Thus, chemical intervention strategies to abolish reactive metabolite formation are often an iterative process, the success of which is heavily dependent on a close working relationship between medicinal chemists, pharmacologists, and biotransformation scientists. Successful case studies involving metabolism-guided design to circumvent reactive metabolite formation in drug discovery are plentiful in the literature. Noteworthy examples are highlighted below.

11.2
Eliminating Reactive Metabolite Formation on Heterocyclic Ring Systems

11.2.1
Mechanism(s) of Thiazole Ring Bioactivation and Rational Chemistry Approaches to Abolish Reactive Metabolite Formation

In an effort to identify novel thrombopoietin (Tpo) receptor mimics for the potential treatment of thrombocytopenia, a series of piperidine-4-carboxylic acids exemplified by compound **1** (Figure 11.1) were disclosed as selective, nonpeptidyl agonists of the Tpo receptor [1]. From a bioactivation perspective, the presence of the 2-carboxamidothiazole motif in **1** raised significant concern because of the potential for thiazole ring opening via the C4–C5 epoxidation → diol pathway, yielding acylthiourea and glyoxal metabolites **2** and **3**, respectively (Figure 11.1), in a manner similar to that discerned for the hepatotoxic nonsteroidal anti-inflammatory drug sudoxicam [2]. Once formed, thioureas can undergo *S*-oxidation to electrophilic sulfenic acid intermediates capable of oxidizing and/or forming adducts with proteins resulting in toxicological consequences [3, 4]. Preclinical safety studies with **1** also appeared to support the potential for reactive metabolite formation. When rats were subjected to single oral doses of **1** (50–500 mg/kg), dramatic increases in liver enzymes (e.g., AST and ALT) were observed at all dose levels [5]. Additionally, when **1** was dosed orally at 100 mg/kg in transgenic mice

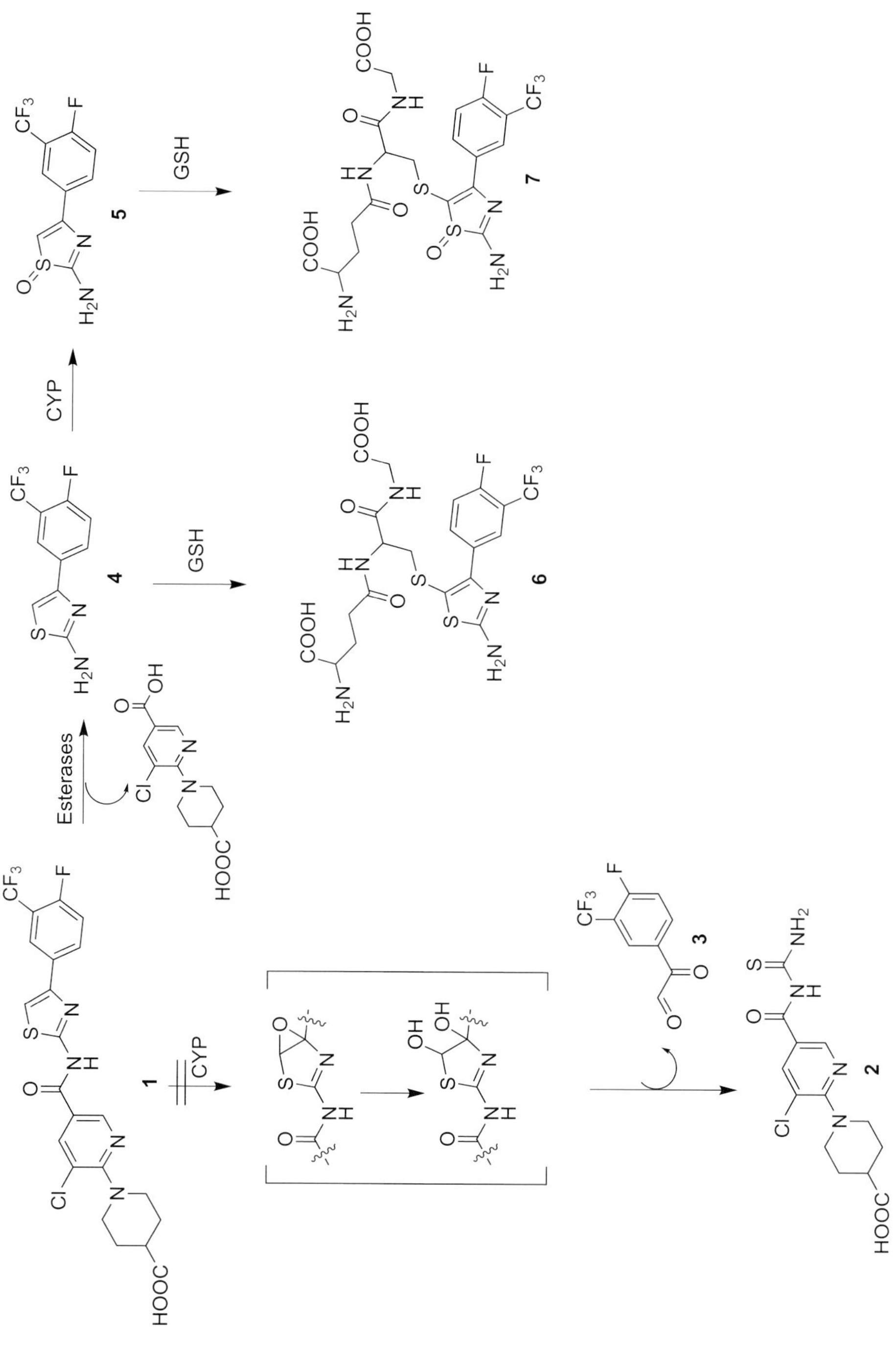

Figure 11.1 Bioactivation of the nonpeptidyl 2-aminothiazole-based Tpo receptor agonist **1**.

expressing the human Tpo receptor, mild elevations in AST were observed, although ALT levels were unchanged [5]. These and other safety evaluations indicated that **1** did not have a safety profile that was commensurate with further development.

Although the thiazole moiety in **1** did not undergo enzyme-catalyzed ring opening to afford reactive acylthiourea and/or glyoxal intermediates, the corresponding 4-(4-fluoro-3-(trifluoromethyl)phenyl)thiazol-2-amine (**4**), a product of carboxylesterase-mediated hydrolysis of **1** in human hepatic tissue and plasma, underwent oxidative bioactivation in HLM (Figure 11.1). Trapping studies with GSH led to the formation of two conjugates **6** and **7**; the molecular weights of **6** and **7** were consistent with the nucleophilic addition of GSH to **4** and a thiazole-*S*-oxide metabolite of **4** (i.e., compound **5**), respectively. Mass spectral fragmentation and ^{1}H NMR analysis indicated that the site of attachment of the glutathionyl moiety in both conjugates was the C5 position in the thiazole ring.

Based on the structures of **6** and **7**, two mechanisms were proposed for reactive metabolite formation with **4**: one involving β-elimination of an initially formed hydroxylamine metabolite (Figure 11.2, *pathway a*) and the other involving a two-electron oxidation of the electron-rich 2-aminothiazole system (Figure 11.2, *pathway b*). The mechanistic insights gained from the metabolism studies influenced subsequent medicinal chemistry strategies, which involved blocking the C5 position with a fluorine atom (compound **8**) or replacing the thiazole ring with a 1,2,4-thiadiazole group (compound **9**) (Figure 11.3). These structural changes not only abrogated the bioactivation liability associated with **1** but also resulted in compound **8** that retained the attractive pharmacological and rat pharmacokinetic attributes (plasma clearance (CL_p), steady-state distribution volume (V_{dss}), half-life ($T_{1/2}$), and oral bioavailability (*F*)) of the prototype agent (Table 11.1) [1]. This differentiation was further manifested in lowered hepatic effects *in vivo* studies with **8** [5]. In contrast with **1**, no changes in either AST or ALT were observed at an oral dose of 50 mg/kg, despite significantly higher systemic exposures of **8**.

The second illustration involves 2-aminothiazole-based protein kinase B (AKT) inhibitors for the potential treatment of cancer [6]. Upon incubation in NADPH-supplemented HLM, 2-aminothiazole **10** underwent substantial CYP-catalyzed bioactivation, a phenomenon that was associated with significant covalent binding to microsomal proteins [6]. On addition of GSH, covalent binding was dramatically reduced and multiple GSH adducts were formed (Figure 11.4). Elucidation of the GSH adduct structure by mass spectrometry and NMR studies provided insights into the bioactivation mechanism (Figure 11.4). All of the metabolites were derived from a common epoxide intermediate **11**, the rate-limiting formation of which is mediated by a CYP-catalyzed epoxidation of the C4–C5 thiazole double bond in **10**. The formation of GSH conjugate **13** can be rationalized from a nucleophilic addition of a GSH molecule on the epoxide ring to form **12** followed by spontaneous dehydration. Alternately, hydrolysis of **11** would lead to the dihydrodiol metabolite **19**, which could then undergo a ring scission to form the glyoxal (**20**) and thiourea (**21**) metabolites. The thiourea **21** is then proposed to cyclize to **22** (characterized as a stable metabolite of **10**) with the accompanying loss of hydrogen sulfide.

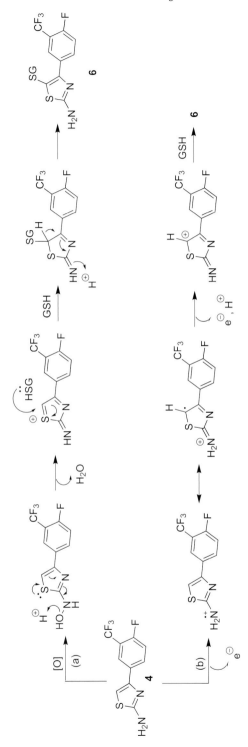

Figure 11.2 Proposed mechanism of bioactivation of the 2-amino-4-arylthiazole metabolite **4**.

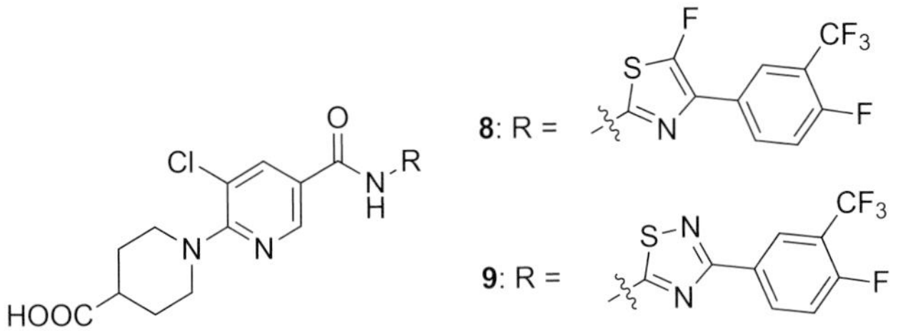

Figure 11.3 Identification of 2-aminothiazole-based Tpo agonists **8** and **9** that are devoid of bioactivation liability.

The formation of the rearranged GSH conjugates **17** and **18** was proposed to occur through the disubstituted thiourea intermediate **14** that can be generated via a ring scission in **12**. Spontaneous cyclization in **14** with the net loss of hydrogen sulfide would lead to the 2-imidazoline intermediate **15**. Nucleophilic attack of an electron lone pair from either secondary amine nitrogen in **16** (the tautomer of intermediate **15**) followed by dehydration would lead to the isobaric GSH conjugates **17** and **18**, respectively.

Apart from the obvious replacement of the thiazole ring in **10** with a thiadiazole motif (compounds **19** and **20**) (Figure 11.5) to eliminate reactive metabolite formation, additional medicinal chemistry efforts were initiated on the synthesis of analogues that would reduce the reactivity of the thiazole ring and destabilize the rate-limiting step involving epoxide formation [6]. Because the oxindole functional group (R^1) in **10** (see Figure 11.5) was directly conjugated with the central thiazole ring through a biaryl bond, modulation of the electronic character of the R^1 substituent was expected to directly influence the electronics of the azole ring and the reactivity at the C4–C5 double bond that was proposed to undergo epoxidation. Indeed, a key finding in the iterative chemistry efforts was that substitution of the R^1 position in **10** (Figure 11.5) with electron-withdrawing fluorine atoms, as well as by electron-deficient aromatics, decreased the electron richness of the biaryl system, thereby diminishing the extent of thiazole ring epoxidation. When electron richness was decreased sufficiently, GSH adduct formation was eliminated (e.g., compounds **21** and **22** in Figure 11.5). A computational model was also developed based on the proposed mechanism and was employed with some degree of success to a priori predict thiazole ring epoxidation with varying R^1 substituents. 2-Amino-thiadiazole **20** and 2-amino-thiazole **22**, which retained AKT potency and selectivity, were also active in *in vivo* animal models of cancer [7, 8].

Table 11.1 *In vitro* Tpo agonist activity and rat pharmacokinetics of 2-aminothiazoles **1**, **8**, and **9**.

Compound	Tpo EC$_{50}$ (µM)	CL$_p$ (ml/min/kg))	V_{dss} (l/kg)	$T_{1/2}$ (h)	Oral F (%)
1	0.087	6.89	0.83	1.34	66.8
8	0.088	2.79	0.34	1.67	73.0
9	0.500	1.49	0.22	1.09	73.5

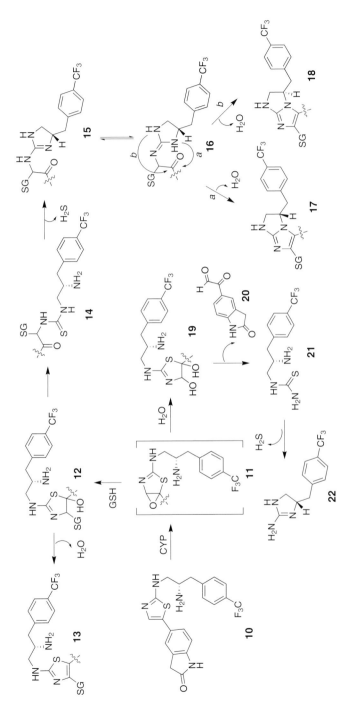

Figure 11.4 Proposed mechanism of bioactivation for the AKT inhibitor **10** in NADPH-supplemented HLM.

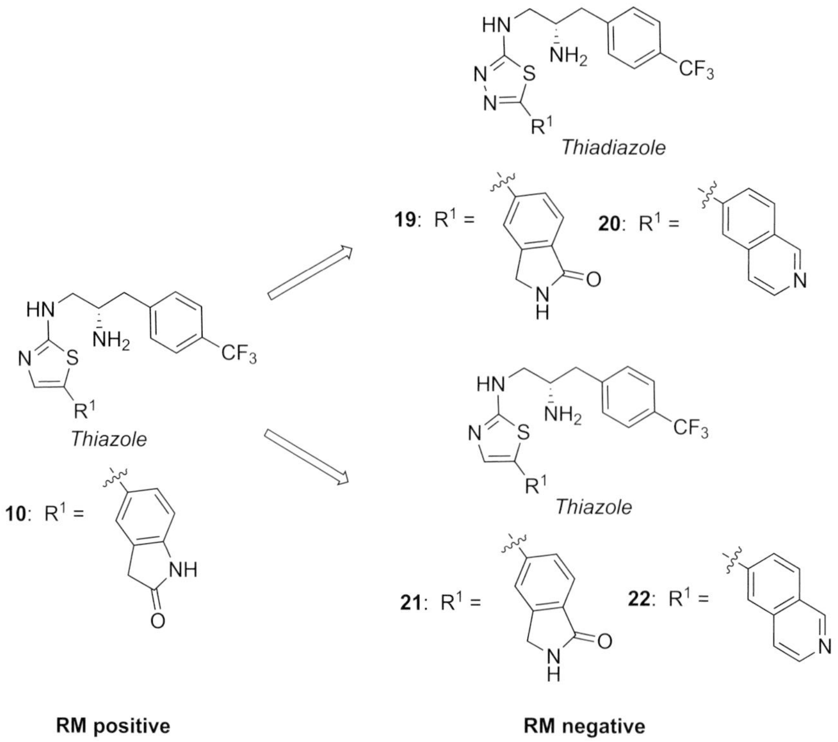

Figure 11.5 Medicinal chemistry strategies to eliminate bioactivation liability of thiazole-based AKT inhibitor **10**.

Yet another illustration of innovative chemistry strategies to mitigate reactive metabolite formation on the thiazole ring system is evident in selective cyclooxygenase-2 (COX-2) inhibitor field. Throughout the last decade, optimization of the selective COX-2 inhibitory attributes of the diarylheterocyclic class of compounds has been actively pursued as a strategy to develop the next generation of nonulcerogenic anti-inflammatory agents [9, 10]. The introduction of diarylheterocycles such as celecoxib, rofecoxib, and valdecoxib as the next generation of nonulcerogenic nonsteroidal anti-inflammatory agents is testimony to the overall efforts [11–13]. The common structural motif in the diarylheterocycle class of COX-2-selective inhibitors is a *cis*-stilbene moiety substituted in one of the pendant phenyl rings with a 4-methylsulfone or sulfonamide substituent [14]. The ring system that is fused to the stilbene framework has been extensively manipulated to include every imaginable heterocyclic and carbocyclic skeleton of varying ring sizes [14]. In one such account, a series of diarylheterocycles, wherein the central ring consisted of an imidazo[2.1-b]thiazole bicyclic system, were reported as potent, and selective COX-2 inhibitors [15]. In the course of metabolism studies, the sulfur atom within the thiazole ring in the lead compound **23** was shown to undergo CYP-mediated oxidation to an electrophilic thiazolo-*S*-oxide metabolite **24**, which

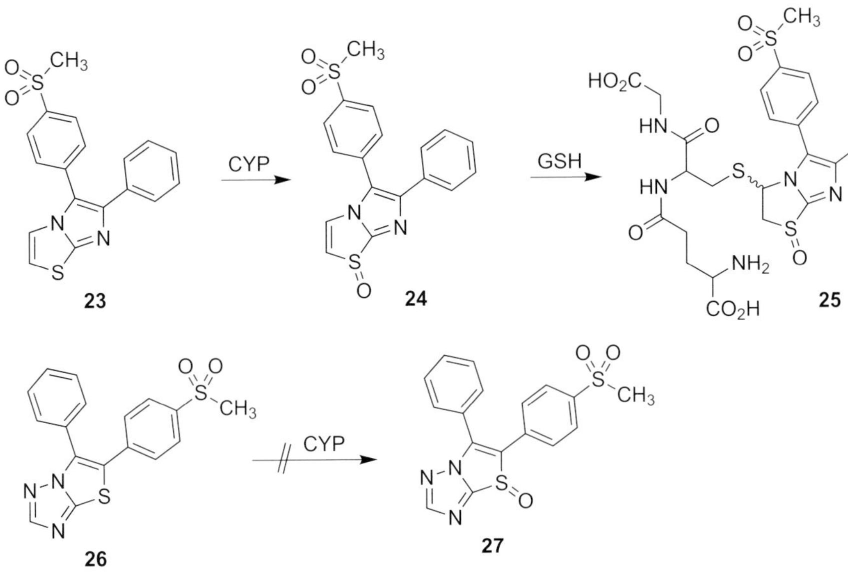

Figure 11.6 Circumventing reactive metabolite formation in the diarylimidazolothiazole derivative **23** through steric hindrance.

was trapped with GSH to yield conjugate **25** (Figure 11.6) [16]. In an elegant medicinal chemistry tactic, the imidazolothiazole motif in **23** was changed to the corresponding fused thiazolotriazole ring system (exemplified with compound **26**). S-Oxidation to **27** was prevented, presumably due to the steric hindrance by the pendant phenyl rings on the thiazole group (see Figure 11.6) [17].

11.2.2
Mechanism(s) of Isothiazole Ring Bioactivation and Rational Chemistry Approaches to Abolish Reactive Metabolite Formation

An account of isothiazole ring bioactivation was disclosed with small molecule inhibitors of mesenchymal–epithelial transition factor (c-Met), a receptor tyrosine kinase that is often deregulated in cancer [18]. In addition to potent c-Met inhibition, the lead compound (isothiazole analogue **27**, Figure 11.7) also displayed attractive pharmacokinetic properties in animals [19]. However, **27** also exhibited very high *in vitro* NADPH-dependent covalent binding to microsomal proteins from animals and humans. The observation that protein covalent binding was significantly reduced in the presence of exogenously added GSH was suggestive of a CYP-catalyzed bioactivation process to reactive metabolite(s) [19]. *In vitro* studies in liver microsomes revealed the formation of a single GSH conjugate, structural details for which were obtained by mass spectrometry and NMR analysis. Spectral data indicated that the GSH conjugate **30** was obtained by the addition of one molecule of GSH on the C4 position on the isothiazole ring in **27** (Figure 11.7). A plausible mechanism for the formation of **30** from **27** is depicted in Figure 11.7 and

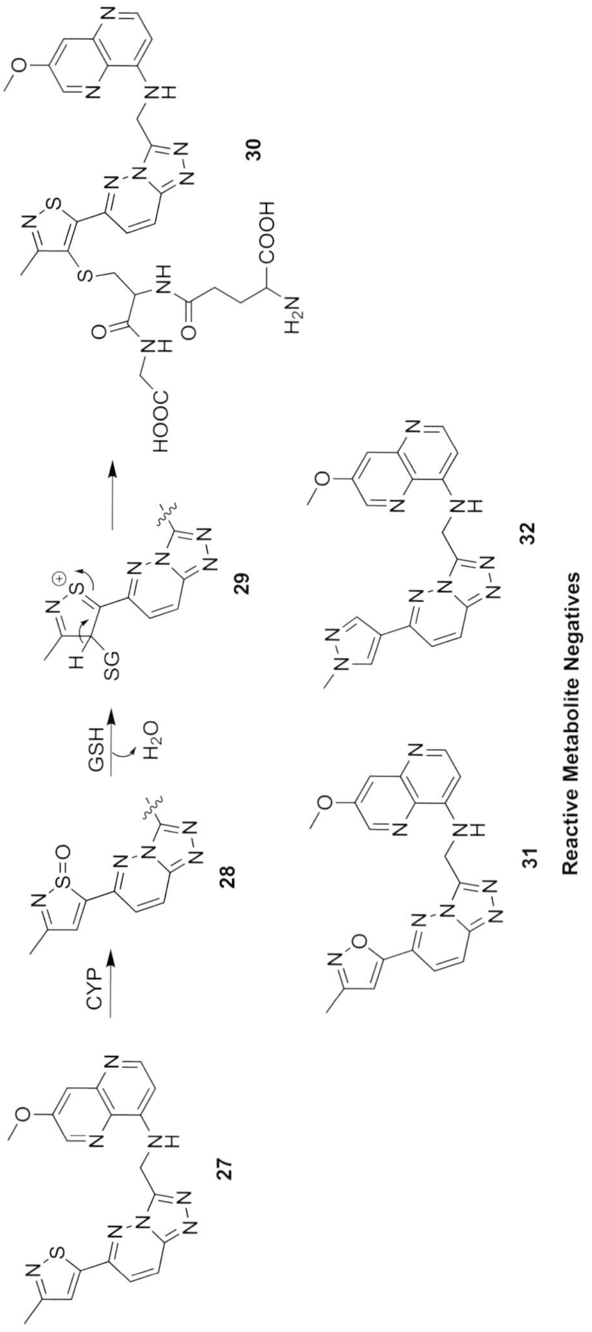

Figure 11.7 Proposed mechanism of CYP-mediated isothiazole ring bioactivation in the c-Met inhibitor **27**.

Table 11.2 *In vitro* c-Met inhibitory potency and rat pharmacokinetics of compounds **27**, **31**, and **32**.

Compound	c-Met IC$_{50}$ (μM)	CL$_p$ (ml/min/kg))	V_{dss} (l/kg)	$T_{1/2}$ (h)	Oral F (%)
27	0.003	3.33	0.2	1.8	42
31	0.015	6.66	0.4	1.5	58
32	0.003	5.00	0.3	1.0	38

involves an initial oxidation of the isothiazole sulfur to the *S*-oxide metabolite **28**. Michael addition of GSH at the C4 position with subsequent loss of water yields the final product **30**.

Iterative structural changes were needed to eliminate the bioactivation liability with the isothiazole class of compounds while maintaining c-Met inhibitory potency and desired pharmacokinetics. Blocking the reactive site often resulted in loss of potency. Therefore, the strategy shifted to substituting the isothiazole with bioisosteric heterocycles, resulting in the isoxazole and pyrazole analogues **31** and **32**, respectively. Both compounds displayed high c-Met potency and desirable pharmacokinetics in rats (Table 11.2). Importantly, compounds **31** and **32** did not produce GSH conjugates when incubated in NADPH- and GSH-supplemented HLM. As such, the lack of GSH conjugation with **31** or **32** can be considered as additional evidence for isothiazole bioactivation via the *S*-oxidation route.

11.3
Medicinal Chemistry Strategies to Mitigate Bioactivation of Electron-Rich Aromatic Rings

Strategies toward eliminating bioactivation of the electron-rich 4-hydroxyaniline motif have been described in detail by Park and coworkers on the antimalarial agent amodiaquine (**33**) (Figure 11.8) [20–25]. The clinical use of amodiaquine is somewhat restricted by several cases of hepatotoxicity and agranulocytosis; the detection of IgG antibodies in patients exposed to the drug is consistent with an immune-mediated hypersensitivity reaction [26, 27]. The immune-mediated toxicity is believed to arise from the metabolism of amodiaquine to a reactive quinone imine species **34** that can covalently bind to cellular proteins or GSH (Figure 11.8). Exchanging the *C'*-4-phenolic OH group with a fluorine results in compound **35** that does not undergo the obligatory two-electron oxidation process to the electrophilic quinone imine species (see Figure 11.8) [22, 23]. An alternate approach to prevent reactive metabolite formation involved the isomerization of the 3' and 4' substituents in amodiaquine; from this exercise emerged analogues **36** and **37** (see Figure 11.8), which are not susceptible to reactive metabolite formation (judged from the lack of formation of GSH conjugates) [24, 25]. Following antimalarial assessment, studies on mechanism of action, and *in vitro* and *in vivo* toxicological assessment, compound **37** was subsequently identified as a candidate for further

Amodiaquine (33) 34 35 36 37

Figure 11.8 Rational design of analogues of the antimalarial agent amodiaquine based on reactive metabolite characterization data.

development studies based on potent activity versus chloroquine-sensitive and -resistant parasites, moderate to excellent *F*, low toxicity in *in vitro* studies, and an acceptable safety profile [25, 28, 29].

In yet another account, the potent and selective inhibition of proline-rich tyrosine kinase 2 (PYK2) by 5-aminooxindoles (e.g., compound **38**) was offset by the finding that the aminooxindole motif was oxidized by CYP3A4 enzyme in HLM to the electrophilic bis-imine species **39** that was trapped with GSH to yield adduct **40** (Figure 11.9) [30]. Reactive metabolite formation was also associated with the mechanism-based inactivation of CYP3A4 activity. Efforts were therefore invested in eliminating the reactive metabolite (and plausible drug–drug interaction and idiosyncratic toxicity) liabilities associated with **38** while retaining or improving PYK2 potency and HLM stability. The cocrystal structure of **38** bound to the ATP-binding pocket of PYK2 suggested that subtle alterations to the lactam ring (in the aminooxindole scaffold) would not adversely affect PYK2 activity. Furthermore, given the propensity of electron-rich aryl rings to undergo CYP-catalyzed reactive metabolite formation, a special emphasis was placed on introducing electron-deficient aniline ring substituents. Several compounds (e.g., **41–44**, Figure 11.9) that resulted from this effort were devoid of reactive metabolite formation, while exhibiting selective PYK2 inhibition and HLM stability similar or superior to their corresponding 5-aminooxindole counterparts [30, 31].

A situation similar to the PYK2 inhibitor case study was encountered with a series of 1,2,4-phenylenetriamine-based FMS (a type III receptor tyrosine kinase) inhibitors [32]. Despite the excellent potency and *in vivo* efficacy of this series, the 1,2,4-phenylenetriamine core in lead compound **45** was considered a liability given its propensity to undergo two-electron oxidation to reactive quinone diimine species with (compound **46**) or without (compound **47**) cleavage of the amide bond (Figure 11.10). In this and other examples, the electrophilic quinones were amenable to trapping with GSH to furnish the corresponding conjugates (e.g., compounds **48** and **49** resulting from GSH adduction to **46** and **47**, respectively) [32].

In the light of these results, lead optimization efforts were directed toward the replacement of the nitrogen substituents at the C2 and C4 positions with carbon substituents in order to eliminate reactive metabolite formation [32]. Structure-based modeling (cocrystallization with FMS protein) provided the framework to efficiently effect this transformation (e.g., compounds **50–52**) and restore potencies to desired levels (Figure 11.11). Needless to say, compounds **50–52** did not appear to undergo reactive metabolite formation (judged from the lack of GSH adduct formation) in liver microsomal incubations.

The third example focuses on pyrazinone-based corticotropin-releasing factor-1 (CRF$_1$) receptor antagonists and potential antidepressant/antianxiolytic drugs [33–36]. In the course of structure–activity relationship investigation pyrazinone **53** (Figure 11.12) was synthesized and was found to have good pharmacokinetic properties in rats as well as efficacy in rodent models of anxiety [33]. However, subsequent *in vivo* disposition studies on **53** in bile duct–cannulated rats revealed extensive oxidative metabolism including the formation of GSH-related adducts [34, 35]. In fact, a major component of the elimination mechanism of **53** in rats (∼40% of

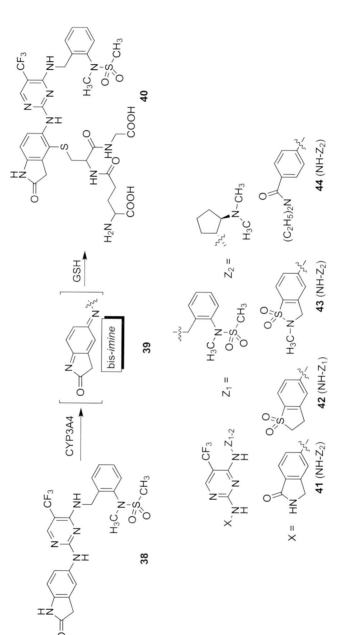

Figure 11.9 Rational design of analogues of the PYK2 inhibitor and 5-aminooxindole derivative **38** based on reactive metabolite characterization data.

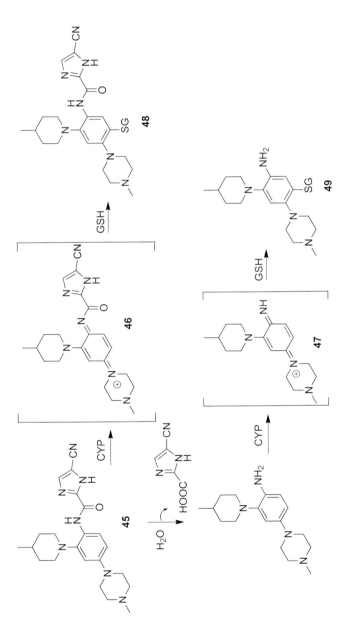

Figure 11.10 Proposed mechanism of bioactivation for the 1,2,4-phenylenetriamine-based inhibitors of the tyrosine kinase FMS.

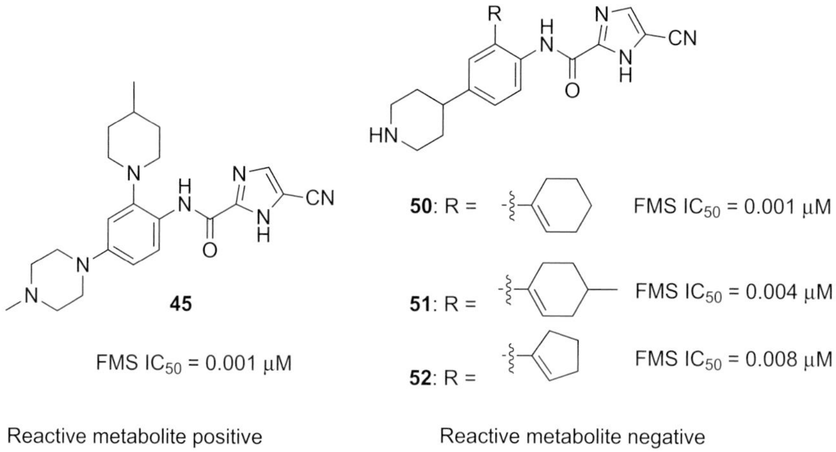

FMS IC$_{50}$ = 0.001 μM

45

50: R = FMS IC$_{50}$ = 0.001 μM

51: R = FMS IC$_{50}$ = 0.004 μM

52: R = FMS IC$_{50}$ = 0.008 μM

Reactive metabolite positive

Reactive metabolite negative

Figure 11.11 Rational design of FMS inhibitors based on structure-based modeling and reactive metabolite formation data.

drug-related material recovered in rat bile) consisted of conjugation with GSH, consistent with reactive metabolite formation *in vivo* [35]. Two distinct bioactivation pathways were deciphered by *in vitro* studies using liver microsomes (see Figure 11.12): (a) oxidative metabolism on the chloropyrazinone ring to yield an electrophilic epoxide **54** that is trapped by GSH to generate adduct **55** and (b) *O*-dealkylation of the difluoromethylphenoxy moiety to yield a phenol metabolite **56**, in which a two-electron oxidation generated the reactive quinone imine species **57** in a manner similar to that discerned with the 2,6-dichloro-4-hydroxyaniline analogues and nonsteroidal anti-inflammatory drugs diclofenac and lumiracoxib [37, 38]. Michael addition of GSH to **57** would lead to the adduct **58**. On the basis of this information, medicinal chemistry strategies were put in place to eliminate reactive metabolite liability in **53**. To eliminate bioactivation of the 2,6-dichloroaniline motif, efforts were directed toward incorporation of a pyridyl group as a bioisosteric replacement. To reduce level of 5-chloropyrazinone ring bioactivation, attempts were made to replace chlorine with the more strongly electron-withdrawing cyano group. Out of this iterative medicinal chemistry exercise emerged **59** (see Figure 11.12) with sufficiently diminished reactive metabolite formation in both rat liver microsomes and HLM [34]. Consistent with the *in vitro* finding, <2–4% of GSH conjugates were recovered in rat bile following *in vivo* administration of **59**. Compound **59** also retained all of the primary pharmacology and pharmacokinetic properties of the lead compound **53** [34, 36].

11.4
Medicinal Chemistry Strategies to Mitigate Bioactivation on a Piperazine Ring System

A unique bioactivation pathway involving ring contraction of a 1,3-disubstituted piperazine to the corresponding imidazoline derivative(s) was recently reported

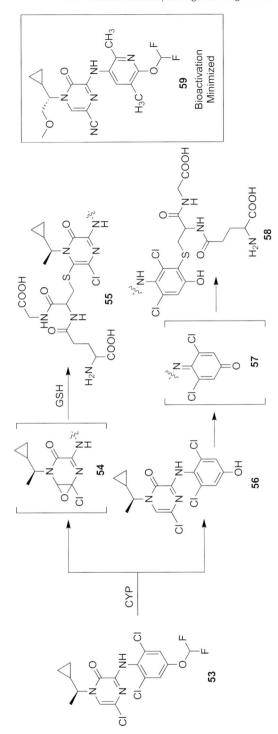

Figure 11.12 Minimization of reactive metabolite formation with a pyrazinone-based corticotropin-releasing factor-1 receptor antagonist **53**.

by Doss *et al.* [39]. The lead compound MB243 (**60**), a potent and selective mela-nocortin receptor agonist for the potential treatment of obesity and erectile dys-function [40], exhibited high levels of covalent binding to liver microsomal proteins from rats and humans. Two thioether adducts **65** and **66** were also detected in GSH-supplemented liver microsomal incubations and in bile duct–cannulated rats dosed with **60**. The two sulfydryl adducts were isolated and their structures were elucidated by mass spectrometry and NMR analysis. A plausible bioactivation pathway for **60** that leads to **65** and **66** is shown in Figure 11.13. A formal six-electron oxidation of the piperazine ring in **60** generates the elec-trophilic conjugated imine–amide intermediate **61**, which is trapped by GSH to yield adduct **62**. Hydrolytic cleavage of the glutamic acid residue in **62** leads to **63**. The free cysteinyl amino group in **63** attacks the thioaminal piperazine ring carbon causing opening of the piperazine ring and formation of a thiazolidine intermediate **64**. Intermediate **64** undergoes ring closure with the concomitant loss of water to form conjugate **65**. Adduct **66** results from further cleavage of the glycine residue in **65**.

Having elucidated the bioactivation pathway of **60**, synthetic efforts were initi-ated to incorporate substituents on the piperazine ring in **60** to decrease bioacti-vation and thereby attenuate the level of nonspecific irreversible binding to microsomal proteins. Various analogues with alkyl substituents on the pipera-zine ring (Figure 11.14) were synthesized, radiolabeled, and tested for covalent binding to microsomal proteins [39]. Alkylpiperazines **67–70** exhibited at least a 10-fold decrease in covalent binding (relative to **60**) while maintaining the phar-macological activity and selectivity against melanocortin receptor [40, 41]. Out of the overall SAR exercise also emerged the orally active bridged isoquinuclidine derivative **71** with superior pharmacokinetics/pharmacodynamics and negligible levels of covalent binding to rat and human microsomal protein when com-pared with **60** (Table 11.3) [42].

11.5
4-Fluorofelbamate as a Potentially Safer Alternative to Felbamate

Finally, against this backdrop, it is noteworthy to comment on the metabolism-guided design of fluorofelbamate (**81**) as a potentially safe alternative to the anticon-vulsant felbamate (**72**). Shortly after the approval of **72** for marketing in 1993 and following >50 cases of aplastic anemia and hepatotoxicity, the US Food and Drug Administration restricted its use to patients already receiving the drug or to those refractory to other epilepsy treatments [43–46]. Evidence linking reactive metabolite formation with felbamate toxicity has been presented in some elegant work by Mac-Donald and coworkers [47–53]. 2-Phenyl-1,3-propanediol monocarbamate (**73**), the product of hydrolysis of **72**, has been observed as a metabolite in preclinical species and humans (Figure 11.15) [54]. Likewise, 3-carbamoyl-2-phenylpropionic acid (**75**), an oxidized metabolite of **73**, has been identified as the major metabolite of felbamate in humans [55]. Thompson *et al.* [47] synthesized the intermediate

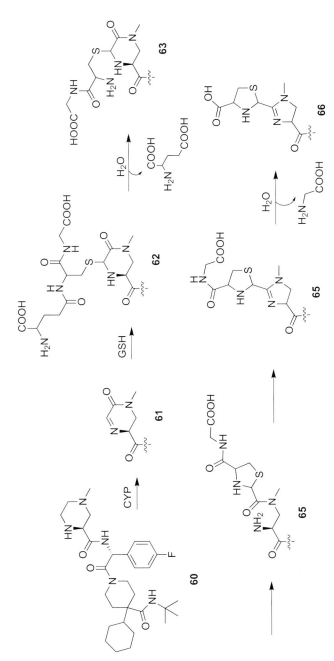

Figure 11.13 Proposed mechanism of bioactivation for the 1,3-disubstituted piperazine derivative **61**, an agonist of the melanocortin receptor.

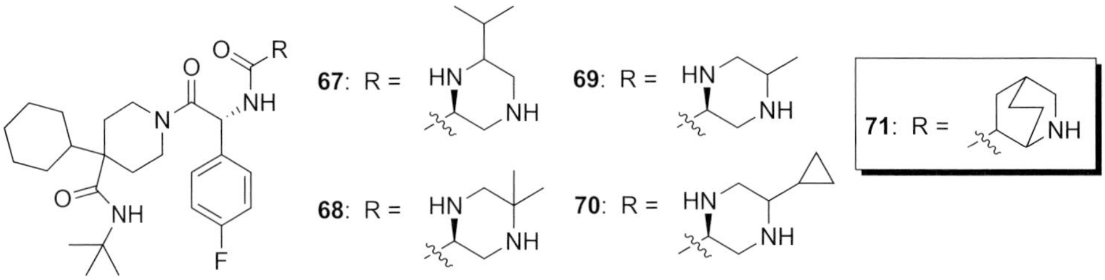

Figure 11.14 Reducing microsomal covalent binding due to reactive metabolite formation with 1,3-disubstituted piperazine derivatives.

3-carbamoyl-2-phenylpropionaldehyde (**74**) and found it to be highly unstable ($T_{1/2}$ <30 s) under physiological conditions. Compound **74** degraded spontaneously to the α,β-unsaturated aldehyde 2-phenylpropenal (**76**) or underwent reversible cyclization to 4-hydroxy-5-phenyltetrahydro-1,3-oxazin-2-one (**77**). Compound **76** (also known as atropaldehyde) was also shown to react with GSH under nonenzymatic conditions (pH 7.4 buffer) and under enzyme-catalyzed conditions (glutathione *S*-transferases A1-1, M1-1, and P1-1) to afford conjugate **78** (Figure 11.15) [47, 51]. Evidence for the occurrence of this pathway *in vivo* has been demonstrated by the characterization of urinary mercapturic acid conjugates **79** and **80** (derived from the reduced and oxidized forms of **76**) following felbamate administration to rats and humans [48–50].

Based on this mechanistic information, **81** (Figure 11.16) was specifically designed to eliminate the reactive metabolite liability of felbamate. The strategic placement of the fluorine atom on the benzylic position prevents the elimination process that affords the α,β-unsaturated aldeyhde **76** from **74** (see Figure 11.16) [56]. The major metabolic fate of **81** in human hepatic tissue involves oxidation to the latent carboxylic acid metabolite **84** (via the alcohol and aldehyde intermediates **82** and **83**, respectively). Whether absence of bioactivation translates into a reduced risk of aplastic anemia and hepatotoxicity remains to be seen in long-term clinical trials. Fluorofelbamate is currently undergoing clinical trials as an antiepileptic agent [57].

Table 11.3 *In vitro* activity against human melanocortin receptors and rat pharmacokinetics of **60** and **71**.

Compound	MC4R EC$_{50}$ (μM)	Microsomal covalent binding (pmol equivalent/mg protein)	CL$_p$ (ml/min/kg))	V$_{dss}$ (l/kg)	T$_{1/2}$ (h)	Oral F (%)
60	0.087	2153	48.7	5.4	1.6	9.0
71	0.0019	26	40	9.6	3.2	32.0

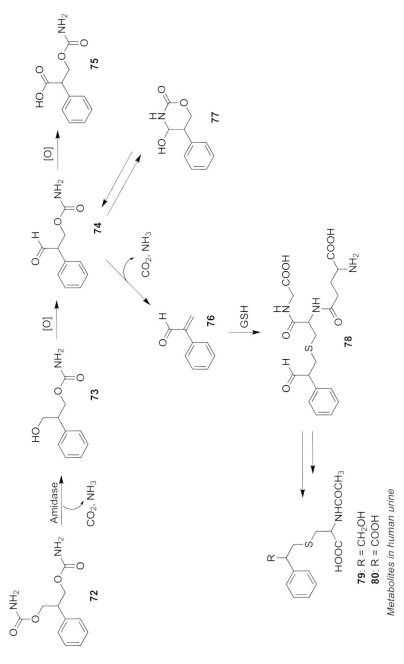

Figure 11.15 Postulated bioactivation mechanism of the anticonvulsant felbamate.

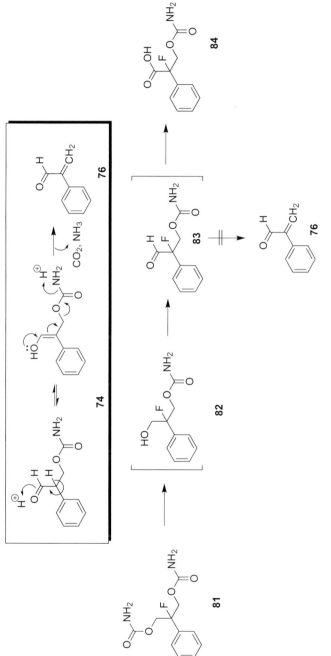

Figure 11.16 A rational chemical approach to circumvent bioactivation liability of felbamate: discovery of fluorofelbamate.

11.6
Concluding Remarks

The detection of conjugates (GSH, amino, and/or cyano) and/or covalent binding to target tissue (e.g., NADPH-supplemented HLM) provides evidence for reactive metabolite formation and usually triggers medicinal chemistry efforts to eliminate the liability in new drug candidates. It is important to point out that absence of reactive metabolite formation in compounds and/or covalent binding to liver microsomal proteins is not a guarantee of their safety. For example, the felbamate metabolic activation process in humans, which leads to the formation of **76**, has never been replicated in human hepatic tissue. At therapeutically relevant concentrations of radiolabeled felbamate in *in vitro* incubations with HLM and human hepatocytes, no GSH adducts and/or covalent binding of felbamate has been discerned [58]. While the reason(s) for this discrepancy remains unclear, in a drug discovery paradigm relying solely on reactive metabolite trapping and liver microsomal covalent binding as means of predicting drug toxicity, felbamate would have passed the hurdle with flying colors.

References

1 Kalgutkar, A.S., Driscoll, J., Zhao, S.X., Walker, G.S., Shepard, R.M., Soglia, J.R., Atherton, J., Yu, Li., Mutlib, A.E., Munchhof, M.J., Reiter, L.A., Jones, C.S., Doty, J.L., Trevena, K.A., Shaffer, C.L., and Ripp, S.L. (2007) A rational chemical intervention strategy to circumvent bioactivation liabilities associated with a nonpeptidyl thrombopoietin receptor agonist containing a 2-amino-4-arylthiazole motif. *Chemical Research in Toxicology*, **20** (12), 1954–1965.

2 Obach, R.S., Kalgutkar, A.S., Ryder, T.F., and Walker, G.S. (2008) In vitro metabolism and covalent binding of enol-carboxamide derivatives and anti-inflammatory agents sudoxicam and meloxicam: insights into the hepatotoxicity of sudoxicam. *Chemical Research in Toxicology*, **21** (9), 1890–1899.

3 Mizutani, T., Yoshida, K., and Kawazoe, S. (1994) Formation of toxic metabolites from thiabendazole and other thiazoles in mice. Identification of thioamides as ring cleavage products. *Drug Metabolism and Disposition*, **22** (5), 750–755.

4 Mizutani, T. and Suzuki, K. (1996) Relative hepatotoxicity of 2-(substituted phenyl)thiazoles and substituted thiobenzamides in mice: evidence for the involvement of thiobenzamides as ring cleavage metabolites in the hepatotoxicity of 2-phenylthiazoles. *Toxicology Letters*, **85** (2), 101–105.

5 Antipas, A.S., Blumberg, L.C., Brissette, W.H., Brown, M.F., Casavant, J.M., Doty, J.L., Driscoll, J., Harris, T.M., Jones, C.S., McCurdy, S.P., McElroy, E., Mitton-Fry, M., Munchhof, M.J., Reim, D.A., Reiter, L.A., Ripp, S.L., Shavnya, A., Smeets, M.I., and Trevena, K.A. (2010) Structure–activity relationships and hepatic safety risks of thiazole agonists of the thrombopoietin receptor. *Bioorganic Medicinal Chemistry Letters*, **20** (14), 4069–4072.

6 Subramanian, R., Lee, M.R., Allen, J.G., Bourbeau, M.P., Fotsch, C., Hong, F.T., Tadesse, S., Yao, G., Yuan, C.C., Surapaneni, S., Skiles, G.L., Wang, X., Wohlhieter, G.E., Zeng, Q., Zhou, Y., Zhu, X., and Li, C. (2010) Cytochrome P450-mediated epoxidation of 2-aminothiazole-based AKT inhibitors: identification of novel GSH adducts and reduction of metabolic activation through structural changes guided by in silico and in vitro

screening. *Chemical Research in Toxicology*, **23** (3), 653–663.

7 Zeng, Q., Bourbeau, M.P., Wohlhieter, G.E., Yao, G., Monenschein, H., Rider, J.T., Lee, M.R., Zhang, S., Lofgren, J., Freeman, D., Li, C., Tominey, E., Huang, X., Hoffman, D., Yamane, H., Tasker, A.S., Dominguez, C., Viswanadhan, V.N., Hungate, R., and Zhang, X. (2010) 2-Aminothiadiazole inhibitors of AKT1 as potential cancer therapeutics. *Bioorganic Medicinal Chemistry Letters*, **20** (5), 1652–1666.

8 Zeng, Q., Allen, J.G., Bourbeau, M.P., Wang, X., Yao, G., Tadesse, S., Rider, J.T., Yuan, C.C., Hong, F.T., Lee, M.R., Zhang, S., Lofgren, J.A., Freeman, D.J., Yang, S., Li, C., Tominey, E., Huang, X., Hoffman, D., Yamane, H.K., Fotsch, C., Dominguez, C., Hungate, R., and Zhang, X. (2010) Azole-based inhibitors of AKT/PKB for the treatment of cancer. *Bioorganic Medicinal Chemistry Letters*, **20** (5), 1559–1564.

9 Kalgutkar, A.S. and Zhao, Z. (2001) Discovery and design of selective cyclooxygenase-2 inhibitors as non-ulcerogenic, anti-inflammatory drugs with potential utility as anti-cancer agents. *Current Drug Targets*, **2** (1), 79–106.

10 Marnett, L.J. and Kalgutkar, A.S. (1998) Design of selective inhibitors of cyclooxygenase-2 as non-ulcerogenic anti-inflammatory agents. *Current Opinion in Chemical Biology*, **2** (4), 482–490.

11 Penning, T.D., Talley, J.J., Bertenshaw, S.R., Carter, J.S., Collins, P.W., Docter, S., Graneto, M.J., Lee, L.F., Malecha, J.W., Miyashiro, J.M., Rogers, R.S., Rogier, D.J., Yu, S.S., Anderson, G.D., Burton, E.G., Cogburn, J.N., Gregory, S.A., Koboldt, C.M., Perkins, W.E., Seibert, K., Veenhuizen, A.W., Zhang, Y.Y., and Isakson, P.C. (1997) Synthesis and biological evaluation of the 1,5-diarylpyrazole class of cyclooxygenase-2 inhibitors: identification of 4-[5-(4-methylphenyl)-3-(trifluoromethyl)-1H-pyrazol-1-yl]benzenesulfonamide (SC-58635, celecoxib). *Journal of Medicinal Chemistry*, **40** (9), 1347–1365.

12 Prasit, P., Wang, Z., Brideau, C., Chan, C.C., Charleson, S., Cromlish, W., Ethier, D., Evans, J.F., Ford-Hutchinson, A.W., Gauthier, J.Y., Gordon, R., Guay, J., Gresser, M., Kargman, S., Kennedy, B., Leblanc, Y., Léger, S., Mancini, J., O'Neill, G.P., Ouellet, M., Percival, M.D., Perrier, H., Riendeau, D., Rodger, I., Tagari, P., Thérien, M., Vickers, P., Wong, E., Xu, L.-J., Young, R.N., and Zamboni, R. (1999) The discovery of rofecoxib [MK 966, Vioxx 4-(4'-methylsulfonylphenyl)-3-phenyl-2(5H)-furanone], an orally active cyclooxygenase-2 inhibitor. *Bioorganic Medicinal Chemistry Letters*, **9** (13), 1773–1778.

13 Talley, J.J., Brown, D.L., Carter, J.S., Graneto, M.J., Koboldt, C.M., Masferrer, J.L., Perkins, W.E., Rogers, R.S., Shaffer, A. F., Zhang, Y.Y., Zweifel, B.S., and Seibert, K. (2000) 4-[5-Methyl-3-phenylisoxazol-4-yl]-benzenesulfonamide, valdecoxib: a potent and selective inhibitor of COX-2. *Journal of Medicinal Chemistry*, **43** (5), 775–777.

14 Talley, J.J. (1999) Selective inhibitors of cyclooxygenase-2 (COX-2). *Progress in Medicinal Chemistry*, **36**, 201–234.

15 Thérien, M., Brideau, C., Chan, C.C., Cromlish, W.A., Gauthier, J.Y., Gordon, R., Greig, G., Kargman, S., Lau, C.K., Leblanc, Y., Chun-Sing, L., O'Neill, G.P., Riendeau, D., Roy, P., Zhaoyin, W., Lijing, X., and Prasit, P. (1997) Synthesis and biological evaluation of 5,6-diarylimidazo [2.1-b]thiazole as selective COX-2 inhibitors. *Bioorganic Medicinal Chemistry Letters*, **7** (1), 47–52.

16 Trimble, L.A., Chauret, N., Silva, J.M., Nicoll-Griffith, D.A., Li, C.-S., and Yergey, J.A. (1997) Characterization of the *in vitro* oxidative metabolites of the COX-2 selective inhibitor L-766,112. *Bioorganic Medicinal Chemistry Letters*, **7** (1), 53–56.

17 Roy, P., Leblanc, Y., Ball, R.G., Brideau, C., Chan, C.C., Chauret, N., Cromlish, W., Ethier, D., Gauthier, J.Y., Gordon, R., Greig, G., Guay, J., Kargman, S., Lau, C. K., O'Neill, G., Silva, J., Thérien, M., van Staden, C., Wong, E., Xu, L., and Prasit, P. (1997) A new series of selective COX-2 inhibitors: 5,6-diarylthiazolo[3,2-b][1,2,4] triazoles. *Bioorganic Medicinal Chemistry Letters*, **7** (1), 57–62.

18 Crosswell, H.E., Dasgupta, A., Alvarado, C.S., Watt, T., Christensen, J.G., De, P., Durden, D.L., and Findley, H.W. (2009) PHA665752, a small-molecule inhibitor of c-Met inhibits hepatocyte growth factor-

stimulated migration and proliferation of c-Met-positive neuroblastoma cells. *BMC Cancer*, **9**, 411.

19 Teffera, Y., Choquette, D., Liu, J., Colletti, A.E., Hollis, L.S., Lin, M.-H.J., and Zhao, Z. (2010) Bioactivation of isothiazoles: minimizing the risk of potential toxicity in drug discovery. *Chemical Research in Toxicology*, **23** (11), 1743–1752.

20 Maggs, J.L., Tingle, M.D., Kitteringham, N.R., and Park, B.K. (1988) Drug–protein conjugates. 14. Mechanisms of formation of protein-arylating intermediates from amodiaquine, a myelotoxin and hepatotoxin in man. *Biochemical Pharmacology*, **37** (2), 303–311.

21 Maggs, J.L., Colbert, J., Winstanley, P.A., Orme, M.L., and Park, B.K. (1987) Irreversible binding of amodiaquine to human liver microsomes: chemical and metabolic factors. *British Journal of Clinical Pharmacology*, **23**, 649.

22 Tingle, M.D., Jewell, H., Maggs, J.L., O'Neill, P.M., and Park, B.K. (1995) The bioactivation of amodiaquine by human polymorphonuclear leucocytes *in vitro*: chemical mechanisms and the effects of fluorine substitution. *Biochemical Pharmacology*, **50** (7), 1113–1119.

23 O'Neill, P.M., Harrison, A.C., Storr, R.C., Hawley, S.R., Ward, S.A., and Park, B.K. (1994) The effect of fluorine substitution on the metabolism and antimalarial activity of amodiaquine. *Journal of Medicinal Chemistry*, **37** (9), 1362–1370.

24 O'Neill, P.M., Mukhtar, A., Stocks, P.A., Randle, L.E., Hindley, S., Ward, S.A., Storr, R.C., Bickley, J.F., O'Neil, I.A., Maggs, J.L., Hughes, R.H., Winstanley, P.A., Bray, P.G., and Park, B.K. (2003) Isoquine and related amodiaquine analogues: a new generation of improved 4-aminoquinoline antimalarials. *Journal of Medicinal Chemistry*, **46** (23), 4933–4945.

25 O'Neill, P.M., Shone, A.E., Stanford, D., Nixon, G., Asadollahy, E., Park, B.K., Maggs, J.L., Roberts, P., Stocks, P.A., Biagini, G., Bray, P.G., Davies, J., Berry, N., Hall, C., Rimmer, K., Winstanley, P.A., Hindley, S., Bambal, R.B., Davis, C.B., Bates, M., Gresham, S.L., Brigandi, R.A., Gomez-de-Las-Heras, F.M., Gargallo, D.V., Parapini, S., Vivas, L., Lander, H., Taramelli, D., and Ward, S.A. (2009) Synthesis, antimalarial activity, and preclinical pharmacology of a novel series of 4′-fluoro and 4′-chloro analogues of amodiaquine. Identification of a suitable "back-up" compound for *N-tert*-butyl isoquine. *Journal of Medicinal Chemistry*, **52** (7), 1828–1844.

26 Neftel, K.A., Woodtly, W., Schmid, M., Frick, P.G., and Fehr, J. (1986) Amodiaquine induced agranulocytosis and liver damage. *British Medical Journal*, **292** (6552), 721–723.

27 Schulthess, H.K., von Felten, A., Gmur, J., and Neftel, K. (1983) Amodiaquine-induced agranulocytosis during suppressive treatment of malaria – demonstration of an amodiaquine-dependent granulocytotoxic antibody. *Schweizer Medizinische Wochenschr*, **113** (50), 1912–1913.

28 Davis, C.B., Bambal, R., Moorthy, G.S., Hugger, E., Xiang, H., Park, B.K., Shone, A.E., O'Neill, P.M., and Ward, S.A. (2009) Comparative preclinical drug metabolism and pharmacokinetic evaluation of novel 4-aminoquinoline anti-malarials. *Journal of Pharmaceutical Sciences*, **98** (1), 362–377.

29 O'Neill, P.M., Park, B.K., Shone, A.E., Maggs, J.L., Roberts, P., Stocks, P.A., Biagini, G.A., Bray, P.G., Gibbons, P., Berry, N., Winstanley, P.A., Mukhtar, A., Bonar-Law, R., Hindley, S., Bambal, R.B., Davis, C.B., Bates, M., Hart, T.K., Gresham, S.L., Lawrence, R.M., Brigandi, R.A., Gomez-delas-Heras, F.M., Gargallo, D.V., and Ward, S.A. (2009) Candidate selection and preclinical evaluation of *N-tert*-butyl isoquine (GSK369796), an affordable and effective 4-aminoquinoline antimalarial for the 21st century. *Journal of Medicinal Chemistry*, **52** (5), 1408–1415.

30 Walker, D.P., Bi, F.C., Kalgutkar, A.S., Bauman, J.N., Zhao, S.X., Soglia, J.R., Aspnes, G.E., Kung, D.W., Klug-McLeod, J., Zawistoski, M.P., McGlynn, M.A., Oliver, R., Dunn, M., Li, J.C., Richter, D.T., Cooper, B.A., Kath, J.C., Hulford, C.A., Autry, C.L., Luzzio, M.J., Ung, E.J., Roberts, W.G., Bonnette, P.C., Buckbinder, L., Mistry, A., Griffor, M.C., Han, S., and Guzman-Perez, A. (2008) Trifluoromethylpyrimidine-based inhibitors of proline-rich tyrosine kinase 2 (PYK2): structure–activity relationships and strategies for the elimination of reactive metabolite formation. *Bioorganic Medicinal Chemistry Letters,* **18** (23), 6071–6077.

31 Sun, H., Sharma, R., Bauman, J., Walker, D.P., Aspnes, G.E., Zawistoski, M.P., and Kalgutkar, A.S. (2009) Differences in CYP3A4 catalyzed bioactivation of 5-aminooxindole and 5-aminobenzsultam scaffolds in proline-rich tyrosine kinase 2 (PYK2) inhibitors: retrospective analysis by CYP3A4 molecular docking, quantum chemical calculations and glutathione adduct detection using linear ion trap/orbitrap mass spectrometry. *Bioorganic Medicinal Chemistry Letters,* **19** (12), 3177–3182.

32 Meegalla, S.K., Wall, M.J., Chen, J., Wilson, K.J., Ballentine, S.K., Desjarlais, R.L., Schubert, C., Crysler, C.S., Chen, Y., Molloy, C.J., Chaikin, M.A., Manthey, C.L., Player, M.R., Tomczuk, B.E., and Illig, C.R. (2008) Structure-based optimization of a potent class of arylamide FMS inhibitors. *Bioorganic Medicinal Chemistry Letters,* **18** (12), 3632–3637.

33 Hartz, R.A., Ahuja, V.T., Rafalski, M., Schmitz, W.D., Brenner, A.B., Denhart, D.J., Ditta, J.L., Deskus, J.A., Yue, E.W., Arvanitis, A.G., Lelas, S., Li, Y.W., Molski, T.F., Wong, H., Grace, J.E., Lentz, K.A., Li, J., Lodge, N.J., Zaczek, R., Combs, A.P., Olson, R.E., Mattson, R.J., Bronson, J.J., and Macor, J.E. (2009) In vitro intrinsic clearance-based optimization of *N*3-phenylpyrazinones as corticotropin-releasing factor-1 (CRF1) receptor antagonists. *Journal of Medicinal Chemistry,* **52** (14), 4161–4172.

34 Hartz, R.A., Ahuja, V.T., Zhuo, X., Mattson, R.J., Denhart, D.J., Deskus, J.A., Vrudhula, V.M., Pan, S., Ditta, J.L., Shu, Y.Z., Grace, J.E., Lentz, K.A., Lelas, S., Li, Y.W., Molski, T.F., Krishnananthan, S., Wong, H., Qian-Cutrone, J., Schartman, R., Denton, R., Lodge, N.J., Zaczek, R., Macor, J.E., and Bronson, J.J. (2009) A strategy to minimize reactive metabolite formation: discovery of (*S*)-4-(1-cyclopropyl-2-methoxyethyl)-6-[6-(difluoromethoxy)-2,5-dimethylpyridin-3-ylamino]-5-oxo-4,5-dihydropyrazine-2-

carbonitrile as a potent, orally bioavailable corticotropin-releasing factor-1 receptor antagonist. *Journal of Medicinal Chemistry,* **52** (23), 7653–7668.

35 Zhuo, X., Hartz, R.A., Bronson, J.J., Wong, H., Ahuja, V.T., Vrudhula, V.M., Leet, J.E., Huang, S., Macor, J.E., and Shu, Y.Z. (2010) Comparative biotransformation of pyrazinone-containing corticotropin-releasing factor receptor-1 antagonists: minimizing the reactive metabolite formation. *Drug Metabolism and Disposition,* **38** (1), 5–15.

36 Hartz, R.A., Ahuja, V.T., Schmitz, W.D., Molski, T.F., Mattson, G.K., Lodge, N.J., Bronson, J.J., and Macor, J.E. (2010) Synthesis and structure–activity relationships of *N*3-pyridylpyrazinones as corticotropin-releasing factor-1 (CRF-1) receptor antagonists. *Bioorganic Medicinal Chemistry letters,* **20** (6), 1890–1894.

37 Tang, W., Stearns, R.A., Wang, R.W., Chiu, S.H., and Baillie, T.A. (1999) Roles of human hepatic cytochrome P450s 2C9 and 3A4 in the metabolic activation of diclofenac. *Chemical Research in Toxicology,* **12** (2), 192–199.

38 Li, Y., Slatter, J.G., Zhang, Z., Li, Y., Doss, G.A., Braun, M.P., Stearns, R.A., Dean, D.C., Baillie, T.A., and Tang, W. (2008) In vitro metabolic activation of lumiracoxib in rat and human liver preparations. *Drug Metabolism and Disposition,* **36** (2), 469–473.

39 Doss, G.A., Miller, R.R., Zhang, Z., Teffera, Y., Nargund, R.P., Palucki, B., Park, M.K., Tang, Y.S., Evans, D.C., Baillie, T.A., and Stearns, R.A. (2005) Metabolic activation of 1,3-disubstituted piperazine derivative: evidence for a novel ring contraction to an imidazoline. *Chemical Research in Toxicology,* **18** (2), 271–276.

40 Palucki, B.L., Park, M.K., Nargund, R.P., Ye, Z., Sebhat, I.K., Pollard, P.G., Kalyani, R.N., Tang, R., Macneil, T., Weinberg, D.H., Vongs, A., Rosenblum, C.I., Doss, G.A., Miller, R.R., Stearns, R.A., Peng, Q., Tamvakopoulos, C., McGowan, E., Martin, W.J., Metzger, J.M., Shepherd, C.A., Strack, A.M., Macintyre, D.E., Van der Ploeg, L.H., and Patchett, A.A. (2005) Discovery of (2*S*)-*N*-[(1*R*)-2-[4-cyclohexyl-4-[[(1,1-dimethylethyl)amino]carbonyl]-1-piperidinyl]-1-[(4-fluorophenyl)methyl]-2-

oxoethyl]-4-methyl-2-piperazinecarboxa-mide (MB243), a potent and selective melanocortin subtype-4 receptor agonist. *Bioorganic Medicinal Chemistry Letters*, **15** (1), 171–175.

41 Palucki, B.L., Park, M.K., Nargund, R.P., Tang, R., MacNeil, T., Weinberg, D.H., Vongs, A., Rosenblum, C.I., Doss, G.A., Miller, R.R., Stearns, R.A., Peng, Q., Tamvakopoulos, C., Van der Ploeg, L.H., and Patchett, A.A. (2005) 2-Piperazinecarboxamides as potent and selective melanocortin subtype-4 receptor agonists. *Bioorganic Medicinal Chemistry Letters*, **15** (8), 1993–1996.

42 Ye, Z., Guo, L., Barakat, K.J., Pollard, P.G., Palucki, B.L., Sebhat, I.K., Bakshi, R.K., Tang, R., Kalyani, R.N., Vongs, A., Chen, A.S., Chen, H.Y., Rosenblum, C.I., MacNeil, T., Weinberg, D.H., Peng, Q., Tamvakopoulos, C., Miller, R.R., Stearns, R.A., Cashen, D.E., Martin, W.J., Metzger, J.M., Strack, A.M., MacIntyre, D.E., Van der Ploeg, L.H., Patchett, A.A., Wyvratt, M.J., and Nargund, R.P. (2005) Discovery and activity of (1*R*,4*S*,6*R*)-*N*-[(1*R*)-2-[4-cyclohexyl-4-[[(1,1-dimethylethyl)amino] carbonyl]-1-piperidinyl]-1-[(4-fluorophenyl)methyl]-2-oxoethyl]-2-methyl-2-azabicyclo[2.2.2]octane-6-carboxamide (3, RY764), a potent and selective melanocortin subtype-4 receptor agonist. *Bioorganic Medicinal Chemistry Letters*, **15** (15), 3501–3505.

43 Pellock, J.M. (1999) Felbamate in epilepsy therapy: evaluating the risks. *Drug Safety*, **21** (3), 225–239.

44 Kaufman, D.W., Kelly, J.P., Anderson, T., Harmon, D.C., and Shapiro, S. (1997) Evaluation of case reports of aplastic anemia among patients treated with felbamate. *Epilepsia*, **38** (12), 1265–1269.

45 O'Neil, M.G., Perdun, C.S., Wilson, M.B., McGown, S.T., and Patel, S. (1996) Felbamate-associated fatal acute hepatic necrosis. *Neurology*, **46** (5), 1457–1459.

46 Nightingale, S.L. (1994) Recommendation to immediately withdraw patients from treatment with felbamate. *JAMA: the Journal of the American Medical Association*, **272** (13), 995.

47 Thompson, C.D., Kinter, M.T., and Macdonald, T.L. (1996) Synthesis and in vitro reactivity of 3-carbamoyl-2-phenylpropionaldeyde and 2-phenylpropenal: putative reactive metabolites of felbamate. *Chemical Research in Toxicology*, **9** (8), 1225–1229.

48 Thompson, C.D., Gulden, P.H., and MacDonald, T.L. (1997) Identification of modified atropaldehyde mercapturic acids in rat and human urine after felbamate administration. *Chemical Research in Toxicology*, **10** (4), 457–462.

49 Thompson, C.D., Barthen, M.T., Hopper, D.W., Miller, T.A., Quigg, M., Hudspeth, C., Montouris, G., Marsh, L., Perhach, J.L., Sofia, R.D., and Macdonald, T.L. (1999) Quantitation in patient urine samples of felbamate and three metabolites: acid carbamate and two mercapturic acids. *Epilepsia*, **40** (6), 769–776.

50 Dieckhaus, C.M., Santos, W.L., Sofia, R.D., and Macdonald, T.L. (2001) The chemistry, toxicology, and identification in rat and urine of 4-hydroxy-5-phenyl-1,3-oxaperhydroin-2-one: a reactive metabolite in felbamate bioactivation. *Chemical Research in Toxicology*, **14** (8), 958–964.

51 Dieckhaus, C.M., Roller, S.G., Santos, W.L., Sofia, R.D., and Macdonald, T.L. (2001) Role of glutathione *S*-transferases A1-1, M1-1, and P1-1 in the detoxification of 2-phenylpropenal, a reactive felbamate metabolite. *Chemical Research in Toxicology*, **14** (5), 511–516.

52 Kapetanovic, I.M., Torchin, C.D., Strong, J.M., Yonekawa, W.D., Lu, C., Li, A.P., Dieckhaus, C.M., Santos, W.L., Macdonald, T.L., Sofia, R.D., and Kupferberg, H.J. (2002) Reactivity of atropaldehyde, a felbamate metabolite in human liver tissue in vitro. *Chemico-Biological Interactions*, **142** (1–2), 119–134.

53 Diekhaus, C.M., Thompson, C.D., Roller, S.G., and MacDonald, T.L. (2002) Mechanisms of idiosyncratic drug reactions: the case of felbamate. *Chemico-Biological Interactions*, **142** (1–2), 99–117.

54 Yang, J.T., Adusumalli, V.E., Wong, K.K., Kucharczyk, N., and Sofia, R.D. (1991) Felbamate metabolism in the rat, rabbit, and dog. *Drug Metabolism and Disposition*, **19** (6), 1126–1134.

55 Adusumalli, V.E., Choi, Y.M., Romanyshyn, L.A., Sparadoski, R.E., Wichmann, J.K., Wong, K.K., Kucharczyk, N., and Sofia, R. D. (1993) Isolation and identification of 3-carbamoyloxy-2-phenylpropionic acid as a major human urinary metabolite of felbamate. *Drug Metabolism and Disposition,* **21** (4), 710–716.

56 Parker, R.J., Hartman, N.R., Roecklein, B. A., Mortko, H., Kupferberg, H.J., Stables, J., and Strong, J.M. (2005) Stability and comparative metabolism of selected felbamate metabolites and postulated fluorofelbamate metabolites by postmitochondrial suspensions. *Chemical Research in Toxicology,* **18** (12), 1842–1848.

57 Roecklein, B.A., Sacks, H.J., Mortko, H., and Stables, J. (2007) Fluorofelbamate. *Neurotherapeutics,* **4** (1), 97–101.

58 Bauman, J.N., Kelly, J.M., Tripathy, S., Zhao, S.X., Lam, W.W., Kalgutkar, A.S., and Obach, R.S. (2009) Can in vitro metabolism-dependent covalent binding data distinguish hepatotoxic from nonhepatotoxic drugs? An analysis using human hepatocytes and liver S-9 fraction. *Chemical Research in Toxicology,* **22** (2), 332–340.

12
Structural Alert and Reactive Metabolite Analysis for the Top 200 Drugs in the US Market by Prescription

Abbreviations

BSEP   Bile salt export pump
CYP   Cytochrome P450
FDA   Food and Drug Administration
GSH   Glutathione
HLM   Human liver microsomes
IADRs   Idiosyncratic adverse drug reactions
NAT   *N*-Acetyltransferase
NSAIDs   Nonsteroidal anti-inflammatory drugs

12.1
Introduction

Reliably predicting the occurrence of idiosyncratic adverse drug reactions (IADRs) for new drug candidates represents a significant challenge in drug discovery/development, despite tremendous strides in the field of chemical toxicology. Several excellent reviews on reactive metabolites have been published that focus on retrospective structure–toxicity relationships and strengthen the structural alert/reactive metabolite hypothesis as a causative factor in drug toxicity (see Chapter 8). These papers reaffirm the notion of general avoidance of structural alerts in drug design as a strategy to minimize IADRs. However, examination of the structural trends with drugs approved over the past approximately five years clearly suggests an overlap between chemical drug space and chemical space occupied by molecules possessing structural alerts. Furthermore, some medicinally important functional groups that are classified as structural alerts, such as the aniline moiety, can be quite challenging to mimic by isosteric replacement. Hence, questions arise such as the following: when is a molecule that contains a structural alert (reactive metabolite positive or negative) a cause for concern? Are some structural alerts more promiscuous than others? In an effort to address these questions, the top 200 most prescribed drugs in the United States in the year 2009 have been examined for: (a) the daily dosing regimen, (b) the presence of structural alerts, (c) evidence

Reactive Drug Metabolites, First Edition. Amit S. Kalgutkar, Deepak Dalvie, R. Scott Obach, and Dennis A. Smith.
© 2012 Wiley-VCH Verlag GmbH & Co. KGaA. Published 2012 by Wiley-VCH Verlag GmbH & Co. KGaA.

for reactive metabolite formation and protein covalent binding, and (d) toxicity mechanism(s) potentially mediated through cellular effects by the parent drug. Structural alerts as outlined in Chapter 5 were identified through a manual inspection of the chemical structures. The phenyl ring was not considered as a structural alert in this analysis; however, phenols, alkoxyaromatic ethers/amines, and alkylaromatic ethers/amines were flagged as alerts because of the greater likelihood of sequential metabolism to quinonoid species (e.g., quinone methides, quinone imines, and imine-methides). For the overall exercise, it was assumed that adequate safety was demonstrated in regulatory preclinical toxicity studies and the reference to toxicity in this analysis relates to the idiosyncratic kind. Table 12.1 lists the top 200 prescribed drugs in the United States in 2009; the list can also be obtained from www.pharmacytimes.com.

12.2
Structural Alert and Reactive Metabolite Analyses for the Top 20 Most Prescribed Drugs in the United States for the Year 2009

Figure 12.1 lists the top 20 drugs prescribed in the United States in 2009. Multiple ranks for a given drug imply that generic forms were marketed by more than one vendor. Of the top 15 drugs by dispensed prescriptions (hydrocodone-/acetaminophen combination, metoprolol, and simvastatin appeared twice in the list, whereas levothyroxine appeared thrice in the list of 20 drugs), 10 (55%) drugs were flagged for the presence of structural alerts and evidence for metabolic activation leading to reactive metabolites has been demonstrated in 5 out of the 10 cases.

12.2.1
Daily Dose Trends

With the exception of acetaminophen (combination with hydrocodone), amoxicillin, azithromycin, and metformin (daily doses range from 2000 to 4000 mg), the maximum recommended daily doses of the top 20 drugs are 100 mg or less (in most cases, the pharmacologically effective doses are significantly lower) (see Figure 12.1). For instance, the maximum recommended daily dose of atorvastatin is 80 mg, but most patients demonstrate significant lowering of cholesterol at 10–20 mg daily doses. This trend presents a significant contrast with the high daily doses of drugs that are associated with toxicity (Figure 12.2) [1].

12.2.2
Presence of Structural Alerts

Among the list of top 20 prescribed medicines, lisinopril, escitalopram, amlodipine, azithromycin, and metformin do not contain structural alerts (Figure 12.1). However, structural alerts (phenol, alkylaromatic ether, hydroxyanilide, anilide, etc.) associated with the formation of electrophilic quinones, quinone imines, and quinone methides were identified as alerts in several instances (highlighted in bold

Table 12.1 Top 200 drugs sold in the US market in 2009 on the basis of dispensed prescriptions.

Drug (Rank)	Drug (Rank)	Drug (Rank)	Drug (Rank)	Drug (Rank)
Hydrocodone/acetaminophen (1, 3, 66)	Valsartan/ hydrochlorothiazide (40)	Losartan (78)	Carvedilol (124)	Irbesartan (168)
Atorvastatin (2)	Trazodone (41, 174)	Propoxyphene N-acetaminophen (79, 163)	Oxycontin (126, 190)	Amphetamine salts (169)
Levothyroxine (4, 12, 18, 103)	Pioglitazone (42)	Valacyclovir (82)	Paroxetine (127)	Ibandronic acid (172)
Lisinopril (5, 32, 74, 81, 150)	Alendronate (43)	Albuterol (84, 129, 132)	Olmesartan/ hydrochlorothiazide (128)	Eszopiclone (173)
Amoxicillin (6)	Sulfamethoxazole/ trimethoprim (44)	Lorazepam (86, 144)	Tadalafil (130)	Ipratropium bromide/salbutamol (176)
Esomeprazole (7)	Lansoprazole (45)	Pantoprazole (89, 139)	Sitagliptin (131)	Folic acid (181)
Clopidogrel (8)	Clonazepam (46)	Amlodipine/benazepril (90)	Ciprofloxacin (133, 180, 182)	Meclizine (185)
Metoprolol (9, 19, 88, 170)	Tramadol (47, 138)	Estrogen vaginal (92)	Amitriptyline (134)	Norethindrone/ ethinylestradiol (188)
Montelukast (10)	Levofloxacin (48)	Oseltamivir (93)	Naproxen (135, 195)	Buprenorphine (189)
Escitalopram (11)	Fluoxetine (49, 121)	Tiotropium bromide (94)	Niacin (136)	Raloxifene (190)
Salbutamol/albuterol (13, 129, 132)	Prednisone (50, 165, 183)	Aripiprazole (95)	Allopurinol (137)	omega-3-acid ethyl esters (191)
Simvastatin (14, 20, 26, 69)	Omeprazole (51, 55, 77, 101)	Methylphenidate (97)	Hydrochlorothiazide/losartan (140)	Lidocaine (194)
Amlodipine (15, 38)	Atenolol (53, 85, 157, 177, 184)	Digoxin (99)	Tolterodine (141)	Ramipril (196)
Azithromycin (16, 29, 98)	Insulin glargine (54)	Fexofenadine (102)	Norgestimate/ethinylestradiol (145)	Benazapril (197)
Metformin (17, 87, 178)		Olmesartan (104)	Penicillin VK (146)	Verapamil (198)
				(continued)

Table 12.1 (*Continued*)

Drug (Rank)	Drug (Rank)	Drug (Rank)	Drug (Rank)	Drug (Rank)
Hydrochlorothiazide (21, 52)	Amoxicillin/potassium clavulanate (56, 91)	Pravastatin (105, 199)	Mineral supplement (147, 187)	Ranitidine (200)
Rosuvastatin (22)	Fenofibrate (59)	Triamterene/hydrochlorothiazide (106, 118)	Codeine/guaifenesin (148)	
	Celecoxib (60)			
Furosemide (23, 96, 152)	Donepezil (61)	Methylprednisolone (107)	Glyburide (149)	
Warfarin (24, 80)	Ezetimibe/simvastatin (62)	Cyclobenzaprine (108, 125)	Fluticasone (151)	
Fluticasone/salmeterol (25)	Cephalexin (63)	Clonidine (109)	Rabeprazole (153)	
Ibuprofen (27, 171)	Mometasone (64)	Risedronate (110)	Lisdexamfetamine (154)	
Sertraline (28)	Drospirenone/ethinylestradiol (65)	Diazepam (111)	Isosorbide mononitrate (155)	
Valsartan (30)	Vitamin D (67)	Carisoprodol (112)	Lamotrigine (156)	
Zolpidem (31, 123)	Ezetimibe (68)	Promethazine (113)	Olanzapine (158)	
Oxycodone/acetaminophen (33, 57, 175)	Gabapentin (70, 186)	Memantine (114)	Lovastatin (159)	
Duloxetine (92)	Pregabalin (71)	Potassium chloride (115, 192)	Ethinylestradiol (161)	
Quetiapine (87)	Sildenafil (72)	Citalopram (116, 142, 193)	Bupropion (162)	
Venlafaxine (93)	Acetaminophen/codeine (73)	Drospirenone (117)	Doxycycline (164)	
Tamsulosin (102)	Fluconazole (75)	Meloxicam (119)	Lisinopril/hydrochlorothiazide (166)	
Alprazolam (39, 58, 83, 122)	Fluticasone (75, 100)	Latanoprost (120)	Enalapril (173)	

Multiple ranks signify that the generic drug is sold by more than one vendor.

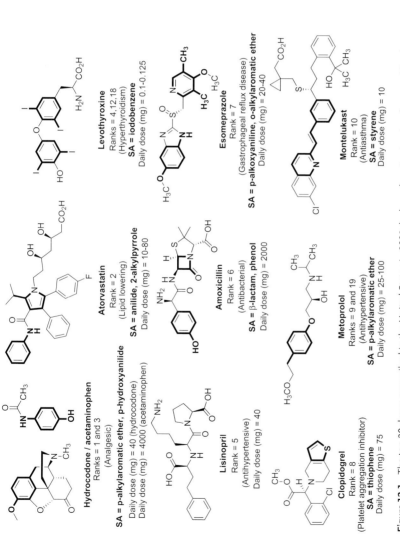

Figure 12.1 The top 20 drugs prescribed in the United States in 2009: hydrocodone/acetaminophen combination, metoprolol, and simvastatin are featured twice in the list, whereas levothyroxine appears thrice in the list of 20 drugs. Multiple ranks for a given drug imply that generic versions are sold by more than one vendor. Structural alerts are highlighted in bold.

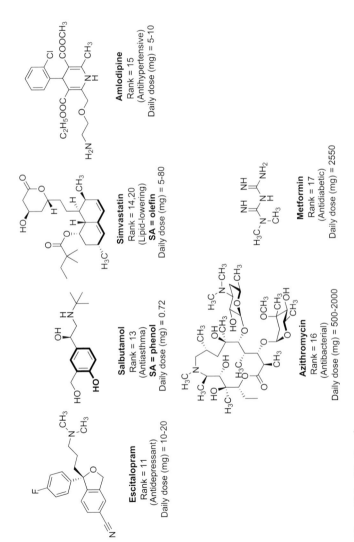

Escitalopram
Rank = 11
(Antidepressant)
Daily dose (mg) = 10–20

Salbutamol
Rank = 13
(Antiasthma)
SA = phenol
Daily dose (mg) = 0.72

Simvastatin
Rank = 14,20
(Lipid-lowering)
SA = olefin
Daily dose (mg) = 5–80

Amlodipine
Rank = 15
(Antihypertensive)
Daily dose (mg) = 5–10

Azithromycin
Rank = 16
(Antibacterial)
Daily dose (mg) = 500–2000

Metformin
Rank = 17
(Antidiabetic)
Daily dose (mg) = 2550

Figure 12.1 (*Continued*)

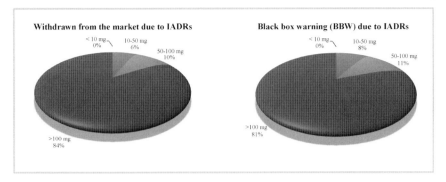

Figure 12.2 Daily dose trends for drugs ($n = 68$) associated with idiosyncratic toxicity.

in Figure 12.1). Two of the most prescribed drugs, esomeprazole and clopidogrel, require metabolic activation for their pharmacology, while amoxicillin is an irreversible covalent inhibitor that does not require bioactivation for acylating its target enzyme.

12.2.3
Evidence for Metabolic Activation to Reactive Metabolites

The most widely dispensed retail prescription in the United States (128 million dispensed prescriptions) in 2009 was the pain reliever Vicodin, which combines the narcotic hydrocodone with acetaminophen. In that same year, a US Food and Drug Administration (FDA) advisory panel voted by a narrow margin to advise the FDA to remove Vicodin and the related painkiller, Percocet (oxycodone/acetaminophen), from the market because of "a high likelihood of overdose from prescription narcotics and acetaminophen products." The FDA panel cited concerns over the potential for liver damage from the acetaminophen component present in these combinations. The acetaminophen–narcotic combination has special hazards if patients develop a tolerance to the narcotic and increase their daily intake of the prescribed medication, leading to a potentially fatal acetaminophen overdose. Each year, acetaminophen overdose is linked to about 400 deaths and 42 000 hospitalizations. At the recommended dosing regimen, the reactive quinone imine metabolite of acetaminophen is detoxified by glutathione (GSH) stores in the liver. However, an acute overdose of acetaminophen depletes the GSH pool, and, as a result, the quinone imine species accumulates in the liver, causing hepatocellular necrosis and possibly damage to other organs [2]. The antidote to acetaminophen overdose is the thiol nucleophile *N*-acetylcysteine (an orally bioavailable antioxidant), which replenishes hepatic GSH and prevents further damage to the liver [3].

In the case of the lipid-lowering agent atorvastatin, cytochrome P450 (CYP) 3A4–catalyzed monohydroxylation(s) on its acetanilide structural alert results in the formation of the corresponding *ortho*- and *para*-hydroxyacetanilide metabolites, which can be potentially oxidized to reactive quinone imine species, similar to acetaminophen (Figure 12.3) [4]. Consistent with this hypothesis, atorvastatin has been

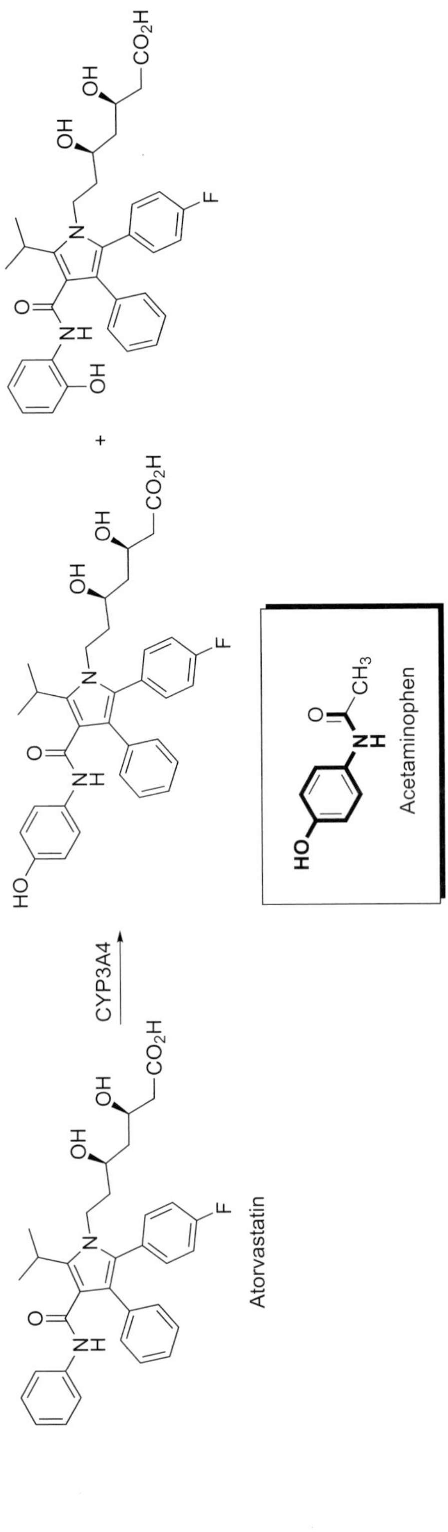

Figure 12.3 Metabolism of atorvastatin to acetaminophen-like metabolites (and potential reactive metabolite precursors).

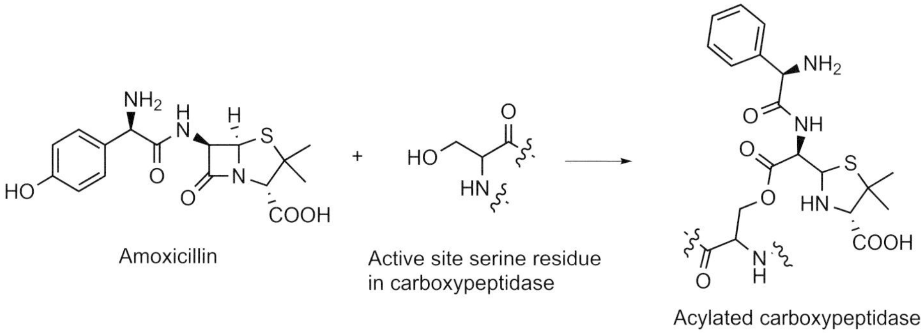

Figure 12.4 Biochemical basis of the antibacterial effects of amoxicillin.

shown to covalently bind to human liver microsomes (HLM) in a NADPH-dependent fashion [5]. Insight into the reactive metabolite structure, which causes microsomal covalent binding, however, has not been determined.

Amoxicillin belongs to the class of β-lactam antibacterial agents whose bacteriocidal action is linked with their ability to react with the serine-type D-ala-D-ala carboxypeptidase. This enzyme is a serine protease involved in the bacterial synthesis of the peptidoglycan layer in the cell wall. All β-lactam antibacterial agents, including amoxicillin, irreversibly acylate the active site serine forming a serine ester–linked adduct (Figure 12.4) [6].

The proton pump inhibitor esomeprazole elicits its pharmacological effects through covalent modification of the gastric ATPase [7]. As such, proton transport by the gastric H^+/K^+-ATPase is the final step in gastric acid secretion. The mechanism of covalent modification by proton pump inhibitors has been extensively studied [8]. As illustrated with esomeprazole, proton pump inhibitors are prodrugs that transform under the acidic environment of the stomach to a spiro intermediate, which then undergoes rearomatization with elimination to a sulfenic acid derivative followed by subsequent dehydration to a tetracyclic sulfenamide analogue. The sulfenamide intermediate reacts irreversibly with an active site cysteine in gastric ATPase to form an adduct and leads to inactivation of the proton pump (Figure 12.5). Besides the formation of the "active" reactive metabolite, it is also interesting to note that omeprazole (the racemic form of esomeprazole) and related proton pump inhibitors are capable of reacting with GSH in HLM in a non-NADPH-dependent fashion [9] indicating that these drugs are intrinsically electrophilic [9]. The detection of the corresponding mercapturic acid analogue (derived from downstream GSH degradation as shown in Figure 12.5) in rat urine following omeprazole administration indicates the existence of this pathway *in vivo* [10]. Conventional alerts, that is, the *para*-alkoxyaniline and *para*-alkylaromatic ether motif found in esomeprazole, do not appear to be susceptible to metabolic activation.

First launched in 1999 in the United States, the blockbuster cardiovascular drug and P2Y12 purinoreceptor antagonist clopidogrel is used in the reduction of atherosclerotic events in patients with stroke, myocardial infarction, or peripheral

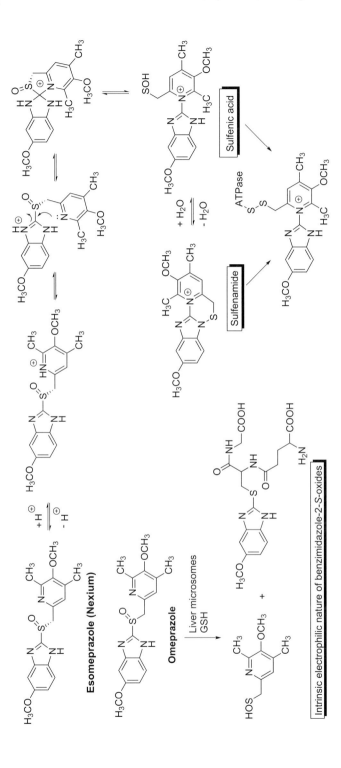

Figure 12.5 Covalent modification of gastric ATPase by a reactive metabolite of esomeprazole and the intrinsic electrophilic nature of the benzimidazole-2-S-oxide motif in the proton pump inhibitors.

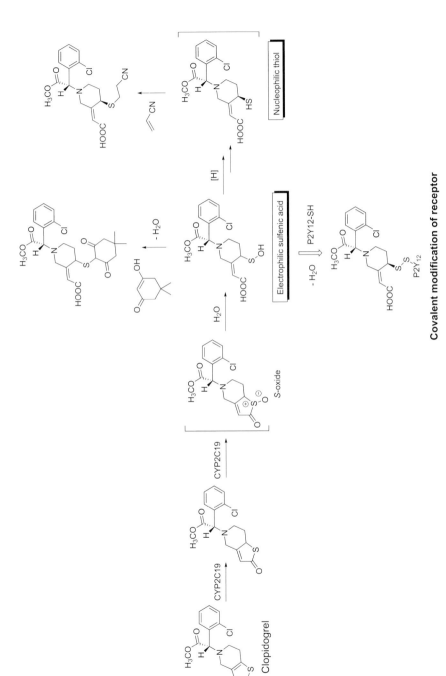

Figure 12.6 Metabolic activation of clopidogrel by CYP2C19 to a reactive metabolite that is responsible for its inhibitory effects on platelet aggregation.

arterial diseases. A prerequisite for clopidogrel pharmacology is its conversion by CYP enzyme(s) to a reactive metabolite that inhibits platelet aggregation by irreversibly inhibiting the P2Y12 receptor in platelets [11]. Based on *in vitro* metabolism studies, it has been speculated that the active metabolite of clopidogrel is a thiol derivative, which forms a covalent disulfide linkage with a cysteinyl residue on the P2Y12 receptor in platelets (Figure 12.6) [12, 13]. However, as shown recently by Dansette *et al.* [14], the molecular species that actually modifies the receptor almost certainly is the sulfenic acid intermediate (an electrophile), and not the thiol, which is nucleophilic in nature. The electrophilic sulfenic acid species derived from a CYP2C19-mediated thiophene ring scission has been trapped in HLM using dimedone as a nucleophilic trapping agent, whereas the nucleophilicity of the thiol metabolite is evident from the characterization of a thioether metabolite following reaction with the exogenously added electrophile acrylonitrile (Figure 12.6).

The antiasthma drug montelukast possesses a styrene motif, which appears to be intrinsically electrophilic, based on evidence of the direct conjugation of montelukast with dansyl-GSH (a fluorescent derivative of GSH) in HLM in the absence of NADPH cofactor [9]. The olefin alerts in simvastatin are the principal sites of oxidative metabolism by CYP3A4 to the corresponding hydroxy and dihydrodiol metabolites [15]; however, there are no GSH trapping data to support the involvement of reactive epoxide intermediates in the course of simvastatin biotransformation. Weak covalent binding to HLM by simvastatin has been demonstrated; the requirement of NADPH further supports the role of CYP3A4 in the bioactivation process [16, 17].

Finally, there is no evidence for reactive metabolite formation with levothyroxine, metoprolol, and salbutamol, all of which possess structural alerts. The thyroid hormone levothyroxine contains the iodobenzene group that, in principle, can form a putative reactive epoxide in a manner similar to bromobenzene; however, the major elimination pathway of this drug involves conjugation of the phenolic OH group to form a sulfate metabolite [18]. The β-blocker metoprolol contains the *para*-alkylaromatic ether architecture that on O-dealkylation can yield a quinone methide precursor. While metoprolol is subject to extensive oxidative metabolism in humans, the biotransformation pathways do not involve reactive metabolite formation and instead proceed via N-demethylation, benzylic hydroxylation, and O-demethylation of the terminal methoxy group [19]. The phenol group in the β2-agonist salbutamol can be oxidized to an *ortho*-quinone via the intermediate catechol metabolite. However, conjugation of the phenol moiety is the principal pathway through which salbutamol is eliminated in humans [20].

12.3
Insights Into the Excellent Safety Records for Reactive Metabolite–Positive Blockbuster Drugs

In general, liver toxicity has been a concern since the initial introduction of statins, but several clinical trials have shown that statins are safe to use for the prevention

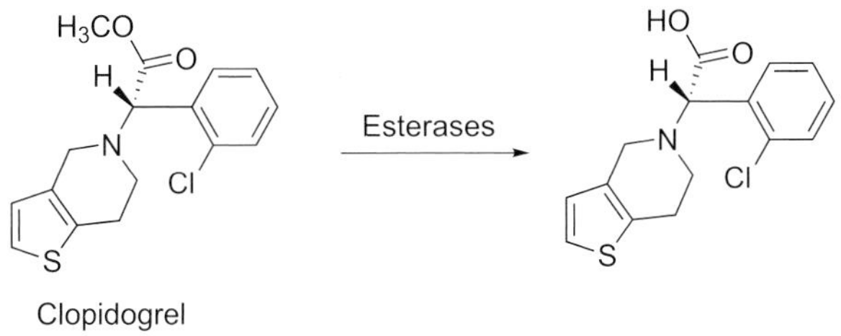

Figure 12.7 Major clearance mechanism of clopidogrel in humans.

of coronary disease and death, even in the setting of chronic liver disease. Irreversible liver damage leading to fatalities or liver transplantation appears to be extremely uncommon with statins. In fact, the incidence of liver enzyme elevations in the statin-treated population has not been consistently different than in placebo-treated patients. Consequently, the excellent safety record of atorvastatin despite the reactive metabolite liability can be potentially explained by its low efficacious daily dose of 10–20 mg, which could reduce the body burden to reactive metabolite exposure. Likewise, reactive metabolite formation with clopidogrel poses a fundamental question from a structure–toxicity perspective: why is clopidogrel not associated with a high incidence of idiosyncratic toxicity despite forming reactive metabolites and despite being administered at a relatively high daily dose of 75 mg? A plausible reason is that the majority (>70%) of the clopidogrel daily dose is rapidly hydrolyzed by human carboxylesterases to the inactive carboxylic acid metabolite (~80–85% of circulating metabolites) (Figure 12.7) [21], which means that only a small percentage of the parent drug (20 mg or less) is theoretically available for conversion to the active reactive metabolite. Indeed, covalent binding to platelets accounts for only 2% of radiolabeled clopidogrel in human mass balance studies (Plavix package insert).

In the case of the proton pump inhibitors such as esomeprazole, the formation of the active reactive species formation is catalyzed by acid and occurs locally at the site of action, so systemic exposure to reactive species (sulfenic acid and sulfenamide) is probably not achieved. Furthermore, it is likely that the GSH displacement reaction discerned with omeprazole in HLM has no toxicological relevance, especially given the low daily efficacious doses and minimal hepatic/systemic exposure of esomeprazole and related proton pump inhibitors in humans.

Finally, while β-lactam antibiotics are generally well tolerated, they are also frequently associated with IADRs such as allergy and anaphylaxis. The acute nature of the treatment most likely aids the tolerability, considering that the daily doses of these agents are very high (>1 g). The IADRs associated with β-lactams such as penicillin have been studied in great detail. In some patients, indiscriminant acylation of free amino and sulfydryl groups on proteins via a nonenzymatic β-lactam ring scission leads to an immune response against the penicillin–protein adduct, and if the antibody response generates sufficient IgE antibodies, a severe allergic reaction such as anaphylaxis can occur [22–24]. On the basis of this knowledge, it was possible to develop a test for penicillin allergy in which penicillin bound to a lysine polymer, when injected on the skin, can cause degranulation of mast cells leading to a local wheal and flare response. The mechanism of penicillin-induced allergic reactions fits the hapten hypothesis where the chemical reactivity of the penicillin allows it to generate a hapten. In fact, one of the principal metabolites of amoxicillin in humans is derived from the hydrolysis of the β-lactam ring [25].

12.4
Structural Alert and Reactive Metabolite Analyses for the Remaining 180 Most Prescribed Drugs

Among the remaining 180 drugs, there are only a handful of cases where incidences of mechanism-independent adverse drug reactions have been noted. Drugs associated with IADRs include lamotrigine, sulfamethoxazole/trimethoprim (co-trimoxole), furosemide, trazodone, fluconazole, amitriptyline, niacin, glyburide, and β-lactam antibiotics exemplified by amoxicillin/potassium clavulanate (Figure 12.8). It is noteworthy to point out that lamotrigine and

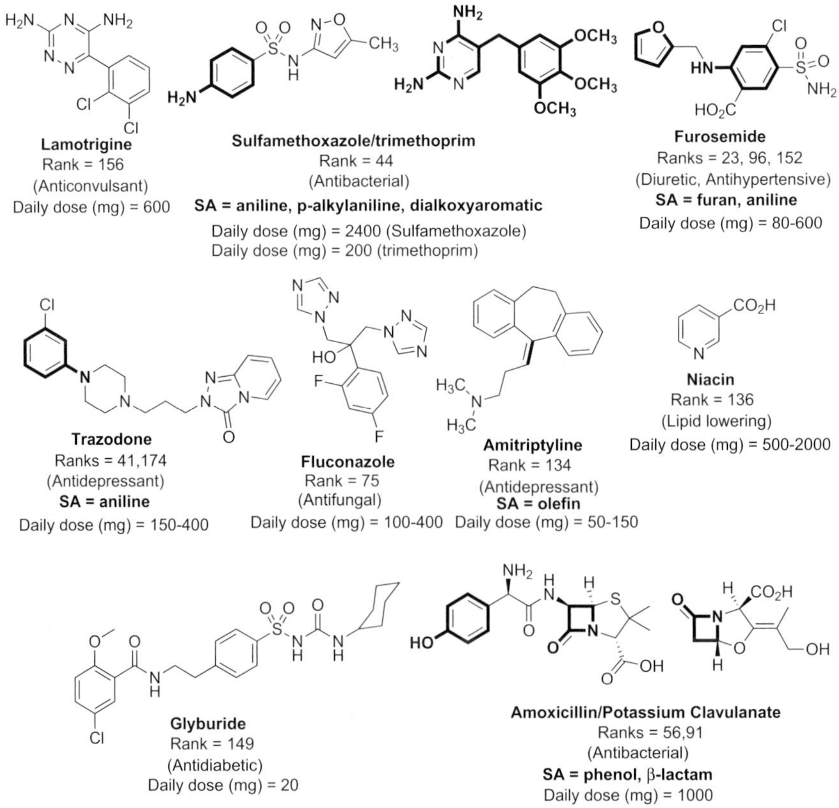

Lamotrigine
Rank = 156
(Anticonvulsant)
Daily dose (mg) = 600

Sulfamethoxazole/trimethoprim
Rank = 44
(Antibacterial)
SA = aniline, p-alkylaniline, dialkoxyaromatic
Daily dose (mg) = 2400 (Sulfamethoxazole)
Daily dose (mg) = 200 (trimethoprim)

Furosemide
Ranks = 23, 96, 152
(Diuretic, Antihypertensive)
SA = furan, aniline
Daily dose (mg) = 80-600

Trazodone
Ranks = 41,174
(Antidepressant)
SA = aniline
Daily dose (mg) = 150-400

Fluconazole
Rank = 75
(Antifungal)
Daily dose (mg) = 100-400

Amitriptyline
Rank = 134
(Antidepressant)
SA = olefin
Daily dose (mg) = 50-150

Niacin
Rank = 136
(Lipid lowering)
Daily dose (mg) = 500-2000

Glyburide
Rank = 149
(Antidiabetic)
Daily dose (mg) = 20

Amoxicillin/Potassium Clavulanate
Ranks = 56,91
(Antibacterial)
SA = phenol, β-lactam
Daily dose (mg) = 1000

Figure 12.8 Widely prescribed drugs associated with idiosyncratic toxicity. Structural alerts are highlighted in bold.

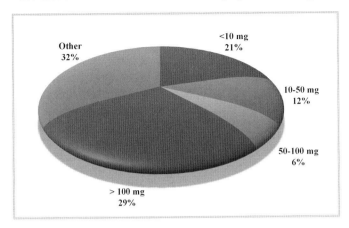

Figure 12.9 Maximum recommended daily doses for the remaining top 180 drugs in the United States based on dispensed prescriptions. "Other" signifies vitamins, biologics, and/or drugs administered via the intravenous route.

sulfamethoxazole/trimethoprim (co-trimoxole) carry black box warnings for skin rashes, blood dyscrasias, and/or hepatotoxicity, but are still widely prescribed. As stated earlier, multiple ranks for the individual drugs indicate that generic versions are marketed by more than one vendor. The daily dose trends for the remaining 180 drugs are shown in Figure 12.9.

Although well tolerated in most patients, the anticonvulsant lamotrigine is associated with a relatively high incidence (>10%) of immune-mediated hypersensitivity reactions including skin rashes, hepatotoxicity, and blood dyscrasias. Although lamotrigine does not contain conventional structural alerts, two separate accounts have demonstrated the formation of an electrophilic epoxide intermediate on the dichlorophenyl ring that can be trapped by GSH (Figure 12.10) [26, 27]. The finding that human epidermal keratinocytes are capable of forming the same GSH conjugate identified in HLM strengthens the link between reactive metabolite formation and the immune-mediated nature of the idiosyncratic cutaneous reactions [28]. Likewise, the relatively high incidence of immune-mediated toxicities (blood dyscrasias, skin rashes, hepatotoxicity) associated with the antibacterial drug sulfamethoxazole have been linked with the oxidative bioactivation of the aniline structural alert to the corresponding hydroxylamine and nitroso intermediates (see Figure 12.10) [29]. The electrophilic nitroso metabolites covalently bind to microsomal protein and human neutrophils, and/or react with GSH to form the corresponding sulfinamide derivatives [30]. Sulfamethoxazole can also be oxidized in keratinocytes, implying that bioactivation and T cell sensitization could occur directly on the skin leading to the severe cutaneous reactions [31]. *N*-Acetylation by *N*-acetyltransferase (NAT) 1 and the polymorphic NAT2 constitutes the major metabolic fate of sulfamethoxazole in humans. Clinical studies with sulfamethoxazole have indicated that patients of the rapid acetylator phenotype require a longer period of time to develop toxicity than those of slow acetylator phenotype, presumably due to the involvement of NAT2 in the elimination of the hydroxylamine

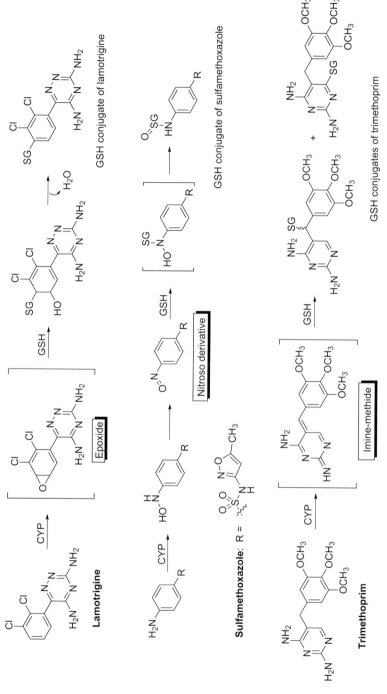

Figure 12.10 Metabolic activation of the anticonvulsant lamotrigine and the antibacterial agents sulfamethoxazole/trimethoprim to reactive metabolites.

metabolites of sulfamethoxazole [32]. Recent studies have revealed the susceptibility of trimethoprim to form a reactive imine-methide species via metabolism of the *para*-alkylaniline alert in HLM (Figure 12.10) [33, 34]. Reactive metabolite arising from the catechol/quinone pathway following *O*-demethylation has also been noted by Uetrecht *et al.* in HLM incubations of trimethoprim [34]. The bioactivation pathways are compatible with the primary metabolic pathways of trimethoprim in humans, which involve *O*-demethylation of the trimethoxybenzene group and hydroxylation of the methylene carbon.

Furosemide is a loop diuretic used in the treatment of edematous states associated with cardiac, renal, and hepatic failure, and for the treatment of hypertension. Furosemide use has been associated with cases of idiosyncratic hepatitis, which have been linked with the bioactivation of its furan structural alert to a reactive epoxide species by CYP enzymes [35, 36]. Similar to acetaminophen, furosemide hepatotoxicity is dependent on dose and can be replicated in rodents [35]. Although the NADPH-dependent microsomal covalent binding of furosemide is significantly attenuated in the presence of GSH [37], the toxicity of furosemide in mice does not result from simple depletion of the thiol antioxidant as is the case with acetaminophen.

Trazodone is a second-generation nontricyclic antidepressant, which is coprescribed with other antidepressants as a sleep-inducing agent because of its sedative side effects. Although trazodone has not served as frontline therapy in the treatment of CNS disorders, there are some reported cases of rare but severe hepatotoxicity associated with its use, which have been linked to its metabolic activation to reactive species (Figure 12.11) [38]. *para*-Hydroxytrazodone, which has been detected as a major urinary metabolite in humans, is bioactivated to a reactive quinone imine species that is trapped with GSH in HLM incubations. Furthermore, the detection of a dihydrodiol metabolite of trazodone in human urine suggests a second bioactivation sequence involving the formation of an electrophilic epoxide on the triazolopyridinone moiety [38]. Consistent with this hypothesis, HLM and recombinant CYP3A4 incubations of trazodone in the presence of GSH have led to the detection of stable dihydrodiol and a thiol conjugate derived from epoxide ring opening (Figure 12.11) [38].

Despite current treatment guidelines that recommend the use of tricyclic antidepressants only in patients with psychosis and treatment resistance, amitriptyline is widely prescribed throughout the world presumably because of its favorable cost/benefit ratio. A causal link between hepatotoxicity and amitriptyline metabolism has been established. Using GSH as a trapping agent in HLM, Wen *et al.* trapped an aromatic ring epoxide, the intermediate that leads to the dihydrodiol metabolite of amitriptyline, which has been detected in human urine (Figure 12.12) [39, 40]. A similar bioactivation pathway has been noted with nortriptyline [39], the *N*-dealkylated metabolite of amitriptyline and a standalone antidepressant agent that is also associated with idiosyncratic hepatotoxicity [41]. As such, the olefin structural alert in amitriptyline is not subject to bioactivation; like lamotrigine, it is the aromatic ring that is metabolized to an electrophilic epoxide intermediate.

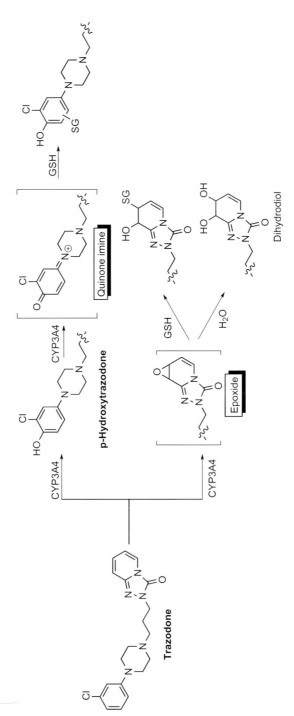

Figure 12.11 Metabolic activation of the antidepressant trazodone.

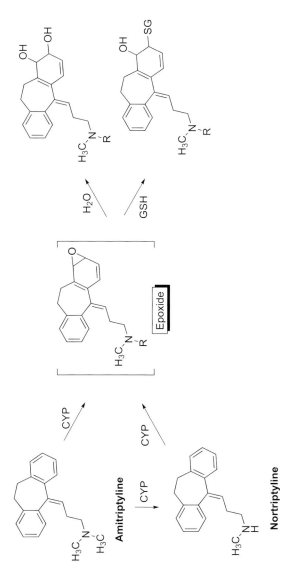

Figure 12.12 Metabolism of the antidepressant amitriptyline and its N-dealkylated metabolite nortriptyline into reactive metabolites.

The antihyperlipidemic drug with the highest potential for hepatic injury is the sustained-release formulation of niacin. Any formulation of niacin can cause hepatotoxicity in daily doses that exceed 2000–3000 mg, but the sustained-release formulation is significantly more hepatotoxic [42]. The immediate-release formulations of niacin in usual therapeutic doses almost never causes serious liver injury. Although niacin does not contain conventional structural alerts, the hepatotoxic effects are believed to be related to its metabolism by a high-affinity, low-capacity amidation pathway that leads to nicotinamide (niacinamide) and N-methyl-2- and N-methyl-4-pyridone-5-carboxamide metabolites; thus, the sustained-release formulation can lead to higher levels of toxic metabolites [43]. The alternative competing metabolic pathway is a low-affinity, high-capacity conjugation pathway (involving the formation of a glycine amide metabolite) that leads to prostaglandin-mediated vasodilation and subsequent cutaneous flushing [43]. The immediate-release formulation overwhelms the higher affinity amidation/oxidation pathway, and the majority of the niacin dose is metabolized via the high-capacity glycine conjugation pathway, leading to a much lower rate of hepatotoxicity. Extended-release niacin has an intermediate rate of dissolution and can be associated with both flushing and hepatotoxicity.

The antidiabetic agent glyburide does not contain structural alerts, but is associated with potent inhibition of the bile salt export pump (BSEP) [44]. In the clinic, glyburide is associated with much greater incidence and severity of hepatic injury than any of the older sulfonyl ureas such as chlorpropamide, which does not inhibit BSEP [45]. Consequently, the inhibitory effects of glyburide against BSEP may be a crucial determinant of its hepatic injury potential despite a low daily dose of 20 mg. BSEP is critically involved in the secretion of bile salts into bile; its impairment may lead to cholestasis and accumulation of cytotoxic bile salts in hepatocytes and, consequently, to liver disease [46]. Genetic studies have shown that polymorphism(s) in the gene coding for BSEP and/or inherited mutations lead to progressive familial intrahepatic cholestasis and severe liver disease [47].

The azole antifungal agent fluconazole also does not contain alerts in its structure, but its use has been associated with severe or lethal hepatotoxicity [48]. The spectrum of hepatic reactions ranges from mild transient elevations in transaminase levels to hepatitis, cholestasis, and fulminant hepatic failure. Fatal reactions can also occur in patients with serious underlying medical illness. Related azole antifungals ketoconazole and itraconazole are potent BSEP inhibitors, which raises the possibility that hepatotoxicity associated with fluconazole is mediated via inhibition of the bile salt transporter [44].

Potassium clavulanate is used in conjunction with amoxicillin (combination sold as augmentin) to destroy penicillin-resistant strains of bacteria. By itself, clavulanate does not possess antibacterial activity. Bacteria produce the serine hydrolase β-lactamase to hydrolyze carboxypeptidase inhibitors, forming a hydrolytically labile serine ester–linked adduct. Reactions between the catalytic serine residue in β-lactamase and specific β-lactamase inhibitors such as clavulanate result in the formation of stable adducts derived from β-lactam ring opening, functionally inactivating the bacterial resistance mechanism. While the rate of hepatic injury with amoxicillin is very low, combination with clavulanate increases this risk [49]. Evidence that clavulanate is principally responsible for hepatotoxicity stems from the observation that clavulanate combined with other β-lactams can also lead to liver injury [50]. A genetic basis for amoxicillin/clavulanate hepatotoxicity has been identified with linkage to the HLA haplotype suggesting that the hepatotoxicity has an immunological component [51]. Furthermore, individuals with GSH transferase null genotypes are known to be at an increased risk of amoxicillin–clavulanate hepatotoxicity, a finding that is consistent with a deficiency in clavulanate detoxification by GSH [52]. All of the current evidence points out to a role for reactive metabolites in clavulanate-mediated hepatotoxicity.

12.4.1
Structural Alert and/or Reactive Metabolite "False Positives"

Out of a shortened list of ∼93 drugs from the most prescribed category (biologics, small molecule injectables, topical agents, vitamins, and mineral supplements have not been considered in the discussion; furthermore, there are several instances where a particular drug is repeated due to its combination with other medications, e.g., the loop diuretic hydrochlorothiazide appears as a single agent, as well as in combination with antihypertensive agents, lisinopril, valsartan, losartan, triamterene, and olmesartan – see Table 12.1), 45 drugs were devoid of structural alerts. Drugs that lack structural alerts include aliphatic compounds with low (e.g., alendronic acid, risedronic acid, and ibandronic acid) to high (e.g., gabapentin, pregabalin, carisoprodol, memantine, isosorbide mononitrate, etc.) daily doses. Additional drugs that lack structural alerts include zolpidem, alprazolam, tramadol, atenolol, celecoxib, valacylcovir, methylphenidate, citalopram, sitagliptin, lisdexamfetamine, bupropion, doxycycline, eszopiclone, meclizine, and so on. Figure 12.13 lists some of the structures of these drugs. There is no description of metabolic activation to reactive metabolites and/or BSEP inhibition for most of these drugs that are devoid of structural alerts. One can only conclude that lack of *in vitro* safety findings tracks with the general clinical safety, despite administration at high daily doses in several cases (e.g., tramadol at 200–300 mg, celecoxib at 200–400 mg, etc.) [1].

Of the 48 drugs that contain structural alerts, evidence for reactive metabolite formation has been presented in ∼19 cases. Foremost among these are prescription strength nonsteroidal anti-inflammatory drugs (NSAIDs) ibuprofen and naproxen that form electrophilic acyl glucuronides as a principal metabolic fate in humans (Figure 12.14) [53, 54]. IADRs such as hepatotoxicity are extremely rare with these NSAIDs despite administration at very high doses and despite the formation of protein-reactive acyl glucuronide metabolites [55, 56]. In contrast with ibuprofen, ibufenac (see Figure 12.14) was withdrawn from commercial use due to several cases of acute hepatotoxicity [57]. The only structural difference in the two drugs is the presence of the extra methyl group in ibuprofen. It has been suggested that the ibufenac acyl glucuronide is more reactive toward proteins than the acyl glucuronide metabolite of ibuprofen, leading to a greater incidence of hepatotoxicity in the clinic [58].

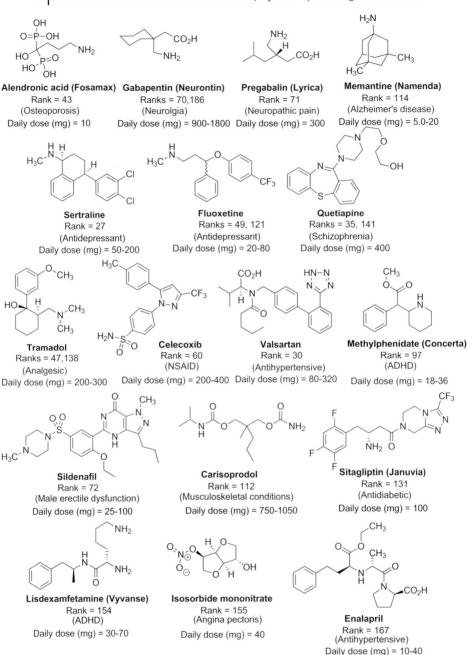

Figure 12.13 Examples of drugs from the "most prescribed" list that do not contain structural alerts and are devoid of idiosyncratic toxicity, some despite high daily doses.

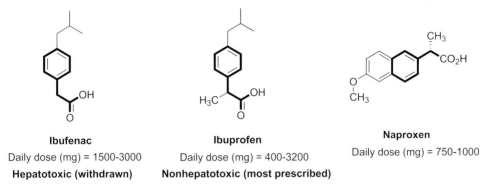

Ibufenac
Daily dose (mg) = 1500-3000
Hepatotoxic (withdrawn)

Ibuprofen
Daily dose (mg) = 400-3200
Nonhepatotoxic (most prescribed)

Naproxen
Daily dose (mg) = 750-1000

Figure 12.14 Structures of NSAIDs naproxen and ibuprofen, which form electrophilic acyl glucuronide metabolites in humans. Ibufenac is an NSAID that was withdrawn due to significant hepatotoxicity incidences.

The list of reactive metabolite–positive drugs also includes the proton pump inhibitors lansoprazole, omeprazole (the racemic form of esomeprazole), pantoprazole, and rabeprazole, which require bioactivation to the electrophilic sulfenamide intermediate for their pharmacological action. In addition, GSH conjugates derived from the reaction of the thiol at the C2 position of the benzimidazole ring have been observed in HLM and in rats, phenomena that reflect the electrophilic nature of the benzimidazole-S-oxide motif in these compounds. Despite the metabolic activation liability, these drugs are widely prescribed, and are generally devoid of idiosyncratic adverse effects. Like esomeprazole, the generic proton pump inhibitors are low daily dose drugs (Figure 12.15).

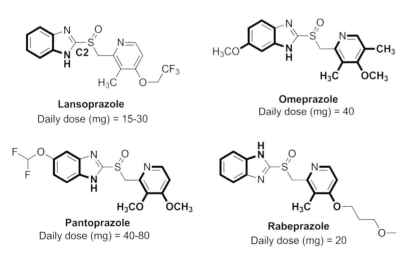

Lansoprazole
Daily dose (mg) = 15-30

Omeprazole
Daily dose (mg) = 40

Pantoprazole
Daily dose (mg) = 40-80

Rabeprazole
Daily dose (mg) = 20

Figure 12.15 Structures of the proton pump inhibitors. Structural alerts are highlighted in bold. The C2 position on the benzimidazole ring is electrophilic.

Paroxetine is a selective serotonin reuptake inhibitor, which contains the 1,3-benzodioxole structural alert. The principal pathway of paroxetine metabolism in humans involves CYP2D6-mediated 1,3-benzodioxole ring scission to a catechol intermediate. This process also leads to mechanism-based inactivation of the CYP isozyme and drug–drug interaction with CYP2D6 substrates in the clinic. *In vitro* studies with [^{3}H]-paroxetine have demonstrated the NADPH-dependent covalent binding to human liver microsomal and S9 proteins, and the characterization of sulfydryl conjugates of reactive quinone metabolites (Figure 12.16) [59]. The observation that GSH and/or *S*-adenosyl methionine dramatically reduced microsomal and S9 covalent binding implied the existence of competing, detoxification pathways of paroxetine metabolism. The likely reason is that the catechol metabolite obtained via ring scission of the 1,3-benzodioxole group can partition between *O*-methylation by catechol-*O*-methyltransferase or undergo oxidation to the reactive *ortho*-quinone intermediate, which is efficiently scavenged by GSH. In humans, the *O*-methylated catechol derivatives constitute the principal metabolic fate of the drug [60]. When coupled with the fact that the clinically effective daily dose of paroxetine is low (20 mg), some insight into the excellent safety record of this drug is obtained, despite the reactive metabolite liability.

Likewise, the 1,3-benzodioxole alert in tadalafil (Figure 12.17) is also metabolized by CYP3A4 to an electrophilic catechol/*ortho*-quinone species, which leads to concomitant enzyme inactivation [61]. However, there are no reports of idiosyncratic toxicity and/or drug–drug interactions associated with tadalafil in erectile dysfunction treatment at the recommended low daily doses between 5 and 20 mg.

In vitro evidence for the formation of reactive quinone species by CYP3A4 has also been gathered with the selective estrogen receptor modulator raloxifene that is used in the treatment of osteoporosis in postmenopausal women. As shown in Figure 12.18, raloxifene is bioactivated on the phenolic structural alerts to yield reactive quinone species that can be trapped with GSH [62, 63]. The process is accompanied by microsomal covalent binding and irreversible inactivation of the CYP3A4 isozyme [62]. However, *in vivo*, glucuronidation of the same phenolic groups, principally in the gut, constitutes the principal elimination mechanism of raloxifene in humans [64]. Thus, the likelihood of raloxifene bioactivation *in vivo* is in question when compared with the efficiency of the glucuronidation in the small intestine, a phenomenon that may provide an explanation for the extremely rare occurrence of toxicity despite a relatively high daily dose of 60 mg.

Cyclobenzaprine is a skeletal muscle relaxant that contains two olefin structural alerts. While the principal metabolic fate of this drug in humans involves *N*-glucuronidation, a significant proportion (∼7–10% of the administered dose) of a dihydrodiol (10,11-dihydroxynortriptyline) metabolite has been detected in human urine, which implies the formation of an electrophilic epoxide intermediate (Figure 12.19) [65]. However, no incidences of toxicity have been reported with this drug at its low daily dose range of 10–30 mg.

In HLM, GSH conjugates believed to arise from the conjugation of the thiol nucleophile to quinone imine intermediates and catechol/*ortho*-quinone species have been reported with the mixed α- and β-adrenergic receptor antagonist and

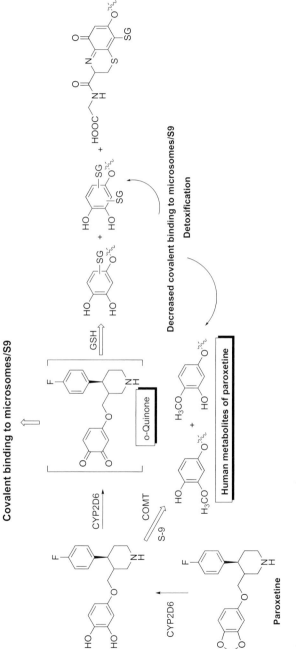

Figure 12.16 Bioactivation and detoxification pathways of the antidepressant paroxetine.

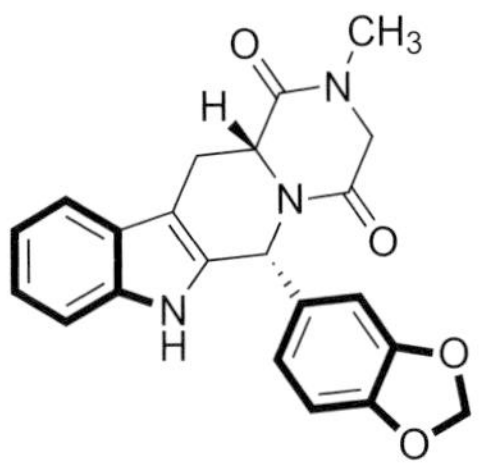

Figure 12.17 Structure of tadalafil, which is metabolized to a catechol derivative by CYP3A4.

antihypertensive drug carvedilol (Figure 12.20) [66]. Formation of the quinone imine species appears to be compatible with the biotransformation pathway of carvedilol that involves aromatic hydroxylation on the carbazole ring to hydroxyaniline-type metabolites. As such, carvedilol is metabolized through *N*-glucuronidation and CYP2D6-mediated oxidative biotransformation pathways, resulting in over 50 metabolites in humans [67]. The clinical dose of carvedilol ranges from 6.25 mg to the maximum recommended daily dose of 100 mg and may provide a rationale for the very rare occurrence of IADRs particularly at the low doses used to treat hypertension.

The loop diuretic hydrochlorothiazide is usually marketed individually or in combination with the angiotensin II receptor antagonists valsartan, losartan, olmesartan, or irbesartan for the treatment of hypertension. Hydrochlorothiazide, losartan, and olmesartan were flagged as structural alert positives. With the exception of losartan, there is no evidence to indicate reactive metabolite formation with hydrochlorothiazide and olmesartan. Hydrochlorothiazide is principally eliminated in humans via renal excretion in the unchanged form, which is facilitated by organic anion transporters [68]. Olmesartan is also eliminated in urine and feces through active hepatobiliary and renal efflux mediated by transport proteins [69]. Losartan undergoes a two-electron oxidation on the 2-alkylimidazole motif to afford a reactive imine-methide species, which is trapped by GSH (Figure 12.21); the bioactivation pathway also leads to HLM covalent binding [70]. However, in humans, there is no evidence for reactive metabolite formation; oxidative metabolism of the primary alcohol moiety leads to an active carboxylic acid metabolite (~15% of the administered losartan dose) (Figure 12.21) [71]. In addition, the majority of a given losartan dose is eliminated in the feces in parent form and as the tetrazole glucuronide conjugate. In contrast with losartan, olmesartan and valsartan do not exhibit microsomal covalent binding.

Lisinopril, benazepril, enalapril, and ramipril (Figure 12.22) are angiotensin-converting enzyme inhibitors, and are used in the treatment of hypertension and/or stroke. Benazepril is the only drug in this group that is structural alert (an anilide functionality) positive. However, in humans, benazepril is principally metabolized through ester hydrolysis followed by glucuronidation [72]. While idiosyncratic toxicity associated with the use of these four drugs is extremely rare, it is interesting to contrast these observations with captopril, the first marketed drug in

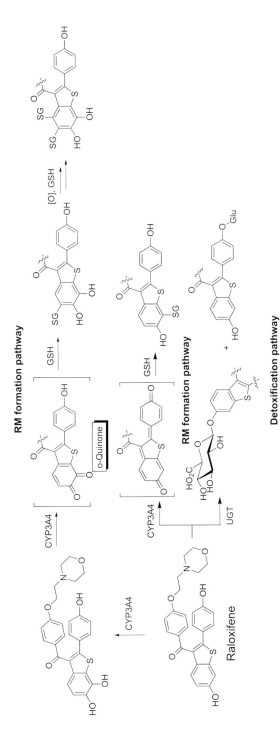

Figure 12.18 Bioactivation pathways of raloxifene.

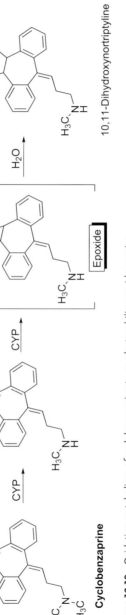

Figure 12.19 Oxidative metabolism of cyclobenzaprine to an electrophilic epoxide species.

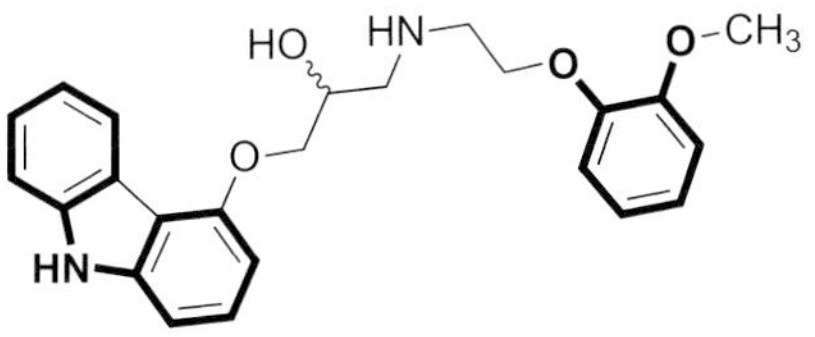

Figure 12.20 Structure of the antihypertensive drug carvedilol.

this category, which contains a free thiol group (Figure 12.22). Unlike the recent angiotensin-converting inhibitors, captopril is a very high-dose drug. When first marketed, captopril was administered at doses up to 1000 mg in severely hypertensive patients. A series of systemic adverse effects including skin rashes, blood dyscrasias, and autoimmune syndromes were reported and the dose dependency of these effects was observed across studies [73]. Conjugates of the free thiol group in captopril with GSH and with cellular proteins have been observed, and have implicated bioactivation of this SH functionality as a plausible cause for toxicity [74].

The anilide structural alert is present in all of the benzodiazepine drugs, clonazepam, lorazepam, and diazepam (Figure 12.23). In addition, clonazepam also contains a *para*-nitroanilide motif. In humans, diazepam and lorazepam are metabolized through innocuous biotransformation pathways (e.g., N-demethylation, aliphatic hydroxylation, O-glucuronidation, etc.) and do not involve aniline ring metabolism. In contrast, the major route of clonazepam metabolism in humans involves the reduction of the *para*-nitroanilide motif to the 7-aminoclonazepam metabolite (presumably via the electrophilic nitroso intermediate), which is then acetylated by polymorphic NAT2 [75]. There are no literature reports on the formation/trapping of reactive species (e.g., nitroso and bis-imine intermediates) in the course of clonazepam metabolism and there is very little evidence for idiosyncratic toxicity with clonazepine. It could be suggested that the low daily dose range of 1.5–20 mg mitigates toxicity risks due to reactive metabolite formation with clonazepam.

In contrast with trovafloxacin, the fluoroquinolone antibiotics, levofloxacin and ciprofloxacin (Figure 12.24), are devoid of idiosyncratic hepatotoxicity despite administration at high daily doses. From a structure–toxicity standpoint, they do not contain the pendant cyclopropylamine functionality at the C7 position of the fluoroquinolone scaffold and cannot form the reactive metabolite, which has been proposed for trovafloxacin [76]. Both levofloxacin and ciprofloxacin contain aniline structural alerts and, in addition, ciprofloxacin also possesses a cyclopropyl group attached to the quinolone nitrogen atom. However, the major clearance pathway(s) in humans occurs via carboxylic acid glucuronidation and/or renal excretion in unchanged form, with little to no contribution from CYP enzymes [77, 78]. Consistent with these *in vivo* observations, levofloxacin does not exhibit covalent binding to HLM [5].

The estrogenic contraceptive ethinylestradiol is sold individually or in combination with other steroidal contraceptives such as drospirenone, norgestimate, and

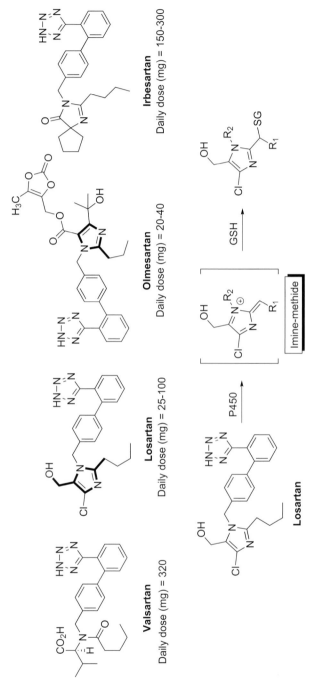

Figure 12.21 Oxidative bioactivation of the antihypertensive agent losartan and structures of related angiotensin II receptor antagonists.

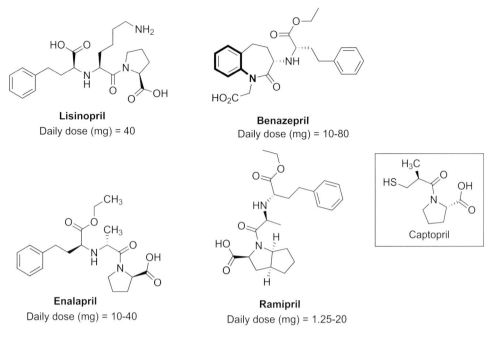

Figure 12.22 Structures of the angiotensin-converting enzyme inhibitors.

norethindrone. Oxidative metabolism of the C-17α terminal alkyne alert present in some of these steroids by CYP3A4 is known to afford a reactive oxirene intermediate, capable of alkylating the heme prosthetic group and/or apoprotein that leads to mechanism-based inactivation of the isozyme (Figure 12.25) [79–81]. In addition, oxidation of the phenol ring in ethinylestradiol also yields an electrophilic *ortho*-quinone species (via the intermediate catechol metabolite) in HLM [82], a process that eventually leads to microsomal covalent binding [5]. Lack of IADRs or drug–drug interactions with CYP3A substrates is most likely due to the very low doses (μg range) of these drugs used in birth control. It is also interesting to note that ethinylestradiol is a potent BSEP inhibitor *in vitro* [44].

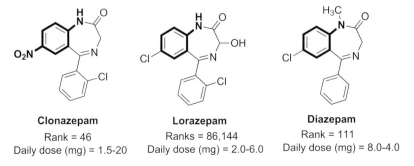

Figure 12.23 Structure of the benzodiazepine drugs that contain an anilide structural alert.

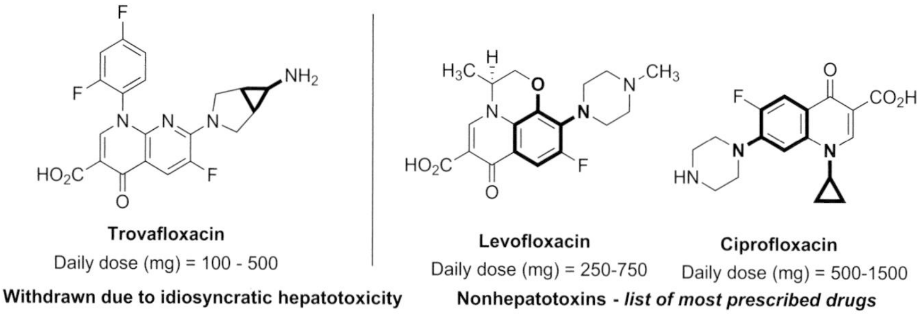

Trovafloxacin
Daily dose (mg) = 100 - 500
Withdrawn due to idiosyncratic hepatotoxicity

Levofloxacin
Daily dose (mg) = 250-750

Ciprofloxacin
Daily dose (mg) = 500-1500

Nonhepatotoxins - *list of most prescribed drugs*

Figure 12.24 Structures of fluoroquinolone antibiotics – hepatotoxic trovafloxacin and nonhepatotoxic ciprofloxacin and levofloxacin.

The opioid analgesic buprenorphine is safely used as a substitution drug in heroin addicts at its recommended daily doses (2–8 mg) (Figure 12.26). However, large overdoses or intravenous misuse can cause hepatotoxicity [83]. NADPH-dependent microsomal covalent binding of buprenorphine and its *N*-dealkylated metabolite norbuprenorphine has been demonstrated [84]. The identity of the reactive metabolite responsible for covalent binding is unclear.

There are several drugs in the "most dispensed" category that possess structural alerts but do not form reactive metabolites and are not associated with significant incidences of idiosyncratic toxicity (Figure 12.27). For example, donepezil is a drug used to treat Alzheimer's disease and contains the *ortho*-dimethoxyphenyl functionality, which on sequential *O*-dealkylation can yield a catechol intermediate. While *O*-demethylation is observed as a metabolic fate in humans, the resulting products are efficiently glucuronidated, and there is no evidence for additional *O*-demethylation and/or aromatic ring hydroxylation that can lead to the formation of electrophilic quinones [85]. Likewise, *O*-demethylation is also observed as a metabolic fate with verapamil, a calcium channel blocker, which contains two *ortho*-dimethoxyphenyl substituents. However, like donepezil, the corresponding metabolites are principally eliminated as glucuronides in humans [86]. The dialkoxyaromatic motif in the selective α1-adrenoceptor blocker tamsulosin also undergoes *O*-dealkylation; however, the corresponding phenolic metabolites are efficiently glucuronidated and sulfated [87].

Oseltamivir, which is used to treat influenza infections, contains a cyclic Michael acceptor motif and, despite administration at a fairly high daily dose of 150 mg, the drug is rarely associated with idiosyncratic toxicity. It is a prodrug and requires enzymatic hydrolysis of its ester linkage to afford the active carboxylic acid metabolite. This metabolic step accounts for >80% metabolism of the drug; no conjugates derived from addition of GSH to the Michael acceptor functionality in either prodrug or active carboxylic acid form have been described [88]. Similar to oseltamivir, prednisolone and methylprednisolone contain a potential Michael acceptor in the A ring of the steroidal architecture. However, in humans, both compounds are metabolized via reduction of the C20 carbonyl group, oxidation of the C20–C21 side chain to carboxylic acid metabolites, and hydroxylation at the 6β-position on

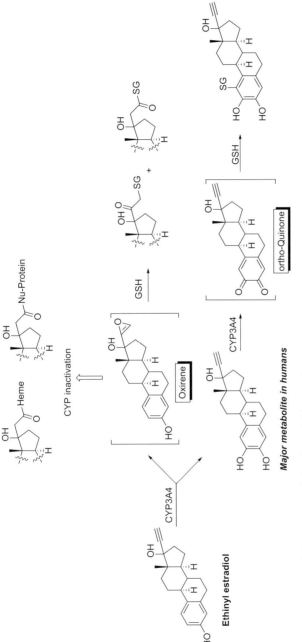

Figure 12.25 Metabolic activation of ethinylestradiol by CYP3A4.

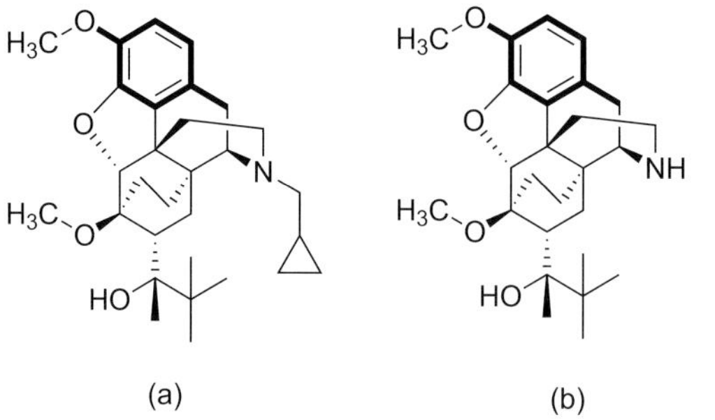

Figure 12.26 Structures of buprenorphine (a) and its *N*-dealkylated metabolite (b) that form reactive metabolites. The *para*-alkylaromatic ether structural alert is highlighted in bold.

the B ring [89]. In addition to the A ring quinone motif, furan and alkylhalide alerts are also discerned in the chemical structure of mometasone, a glucocorticoid used in the treatment of topical dermatological disorders and allergic rhinitis. There is very limited information on the pharmacokinetics of mometasone after oral inhalation at the efficacious dose of 0.2 mg. However, based on the limited available information, it appears that 6β-hydroxylation is a key metabolic fate with no detectable metabolism on the quinone, furan, and/or alkylhalide functionalities [90]. The furan structural alert in the H2 antagonist ranitidine also does not appear to be problematic from a toxicological standpoint, despite the requirement of a high daily dose of 300 mg. Approximately 65–70% of the clearance mechanism of ranitidine in humans involves urinary excretion mediated through transport proteins [91]. Likewise, the principle clearance mechanism of the inhaled bronchodilator tiotropium in humans involves renal excretion. Potential toxicity risks due to pendant thiophenes and epoxide motif do not appear to be a cause for concern especially when considering a low inhalation dose of ~18 μg/day [92]. The selective cholesterol absorption inhibitor ezetimibe contains phenol and an aniline structural alert, which could lead to quinone species on oxidative metabolism. However, the primary route of elimination in humans is via phenol glucuroniation with virtually no contribution from CYP enzymes [93]. Like simvastatin, lovastatin and pravastatin are low daily dose statins (10–20 mg effective dose range) and relatively safe with over a decade of clinical experience despite containing the olefin structural alerts.

12.5
Structure Toxicity Trends

Meloxicam, zolpidem, and quetiapine are noteworthy examples of drugs in the most prescribed list whose predecessors sudoxicam, alpidem, and clozapine, respectively, have been associated with significant incidences of IADRs [1]. The NSAID sudoxicam and the anxiolytic agent alpidem have been withdrawn due to hepatotoxicity, whereas the antipsychotic agent clozapine carries a black box warning associated with a high incidence of blood dyscrasias and hepatotoxicity.

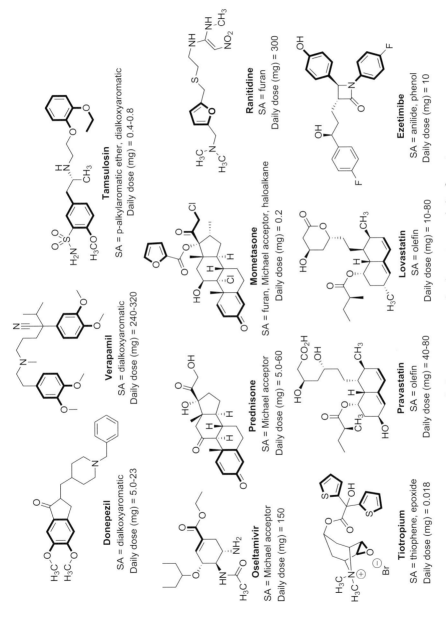

Figure 12.27 Structural alert-positive drugs, which are not associated with reactive metabolite formation.

12.5.1
Meloxicam versus Sudoxicam

In the case of sudoxicam, CYP-catalyzed thiazole ring scission in HLM generates an acylthiourea metabolite (Figure 12.28), which on hydrolysis would afford the thiourea metabolite, capable of oxidizing GSH and proteins [93]. The bioactivation pathway leading to the acylthiourea also represents the major metabolic fate of sudoxicam in animals and humans [94]. The structurally related NSAID meloxicam does not possess the hepatotoxic liability associated with sudoxicam despite administration at comparable doses. Although introduction of a methyl group at the C5 position on the thiazole ring in meloxicam is the only structural difference, the change dramatically alters the metabolic profile. Oxidation of the C5 methyl group to the alcohol (and carboxylic acid) metabolite(s) constitutes the major metabolic fate of meloxicam in humans (Figure 12.28) [93]. It is noteworthy to point out that the C5 methyl group on the aminothiazole ring in meloxicam was essential for selective cyclooxygenase (COX)-2 inhibitory potency and was not specifically introduced to eliminate reactive metabolite formation [95].

12.5.2
Zolpidem versus Alpidem

Alpidem was withdrawn from commercial use within the first year of its introduction due to several cases of severe hepatotoxicity. Although alpidem is devoid of a prototypic structural alert, evidence has been presented for oxidative bioactivation of the chloro-imidazopyridine ring to an electrophilic epoxide that reacts with GSH or microsomal protein [70, 96]. The detection of mercapturic acid conjugates in human excreta provides evidence for the existence of this pathway *in vivo* (Figure 12.28) [96]. Interestingly, the structural analogue of alpidem, that is, zolpidem, is not hepatotoxic. A key structural difference between the two drugs is the replacement of the two chlorine atoms in alpidem with two methyl groups in zolpidem. Zolpidem is metabolized via oxidation of both methyl groups to the corresponding alcohol and carboxylic acid metabolites and is not subject to bioactivation [96]. In addition, alpidem exhibits potent inhibition of mitochondrial respiration and depletes GSH in primary hepatocyte cultures, liabilities that are not observed with zolpidem even at high concentrations [97].

12.5.3
Quetiapine versus Olanzapine versus Clozapine

Clozapine exhibits covalent binding to human neutrophil proteins *in vitro*, via a myeloperoxidase-catalyzed oxidation of its dibenzodiazepine ring to a reactive iminium species, which covalently binds to the target tissues and also reacts with GSH (Figure 12.28) [98, 99]. Proteins covalently modified with clozapine have been observed in neutrophils of patients being treated with clozapine, which reaffirms the relevance of the *in vitro* studies. Quetiapine is not associated with IADRs

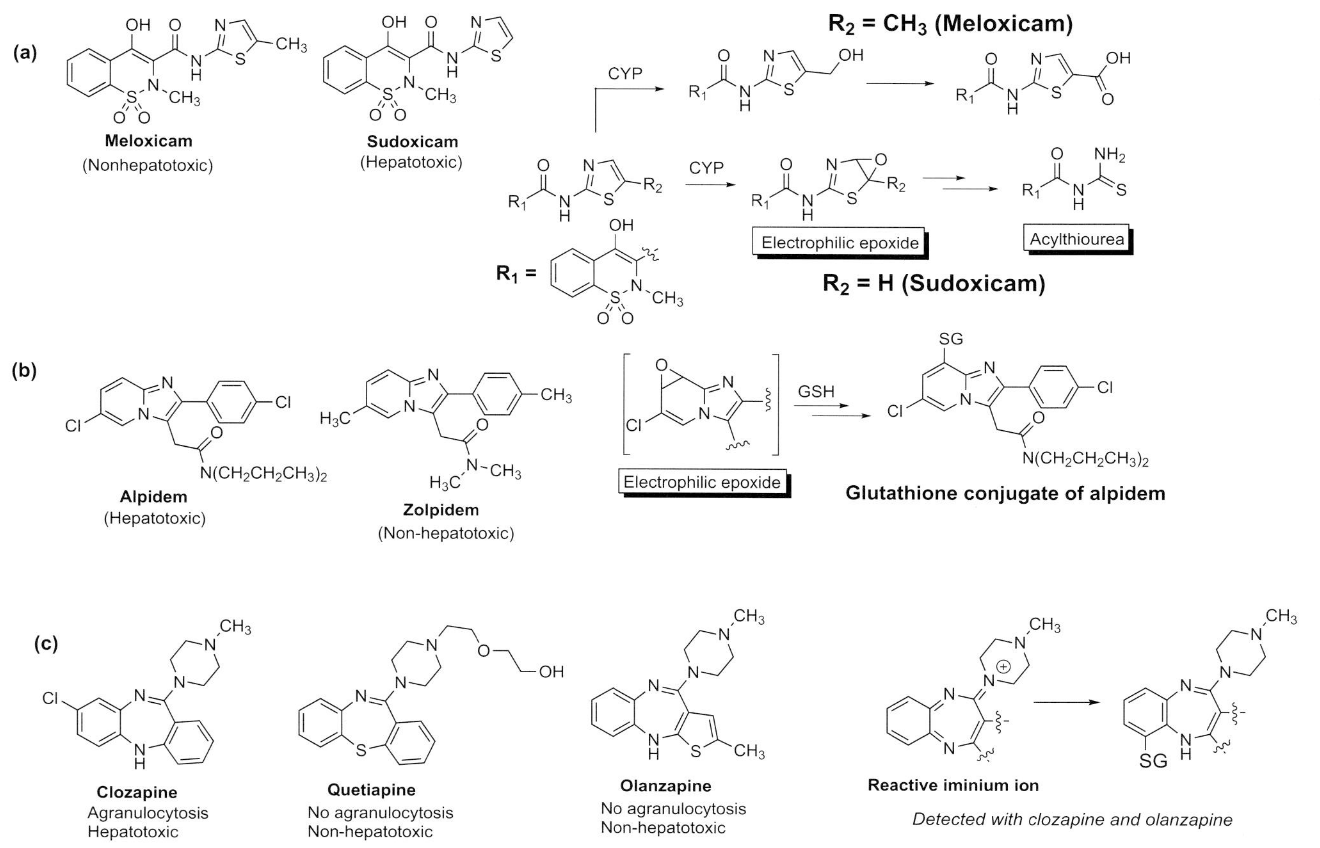

Figure 12.28 Structure toxicity relationships: (a) meloxicam and sudoxicam, (b) zolpidem and alpidem, and (c) quetiapine, clozapine, and olanzapine.

despite administration at high doses (400–800 mg). In fact, quetiapine (Table 12.1) was ranked 35th in terms of dispensed prescriptions in 2009. The bridging nitrogen atom in quetiapine is replaced with a sulfur; consequently, this drug cannot form a reactive iminium. In contrast, olanzapine (ranked 158th, Table 12.1) forms a reactive iminium metabolite very similar to the one observed with clozapine, yet olanzapine is not associated with a significant incidence of blood dyscrasias. One difference between the two drugs is the daily dose; the maximum recommended daily doses of clozapine and olanzapine are 900 and 10 mg, respectively.

References

1 Stefan, A.F., Walker, D.P., Bauman, J., Price, D.A., Baillie, T.A., Kalgutkar, A.S., and Aleo, M.D. (2011) Structural alert/reactive metabolite concept as applied in medicinal chemistry to mitigate the risk of idiosyncratic drug toxicity: a perspective based on the critical examination of trends in the top 200 drugs marketed in the United States. *Chemical Research in Toxicology,* **24** (9), 1345–1410.

2 Park, B.K., Kitteringham, N.R., Maggs, J.L., Pirmohamed, M., and Williams, D.P. (2005) The role of metabolic activation in drug-induced hepatotoxicity. *Annual Reviews in Pharmacology and Toxicology,* **45**, 177–202.

3 Ferner, R.E., Dear, J.W., and Bateman, D.N. (2011) Management of paracetamol poisoning. *British Medical Journal,* **342**, d2218.

4 Lennernas, H. (2003) Clinical pharmacokinetics of atorvastatin. *Clinical Pharmacokinetics,* **42** (13), 1141–1160.

5 Nakayama, S., Atsumi, R., Takakusa, H., Kobayashi, Y., Kurihara, A., Nagai, Y., Nakai, D., and Okazaki, O. (2009) A zone classification system for risk assessment of idiosyncratic drug toxicity using daily dose and covalent binding. *Drug Metabolism and Disposition,* **37** (9), 1970–1977.

6 Lu, W.P., Kincaid, E., Sun, Y., and Bauer, M.D. (2001) Kinetics of beta-lactam interactions with penicillin-susceptible and -resistant penicillin-binding protein 2x proteins from *Streptococcus pneumoniae.* Involvement of acylation and deacylation in beta-lactam resistance.

Journal of Biological Chemistry, **276** (34), 31494–31501.

7 Besancon, M., Simon, A., Sachs, G., and Shin, J.M. (1997) Sites of reaction of the gastric H, K-ATPase with extracytoplasmic thiol reagents. *Journal of Biological Chemistry,* **272** (36), 22438–22446.

8 Shin, J.M., Cho, Y.M., and Sachs, G. (2004) Chemistry of covalent inhibition of the gastric (H+K+)-ATPase by proton pump inhibitors. *Journal of the American Chemical Society,* **126** (25), 7800–7811.

9 Gan, J., Ruan, Q., He, B., Zhu, M., Shyu, W.C., and Humphreys, W.G. (2009) In vitro screening of 50 highly prescribed drugs for thiol adduct formation – comparison of potential for drug-induced toxicity and extent of adduct formation. *Chemical Research in Toxicology,* **22** (4), 690–698.

10 Weidolf, L., Karlsson, K.E., and Nilsson, I.A. (1992) Metabolic route of omeprazole involving conjugation with GSH identified in the rat. *Drug Metabolism and Disposition,* **20** (2), 262–267.

11 Savi, P., Pereillo, J.M., Uzabiaga, M.F., Combalbert, J., Picard, C., Maffrand, J.P., Pascal, M., and Herbert, J.M. (2000) Identification and biological activity of the active metabolite of clopidogrel. *Thrombosis and Haemostasis,* **84** (5), 891–896.

12 Pereillo, J.M., Maftouh, M., Andrieu, A., Uzabiaga, M.F., Fedeli, O., Savi, P., Pascal, M., Herbert, J.M., Maffrand, J.P., and Picard, C. (2002) Structure and stereochemistry of the active metabolite of clopidogrel. *Drug Metabolism and Disposition,* **30** (11), 1288–1295.

13 Savi, P., Zachayus, J.L., Delesque-Touchard, N., Labouret, C., Herve, C., Uzabiaga, M.F., Pereillo, J.M., Culouscou, J.M., Bono, F., Ferrara, P., and Herbert, J. M. (2006) The active metabolite of clopidogrel disrupts P2Y12 receptor oligomers and partitions them out of lipid rafts. *Proceedings of the National Academy of Sciences of the United States of America*, **103** (29), 11069–11074.

14 Dansette, P.M., Libraire, J., Bertho, G., and Mansuy, D. (2009) Metabolic oxidative cleavage of thioesters: evidence for the formation of sulfenic acid intermediates in the bioactivation of the antithrombotic prodrugs ticlopidine and clopidogrel. *Chemical Research in Toxicology*, **22** (2), 369–373.

15 Prueksaritanont, T., Gorham, L.M., Ma, B., Liu, L., Yu, X., Zhao, J.J., Slaughter, D. E., Arison, B.H., and Vyas, K.P. (1997) In vitro metabolism of simvastatin in humans. Identification of metabolizing enzymes and effect of the drug on hepatic P450s. *Drug Metabolism and Disposition*, **25** (10), 1191–1199.

16 Bauman, J.N., Kelly, J.M., Tripathy, S., Zhao, S.X., Lam, W.W., Kalgutkar, A.S., and Obach, R.S. (2009) Can in vitro metabolism-dependent covalent binding data distinguish hepatotoxic from nonhepatotoxic drugs? An analysis using human hepatocytes and liver S-9 fraction. *Chemical Research in Toxicology*, **22** (2), 332–340.

17 Obach, R.S., Kalgutkar, A.S., Soglia, J.R., and Zhao, S.X. (2008) Can in vitro metabolism-dependent covalent binding data in liver microsomes distinguish hepatotoxic from nonhepatotoxic drugs? An analysis of 18 drugs with consideration of intrinsic clearance and daily dose. *Chemical Research in Toxicology*, **21** (9), 1814–1822.

18 LoPresti, J.S. and Nicoloff, J.T. (1994) 3,5,3′-Triiodothyronine (T3) sulfate: a major metabolite in T3 metabolism in man. *Journal of Clinical Endocrinology and Metabolism*, **78** (3), 688–692.

19 Murthy, S.S., Shetty, H.U., Nelson, W.L., Jackson, P.R., and Lennard, M.S. (1990) Enantioselective and diastereoselective aspects of the oxidative metabolism of metoprolol. *Biochemical Pharmacology*, **40** (7), 1637–1644.

20 Morgan, D.J. (1990) Clinical pharmacokinetics of β-agonists. *Clinical Pharmacokinetics*, **18** (4), 270–274.

21 Farid, N.A., Kurihara, A., and Wrighton, S. A. (2010) Metabolism and disposition of the thienopyridine antiplatelet drugs ticlopidine, clopidogrel, and prasugrel in humans. *Journal of Clinical Pharmacology*, **50** (2), 126–142.

22 Zhao, Z., Baldo, B.A., and Rimmer, J. (2002) beta-Lactam allergenic determinants: fine structural recognition of a cross-reacting determinant on benzylpenicillin and cephalothin. *Clinical and Experimental Allergy*, **32** (11), 1644–1650.

23 Levine, B.B. (1960) Formation of D-penicillamine–cysteine mixed disulfide by reaction of D-benzylpenicilloic acid with cysteine. *Nature*, **187**, 940–941.

24 Levine, B.B. and Ovary, Z. (1961) Studies on the mechanism of the formation of the penicillin antigen. III. The *N*-(D-alpha-benzylpenicilloyl) group as an antigenic determinant responsible for hypersensitivity to penicillin G. *Journal of Experimental Medicine*, **114**, 875–904.

25 Connor, S.C., Everett, J.R., Jennings, K.R., Nicholson, J.K., and Woodnut, G. (1994) High resolution ^{1}H NMR spectroscopic studies of the metabolism and excretion of ampicillin in rats and amoxycillin in rats and man. *Journal of Pharmacy and Pharmacology*, **46** (2), 128–134.

26 Maggs, J.L., Naisbitt, D.J., Tettey, J.N., Pirmohamed, M., and Park, B.K. (2000) Metabolism of lamotrigine to a reactive arene oxide intermediate. *Chemical Research in Toxicology*, **13** (11), 1075–1081.

27 Chen, H., Grover, S., Yu, L., Walker, G., and Mutlib, A. (2010) Bioactivation of lamotrigine in vivo in rat and in vitro in HLM, hepatocytes, and epidermal keratinocytes: characterization of thioether conjugates by liquid chromatography/mass spectrometry and high field nuclear magnetic resonance spectroscopy. *Chemical Research in Toxicology*, **23** (1), 159–170.

28 Naisbitt, D.J., Farrell, J., Wong, G., Depta, J.P., Dodd, C.C., Hopkins, J.E.,

Gibney, C.A., Chadwick, D.W., Pichler, W. J., Pirmohamed, M., and Park, B.K. (2003) Characterization of drug-specific T cells in lamotrigine hypersensitivity. *Journal of Allergy and Clinical Immunology*, **111** (6), 1393–1403.

29 Cribb, A.E., Miller, M., Leeder, J.S., Hill, J., and Spielberg, S.P. (1991) Reactions of the nitroso and hydroxylamine metabolites of sulfamethoxazole with reduced GSH. Implications for idiosyncratic toxicity. *Drug Metabolism and Disposition*, **19** (5), 900–906.

30 Callan, H.E., Jenkins, R.E., Maggs, J.L., Lavergne, S.N., Clarke, S.E., Naisbitt, D.J., and Park, B.K. (2009) Multiple adduction reactions of nitroso sulfamethoxazole with cysteinyl residues of peptides and proteins: implications for hapten formation. *Chemical Research in Toxicology*, **22** (5), 937–948.

31 Reilly, T.P., Lash, L.H., Doll, M.A., Hein, D.W., Woster, P.M., and Svensson, C.K. (2000) A role for bioactivation and covalent binding within epidermal keratinocytes in sulfonamide-induced cutaneous drug reactions. *Journal of Investigative Dermatology*, **114** (6), 1164–1173.

32 Makarova, S.I. (2008) Human *N*-acetyltransferases and drug-induced hepatotoxicity. *Current Drug Metabolism*, **9** (6), 538–545.

33 Damsten, M.C., de Vlieger, J.S., Niessen, W.M., Irth, H., Vermeulen, N.P., and Commandeur, J.N. (2008) Trimethoprim: novel reactive intermediates and bioactivation pathways by cytochrome p450s. *Chemical Research in Toxicology*, **21** (11), 2181–2187.

34 Lai, W.G., Zahid, N., and Uetrecht, J.P. (1999) Metabolism of trimethoprim to a reactive iminoquinone methide by activated human neutrophils and hepatic microsomes. *Journal of Pharmacology and Experimental Therapeutics*, **29** (1), 292–299.

35 Mitchell, J.R., Potter, W.Z., Hinson, J.A., and Jollow, D.J. (1974) Hepatic necrosis caused by furosemide. *Nature*, **251** (5475), 508–511.

36 Mitchell, J.R., Snodgrass, W.R., and Gillette, J.R. (1976) The role of biotransformation in chemical-induced liver injury. *Environmental Health Perspectives*, **15**, 27–38.

37 Masubuchi, N., Makino, C., and Murayama, N. (2007) Prediction of in vivo potential for metabolic activation of drugs into chemically reactive intermediate: correlation of in vitro and in vivo generation of reactive intermediates and in vitro GSH conjugate formation in rats and humans. *Chemical Research in Toxicology*, **20** (3), 455–464.

38 Kalgutkar, A.S., Henne, K.R., Lame, M.E., Vaz, A.D.N., Collin, C., Soglia, J.R., Zhao, S.X., and Hop, C.E.C.A. (2005) Metabolic activation of the nontricyclic antidepressant trazodone to electrophilic quinone-imine and epoxide intermediates in HLM and recombinant P4503A4. *Chemico-Biological Interactions*, **155** (1–2), 10–20.

39 Wen, B., Ma, L., and Zhu, M. (2008) Bioactivation of the tricyclic antidepressant amitriptyline and its metabolite nortriptyline to arene oxide intermediates in HLM and recombinant P450s. *Chemico-Biological Interactions*, **173** (1), 59–67.

40 Prox, A. and Breyer-Pfaff, U. (1987) Amitriptyline metabolites in human urine. Identification of phenols, dihydrodiols, glycols, and ketones. *Drug Metabolism and Disposition*, **15** (6), 890–896.

41 Pedersen, A.M. and Enevoldsen, H.K. (1996) Nortriptyline-induced hepatic failure. *Therapeutic Drug Monitoring*, **18** (1), 100–102.

42 McKenney, J.M., Proctor, J.D., Harris, S., and Chinchili, V.M. (1994) A comparison of the efficacy and toxic effects of sustained- vs immediate-release niacin in hypercholesterolemic patients. *JAMA: the Journal of the American Medical Association*, **271** (9), 672–677.

43 Pieper, J.A. (2003) Overview of niacin formulations: differences in pharmacokinetics, efficacy, and safety. *American Journal of Health-System Pharmacy*, **60** (13 Suppl. 2), S9–S14.

44 Morgan, R.E., Trauner, M., van Staden, C.J., Lee, P.H., Ramachandran, B., Eschenberg, M., Afshari, C.A., Qualls, C. W. Jr., Lightfoot-Dunn, R., and Hamadeh,

H.K. (2010) Interference with bile salt export pump function is a susceptibility factor for human liver injury in drug development. *Toxicological Sciences*, **118** (2), 485–500.

45 Goodman, R., Dean, P., Radparvar, A., and Kitabchi, A. (1987) Glyburide-induced hepatitis. *Annals of Internal Medicine*, **106** (6), 837–839.

46 Stieger, B. (2010) Role of the bile salt export pump, BSEP, in acquired forms of cholestasis. *Drug Metabolism Reviews*, **42** (3), 437–445.

47 Lam, P., Soroka, C.J., and Boyer, J.L. (2010) Genetic determinants of drug-induced cholestasis and intrahepatic cholestasis of pregnancy. *Seminars in Liver Disease*, **30** (2), 147–159.

48 Trujillo, M.A., Galgiani, J.N., and Sampliner, R.E. (1994) Evaluation of hepatic injury arising during fluconazole therapy. *Archives of Internal Medicine*, **154** (1), 102–104.

49 Drawz, S.M. and Bonomo, R.A. (2010) Three decades of beta-lactamase inhibitors. *Clinical Microbiology Reviews*, **23** (1), 160–201.

50 Van der Auwerea, P. and Legrand, J.C. (1985) Ticarcillin clavulanic acid therapy in severe infections. *Drugs under Experimental and Clinical Research*, **11** (11), 805–813.

51 Hautekeete, M.L., Horsmans, Y., Van Waeyenberge, C., Demanet, C., Henrion, J., Verbist, L., Brenard, R., Sempoux, C., Michielsen, P.P., Yap, P.S., Rahier, J., and Geubel, A.P. (1999) HLA association of amoxicillin–clavulanate induced hepatitis. *Gastroenterology*, **117** (5), 1181–1186.

52 Lucena, M.I., Andrade, R.J., Martinez, C., Ulzurrun, E., Garcia-Martin, E., Borraz, Y., Fernandez, M.C., Romero-Gomez, M., Castiella, A., Planas, R., Costa, J., Anzola, S., and Agundez, J.A.G. (2008) GSH *S*-transferase M1 and T1 null genotypes increase susceptibility to idiosyncratic drug-induced liver injury. *Hepatology*, **48** (2), 588–596.

53 Davies, N.M. (1998) Clinical pharmacokinetics of ibuprofen. The first 30 years. *Clinical Pharmacokinetics*, **34** (2), 101–154.

54 Davies, N.M. and Anderson, K.E. (1997) Clinical pharmacokinetics of naproxen. *Clinical Pharmacokinetics*, **32** (4), 268–293.

55 Castillo, M. and Smith, P.C. (1995) Disposition and covalent binding of ibuprofen and its acyl glucuronide in the elderly. *Clinical Pharmacology and Therapeutics*, **57** (6), 636–644.

56 Olsen, J., Bjornsdottir, I., Tjornelund, J., and Honore Hansen, S. (2002) Chemical reactivity of the naproxen acyl glucuronide and the naproxen coenzyme A thioester towards bionucleophiles. *Journal of Pharmaceutical and Biomedical Analysis*, **29** (1–2), 7–15.

57 Goldkind, L. and Laine, L. (2006) A systematic review of NSAIDs withdrawn from the market due to hepatotoxicity: lessons learned from the bromfenac experience. *Pharmacoepidemiological Drug Safety*, **15** (4), 213–220.

58 Walker, G.S., Atherton, J., Bauman, J., Kohl, C., Lam, W., Reily, M., Lou, Z., and Mutlib, A. (2007) Determination of degradation pathways and kinetics of acyl glucuronides by NMR spectroscopy. *Chemical Research in Toxicology*, **20** (6), 876–886.

59 Venkatakrishnan, K. and Obach, R.S. (2005) In vitro–in vivo extrapolation of CYP2D6 inactivation by paroxetine: prediction of nonstationary pharmacokinetics and drug interaction magnitude. *Drug Metabolism and Disposition*, **33** (6), 845–852.

60 Zhao, S.X., Dalvie, D.K., Kelly, J.M., Soglia, J.R., Frederick, K.S., Smith, E.B., Obach, R.S., and Kalgutkar, A.S. (2007) NADPH-dependent covalent binding of [3H]paroxetine to HLM and S-9 fractions: identification of an electrophilic quinone metabolite of paroxetine. *Chemical Research in Toxicology*, **20** (11), 1649–1657.

61 Ring, B.J., Patterson, B.E., Mitchell, M.I., Vandenbranden, M., Gillespie, J., Bedding, A.W., Jewell, H., Payne, C.D., Forgue, S.T., Eckstein, J., Wrighton, S.A., and Phillips, D.L. (2005) Effect of tadalafil on cytochrome P450 3A4-mediated clearance: studies in vitro and in vivo. *Clinical Pharmacology and Therapeutics*, **77** (1), 63–75.

62 Chen, Q., Ngui, J.S., Doss, G.A., Wang, R. W., Cai, X., DiNinno, F.P., Blizzard, T.A., Hammond, M.L., Stearns, R.A., Evans, D. C., Baillie, T.A., and Tang, W. (2002) Cytochrome P450 3A4-mediated bioactivation of raloxifene: irreversible enzyme inhibition and thiol adduct formation. *Chemical Research in Toxicology*, **15** (7), 907–914.

63 Yu, L., Liu, H., Li, W., Zhang, F., Luckie, C., van Breemen, R.B., Thatcher, G.R.J., and Bolton, J.L. (2004) Oxidation of raloxifene to quinoids: potential toxic pathways via a diquinone methide and *o*-quinones. *Chemical Research in Toxicology*, **17** (7), 879–888.

64 Dalvie, D., Kang, P., Zientek, M., Xiang, C., Zhou, S., and Obach, R.S. (2008) Effect of intestinal glucuronidation in limiting hepatic exposure and bioactivation of raloxifene in humans and rats. *Chemical Research in Toxicology*, **21** (12), 2260–2271.

65 Hucker, H.B., Stauffer, S.C., Balletto, A.J., White, S.D., Zacchei, A.G., and Arison, B.H. (1978) Physiological disposition and metabolism of cyclobenzaprine in the rat, dog, rhesus monkey, and man. *Drug Metabolism and Disposition*, **6** (6), 659–672.

66 Lim, H.-K., Chen, J., Sensenhauser, C., Cook, K., and Subrahmanyam, V. (2007) Metabolite identification by data-dependent accurate mass spectrometric analysis at resolving power of 60000 in external calibration mode using an LTQ/orbitrap. *Rapid Communications in Mass Spectrometry*, **21** (12), 1821–1832.

67 Zhou, H.-H. and Wood, A.J.J. (1995) Stereoselective disposition of carvedilol is determined by CYP2D6. *Clinical Pharmacology and Therapeutics*, **57** (5), 518–524.

68 Kondrack, R. and Mohiuddin, S. (2009) Valsartan/hydrochlorothiazide: pharmacology and clinical efficacy. *Expert Opinion in Drug Metabolism and Toxicology*, **5** (9), 1125–1134.

69 Yamada, A., Maeda, K., Kamiyama, E., Sugiyama, D., Kondo, T., Shiroyanagi, Y., Nakazawa, H., Okano, T., Adachi, M., Schuetz, J.D., Adachi, Y., Hu, Z., Kusuhara, H., and Sugiyama, Y. (2007) Multiple human isoforms of drug transporters contribute to the hepatic and renal transport of olmesartan, a selective antagonist of the angiotensin II AT1-receptor. *Drug Metabolism and Disposition*, **35** (12), 2166–2176.

70 Usui, T., Mise, M., Hashizume, T., Yabuki, M., and Komuro, S. (2009) Evaluation of the potential for drug-induced liver injury based on in vitro covalent binding to human liver proteins. *Drug Metabolism and Disposition*, **37** (12), 2383–2392.

71 Schmidt, B. and Schieffer, B. (2003) Angiotensin II AT1 receptor antagonists. Clinical implications of active metabolites. *Journal of Medicinal Chemistry*, **46** (12), 2261–2270.

72 Waldmeier, F., Kaiser, G., Ackermann, R., Faigle, J.W., Wagner, J., Barner, A., and Lasseter, K.C. (1991) The disposition of [^{14}C]-labelled benazepril HCl in normal adult volunteers after single and repeated oral dose. *Xenobiotica*, **21** (2), 251–261.

73 Wilkin, J.K., Hammond, J.J., and Kirkendall, W.M. (1980) The captopril-induced eruption. A possible mechanism: cutaneous kinin potentiation. *Archives of Dermatology*, **116** (8), 902–905.

74 Yeung, J.H., Breckenridge, A.M., and Park, B.K. (1983) Drug protein conjugates – VI. Role of GSH in the metabolism of captopril and captopril plasma protein conjugates. *Biochemical Pharmacology*, **32** (23), 3619–3625.

75 Olivera, M., Martinez, C., Gervasini, G., Carrillo, J.A., Ramos, S., Benitez, J., Garcia-Martin, E., and Agundez, J.A. (2007) Effect of common NAT2 variant alleles in the acetylation of the major clonazepam metabolite, 7-aminoclonazepam. *Drug Metabolism Letters*, **1** (1), 3–5.

76 Sun, Q., Zhu, R., Foss, F.W. Jr., and Macdonald, T.L. (2008) In vitro metabolism of a model cyclopropylamine to reactive intermediate: insights into trovafloxacin-induced hepatotoxicity. *Chemical Research in Toxicology*, **21** (3), 711–719.

77 Fish, D.N. and Chow, A.T. (1997) The clinical pharmacokinetics of levofloxacin. *Clinical Pharmacokinetics*, **32** (2), 101–119.

78 Vance-Bryan, K., Guay, D.R., and Rotschafer, J.C. (1990) Clinical pharmacokinetics of ciprofloxacin. *Clinical Pharmacokinetics*, **19** (6), 434–461.

79 Ortiz de Montellano, P.R., Kunze, K.L., Yost, G.S., and Mico, B.A. (1979) Self-catalyzed destruction of cytochrome P450: covalent binding of ethynyl sterols to prosthetic heme. *Proceedings of the National Academy of Sciences of the United States of America*, **76** (2), 746–749.

80 Guengerich, F.P. (1990) Metabolism of 17a-ethynylestradiol in humans. *Life Science*, **47** (22), 1981–1988.

81 Lin, H.-L., Kent, U.M., and Hollenberg, P. F. (2002) Mechanism-based inactivation of cytochrome P4503A4 by 17α-ethynylestradiol: evidence for heme destruction and covalent binding to protein. *Journal of Pharmacology and Experimental Therapeutics*, **301** (1), 160–167.

82 Purba, H.S., Maggs, J.L., Orme, M.L., Back, D.J., and Park, B.K. (1987) The metabolism of 17α-ethinyloestradiol by HLM: formation of catechol and chemically reactive metabolites. *British Journal of Clinical Pharmacology*, **23** (4), 447–453.

83 Herve, S., Riachi, G., Noblet, C., Guillement, N., Tanasescu, S., Goria, O., Thuillez, C., Tranvouez, J.L., Ducrotte, P., and Lerebours, E. (2004) Acute hepatitis dues to buprenorphine administration. *European Journal of Gastroenterology and Hepatology*, **16** (10), 1033–1037.

84 Berson, A., Fau, D., Fornacciari, R., Degove-Goddard, P., Sutton, A., Descatoire, V., Haouzi, D., Letteron, P., Moreau, A., Feldmann, G., and Pessayre, D. (2001) Mechanisms for experimental buprenorphine hepatotoxicity: major role of mitochondrial dysfunction versus metabolic activation. *Journal of Hepatology*, **34** (2), 261–269.

85 Tiseo, P.J., Perdomo, C.A., and Friedhoff, L.T. (1998) Metabolism and elimination of ^{14}C-donepezil in healthy volunteers. *British Journal of Clinical Pharmacology*, **46** (Suppl. 1), 19–24.

86 Borlak, J., Walles, M., Elend, M., Thum, T., Preiss, A., and Levsen, K. (2003) Verapamil: identification of novel metabolites in cultures of primary human hepatocytes and human urine by LC-MS[n] and LC-NMR. *Xenobiotica*, **33** (6), 655–676.

87 Soeishi, Y., Matsuhima, H., Watanabe, T., Higuchi, S., Cornelissen, K., and Ward, J. (1996) Absorption, metabolism and excretion of tamsulosin hydrochloride in man. *Xenobiotica*, **26** (6), 637–645.

88 He, G., Massarella, J., and Ward, P. (1999) Clinical pharmacokinetics of the prodrug oseltamivir and its active metabolite Ro 64-0802. *Clinical Pharmacokinetics*, **37** (6), 471–484.

89 Vree, T.B., Lagerwerf, A.J., Verwey-van Wissen, C.P., and Jongen, P.J. (1999) High-performance liquid-chromatography analysis, preliminary pharmacokinetics, metabolism and renal excretion of methylprednisolone with its C6 and C20 hydroxy metabolites in multiple sclerosis patients receiving high-dose pulse therapy. *Journal of Chromatography. B, Biomedical Sciences and Applications*, **732** (2), 337–348.

90 Sahasranaman, S., Issar, M., and Hochhaus, G. (2006) Metabolism of mometasone furoate and biological activity of the metabolites. *Drug Metabolism and Disposition*, **34** (2), 225–233.

91 Bell, J.A., Dallas, F.A., Jenner, W.N., and Marin, L.E. (1980) The metabolism of ranitidine in animals and man. *Biochemical Society Transactions*, **8** (1), 93.

92 Price, D., Sharma, A., and Cerasoli, F. (2009) Biochemical properties, pharmacokinetics and pharmacological response of tiotropium in chronic obstructive pulmonary disease patients. *Expert Opinion in Drug Metabolism and Toxicology*, **5** (4), 417–424.

93 Obach, R.S., Kalgutkar, A.S., Ryder, T.F., and Walker, G.S. (2008) In vitro metabolism and covalent binding of enol-carboxamide derivatives and anti-inflammatory agents sudoxicam and meloxicam: insights into the hepatotoxicity of sudoxicam. *Chemical Research in Toxicology*, **21** (9), 1890–1899.

94 Woolf, T.F. and Radulovic, L.L. (1989) Oxicams: metabolic disposition in man and animals. *Drug Metabolism Reviews*, **21** (2), 255–276.

95 Lazer, E.S., Miao, C.K., Cywin, C.L., Sorcek, R., Wong, H.C., Meng, Z.,

Potocki, I., Hoermann, M., Snow, R.J., Tschantz, M.A., Kelly, T.A., McNeil, D.W., Coutts, S.J., Churchill, L., Graham, A.G., David, E., Grob, P.M., Engel, W., Meier, H., and Tummlitz, G. (1997) Effect of structural modification of enol-carboxamide-type nonsteroidal anti-inflammatory drugs on COX-2/COX-1 selectivity. *Journal of Medicinal Chemistry,* **40** (6), 980–989.

96 Durand, A., Thénot, J.P., Bianchetti, G., and Morselli, P.L. (1992) Comparative pharmacokinetic profile of two imidazopyridine drugs: zolpidem and alpidem. *Drug Metabolism Reviews,* **24** (2), 239–266.

97 Berson, A., Descatoire, V., Sutton, A., Fau, D., Maulny, B., Vadrot, N., Feldmann, G., Berthon, B., Tordjmann, T., and Pessayre, D. (2001) Toxicity of alpidem, a peripheral benzodiazepine receptor ligand, but not zolpidem, in rat hepatocytes: role of mitochondrial permeability transition and metabolic activation. *Journal of Pharmacology and Experimental Therapeutics,* **299** (2), 793–800.

98 Liu, Z.C. and Uetrecht, J.P. (1995) Clozapine is oxidized by activated human neutrophils to a reactive nitrenium ion that irreversibly binds to the cells. *Journal of Pharmacology and Experimental Therapeutics,* **275** (3), 1476–1483.

99 Uetrecht, J.P., Zahid, N., Tehim, A., Fu, J.M., and Rakhit, S. (1997) Structural features associated with reactive metabolite formation in clozapine analogues. *Chemico-Biological Interactions,* **104** (2–3), 117–129.

13
Mitigating Toxicity Risks with Affinity Labeling Drug Candidates

Abbreviations

COX	Cyclooxygenase
DPP IV	Dipeptidyl peptidase
EGFR	Epidermal growth factor receptor
GSH	Glutathione
LC/MS–MS	Liquid chromatography tandem mass spectrometry
VEGFR2	Vascular endothelial growth factor receptor 2

13.1
Introduction

The primary focus in the development of small molecules as drugs is on discovering candidates, which are highly selective for a given pharmacological target and possess an attractive toxicity profile. For this reason, most compounds are designed to interact with their target proteins (enzymes and/or receptors) via noncovalent interactions. Another approach to inhibiting enzymes, which is gaining popularity, involves covalent inhibition via irreversible modification of proteins. These "affinity labels" or "targeted covalent drugs" do not merely bind to a protein, but they form a durable covalent bond, which shuts down the activity of the protein molecule throughout the life of the protein, which is usually between a few hours to a few days [1]. The concept of irreversible inhibition is not new and has been a proven technique for inhibiting enzymes with several classes of drugs [1, 2]. Representative examples of drugs that modulate their target through a covalent interaction are shown in Figure 13.1.

13.2
Designing Covalent Inhibitors

Despite the fact that the concept of covalent inhibitors is a very attractive one, it is hard to achieve this in practice. This is because it is difficult to strike a right balance

Reactive Drug Metabolites, First Edition. Amit S. Kalgutkar, Deepak Dalvie, R. Scott Obach, and Dennis A. Smith.
© 2012 Wiley-VCH Verlag GmbH & Co. KGaA. Published 2012 by Wiley-VCH Verlag GmbH & Co. KGaA.

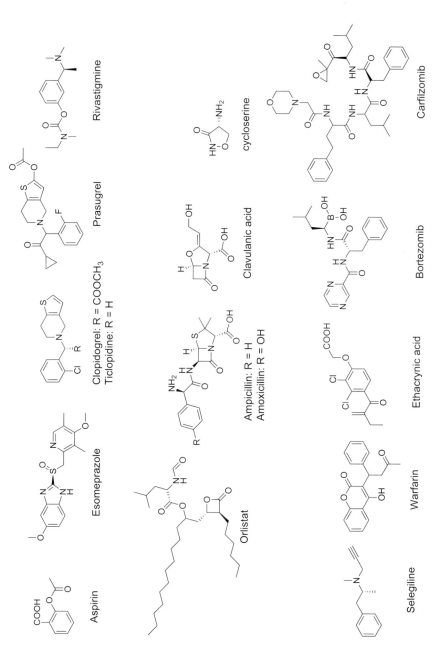

Figure 13.1 Examples of irreversible inhibitors that form a covalent bond with their respective enzyme targets.

between indiscriminate chemical reactivity and selectivity for the desired pharmacological target. All covalent inhibitors contain a reactive motif (a substructure), which is referred to as a "warhead." For covalent modification, the warhead has to be electrophilic and reactive in nature [3]. It is known that compounds with reactive functionalities tend to bind covalently to biological macromolecules (proteins and DNA). The presence of an electrophilic species increases the potential of these molecules to randomly react with macromolecules *in vivo* and can possibly lead to deleterious effects such as cell damage, cytotoxicity, mutagenesis, and tumorigenicity. Hence, there is consensus that nonspecific covalent binding should be avoided or minimized when optimizing drug properties [4–9]. For this reason, incorporation of electrophilic moieties is generally avoided in drug development. However, in cases where selectivity with respect to modification of the target can be achieved, these compounds can prove to be effective therapeutic agents. These inhibitors can have many desirable features, including increased biochemical efficiency of target disruption, less sensitivity toward pharmacokinetic parameters, increased duration of action that outlasts the pharmacokinetics of the compound, and the potential to overcome resistance due to mutations by virtue of time-dependent inactivation [10, 11].

When designing a selective covalent modifier, it is important that the reactivity of the molecule be managed to circumvent potential toxicological consequences. In an ideal case, the warhead should not react under physiological conditions but should be reactive enough to form a covalent bond with the nucleophile within the target protein. This will lead to a high degree of specificity and will possibly reduce unwanted nonspecific interactions with proteins, thus mitigating the likelihood of toxicity occurrence. Since this is practically infeasible, an alternative is to incorporate a warhead that has very low intrinsic reactivity. Thus, the reactivity of the warhead will only come into play when the molecule binds to the active site of the receptor/enzyme with the nucleophilic sites in close proximity for covalent bond formation. To accomplish this, two factors must be considered in the design strategy. First, the inhibitor must have high binding affinity for the receptor (as reflected by its dissociation constant (K_i); Figure 13.2) and should be selective toward the desired target. The noncovalent affinity (K_i) of the inhibitor must be high enough to ensure that the compound binds selectively to the desired target and achieves a residence time that is sufficient for a covalent reaction. The strategy applied here is similar to the one applied in the design of selective reversible inhibitors. Second, it

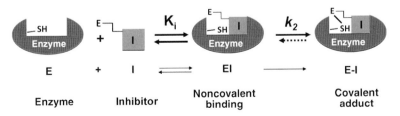

Figure 13.2 Schematic diagram of the interaction of covalent inhibitor and the enzyme.

is essential to "fine-tune" the reactivity of the warhead in the molecule [12]. Understanding reactivity and being able to characterize the electrophilic potential enables the rational design of irreversible covalent drugs. The reaction rate of the bound inhibitor (k_2) must be high enough to give a high probability that the reaction will occur within the lifetime of the noncovalent complex that is formed in the initial step of the reaction but not high enough that it leads to binding with nonspecific proteins. Thus, a successful covalent modifier can be envisioned as one that consists of two moieties: "a specificity group" and a bonding group, that is, the warhead (Figure 13.2) [12, 13]. The specificity group undergoes specific, noncovalent orientation within the enzyme active site and positions the warhead near the target amino acid. This will allow the warhead to be positioned in close proximity to the nucleophilic residue and will ensure that the reaction between the warhead and this amino acid occurs readily, forming a covalent bond with the protein. It is well known that an intimate proximity between reacting groups can accelerate the rate of reaction by many orders of magnitude, and this can allow efficient bonding between reactants for which the intrinsic bimolecular reaction rate is negligible [14]. An additional factor that helps in the bond formation is high local concentration of the warhead in the neighborhood of the target amino acid residue.

13.2.1
Selection of Warheads

The first step in the optimization of warhead reactivity is proper selection of the electrophilic moiety. Most warheads incorporated into covalent inhibitors interact with their target proteins via an alkylation or acylation reaction. Some important moieties include alkylating agents such as halomethyl-, diazomethyl-, and acyloxymethyl ketones, epoxides, aziridine derivatives, and conjugated enones (α,β-unsaturated carbonyl derivatives) or enones such as vinyl sulfones or acrylonitriles (Figure 13.3). These groups exhibit very little biological utility because of their high indiscriminate reactivity with biological nucleophiles including the endogenous antioxidant glutathione (GSH) leading to toxicity.

Despite their high reactivity, α,β-unsaturated carbonyl groups are the most popular warheads that have been incorporated into covalent inhibitors. Typically referred to as Michael acceptors, these groups react with nucleophiles at the electrophilic β-position of the unsaturated system (Figure 13.4).

Among the different nucleophiles (oxygen-, nitrogen-, or sulfur-based nucleophiles) encountered in proteins, Michael acceptors primarily react with sulfhydryl group of cysteine and this specificity is what makes these warheads an attractive functional group in the design of irreversible covalent modifiers. The electrophilicity at the β-position is influenced by the type of carbonyl group in the α,β-unsaturated carbonyl unit. High carbonyl activities found in aldehydes and esters generally translate into high Michael acceptor reactivities often leading to mutagenicity, skin sensitization, or liver toxicity [15–17]. On the other hand, carboxylic acids, amides, and ketones are typically less prone to such pathogenic behavior. Several naturally occurring cytotoxic compounds that have

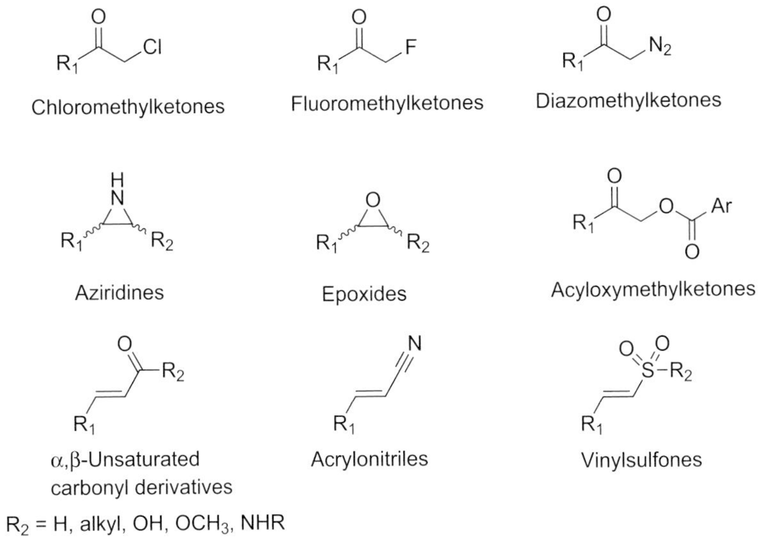

Chloromethylketones Fluoromethylketones Diazomethylketones

Aziridines Epoxides Acyloxymethylketones

α,β-Unsaturated carbonyl derivatives Acrylonitriles Vinylsulfones

R₂ = H, alkyl, OH, OCH₃, NHR

Figure 13.3 Irreversible warhead inhibitors.

been used as drugs contain Michael acceptors and these groups are essential for their disease-fighting activity (Figure 13.5) [12, 18].

In the past decade, Michael acceptors have been incorporated into compounds that inhibit epidermal growth factor receptor (EGFR) family of kinases [19–23]. These compounds were rationally designed by appending an acrylamide as an electrophilic warhead (which is reactive toward the electron-rich sulfur present in the cysteine residue) to the well-characterized EGFR-selective 4-anilinoquinazoline and 4-anilinoquinoline-3-carbonitrile scaffolds. Using the known reversible inhibitors complexed with EGFR such as erlotinib, gefitinib, and lapatinib (Figure 13.6), it was possible to predict the optimal site for electrophile attachment.

The resulting inhibitors undergo a Michael addition reaction in which the solvent-exposed cysteine residue that is present in EGFR (Cys773) or ERB2 (Cys805) forms a covalent bond with the inhibitor. The unique benefit of these "targeted covalent inhibitors" of EGFR tyrosine kinase is their exceptional potency in overcoming endogenous ATP competition and selectivity that is largely orthogonal to that afforded by conventional, noncovalent inhibitors. In addition, sustained

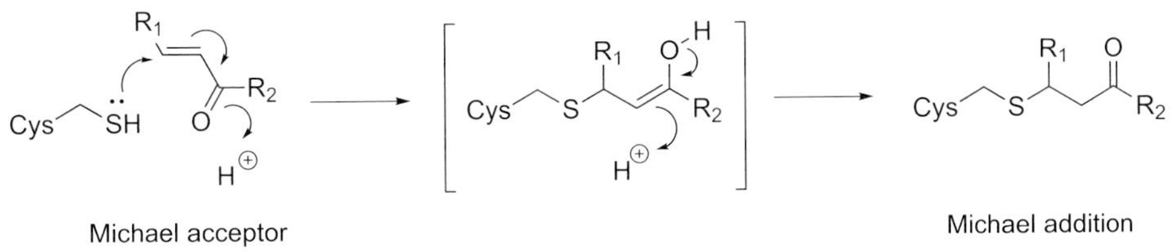

Michael acceptor Michael addition

Figure 13.4 Nucleophilic addition of a cysteine thiol to α,β-unsaturated carbonyl derivatives.

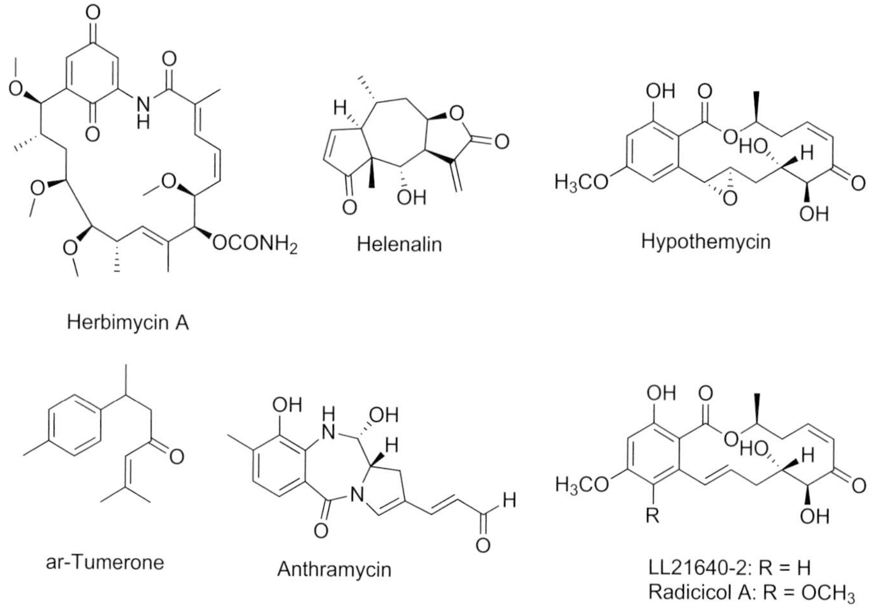

Figure 13.5 Structures of natural products containing Michael acceptors.

potency in the face of resistance mutations has also emerged as an important attribute of this mechanism. The consequence is complete inhibition of EGFR signaling and more durable inhibition of the target until the return of its activity, which is
dependent on protein resynthesis. These compounds exhibit low reactivity with
GSH in cellular assays and exhibit low reactivity with dithiothreotol in enzyme

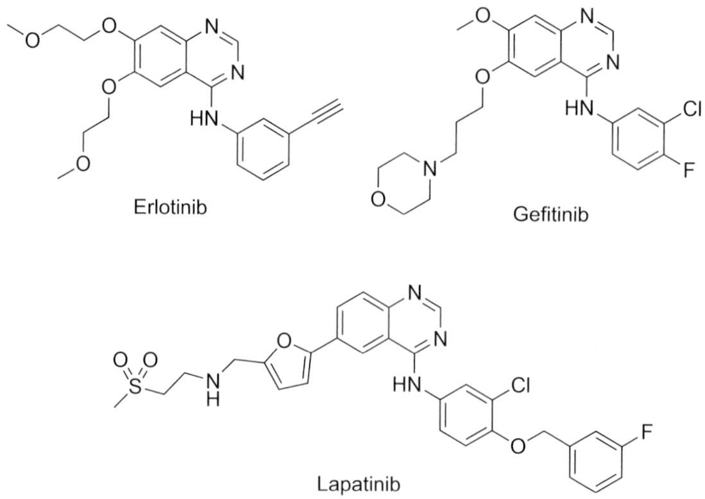

Figure 13.6 Structures of reversible kinase inhibitors.

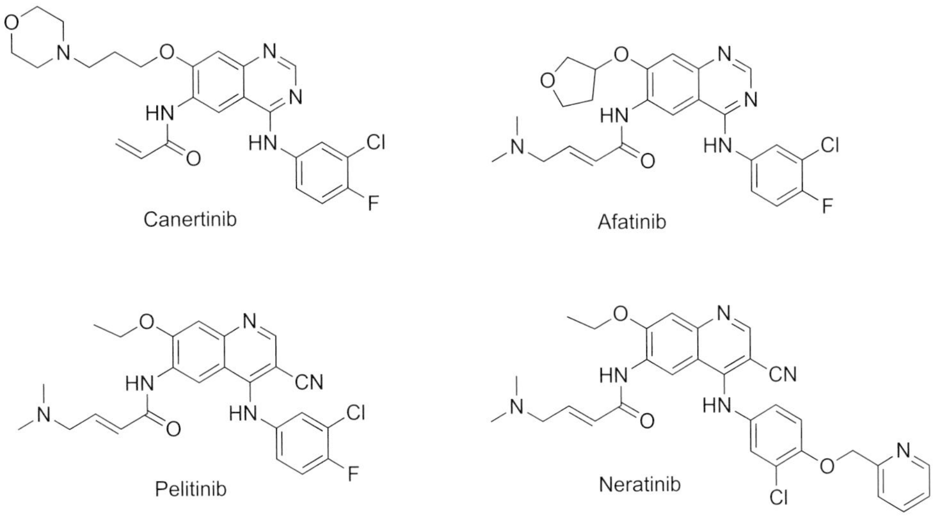

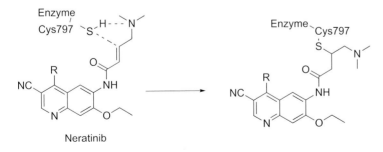

Figure 13.7 Covalent EGFR inhibitors in clinical development.

assays, strongly suggesting that their reactivity toward nonspecific thiol nucleophiles is low. To date, a few irreversible kinase inhibitors, canertinib, afatinib/BIBW2992, neratinib, pelitinib, and PF-0299804 (structure not disclosed), have been introduced into clinical study (Figure 13.7) [24–28].

While canertinib is an unsubstituted acrylamide, afatinib, neratinib, and pelitinib are substituted acrylamides with an *N,N*-dimethylaminomethyl substituent at the β-position to the carbonyl group in the warhead. The substitution at the β-position helps in modulating the reactivity of the unit. The presence of a general base at an adjacent site on the inhibitor helps in achieving selectivity and accelerates covalent bond formation between the warhead and the cysteine residue (Figure 13.8). A similar concept has also been used against other kinases such as vascular endothelial growth factor receptor 2 (VEGFR2) and the Tec family kinase, BTK (PCI-32765) (Figure 13.9) [23, 29–31]. Likewise, rupintrivir (AG7088) (Figure 13.9), a highly potent and specific 3C protease inhibitor designed as an antiviral agent to treat

Figure 13.8 Interaction of cysteine-797 in EGFR with neratinib.

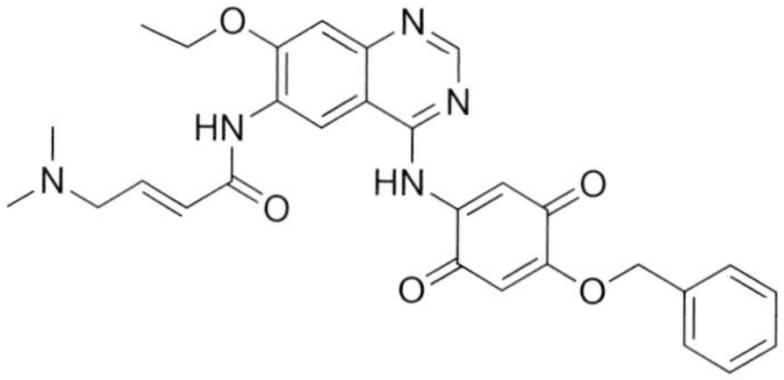

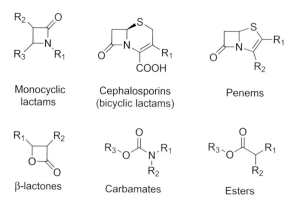

Inhibitor 19
(EGFR and VEGFR2 Inhibitor)

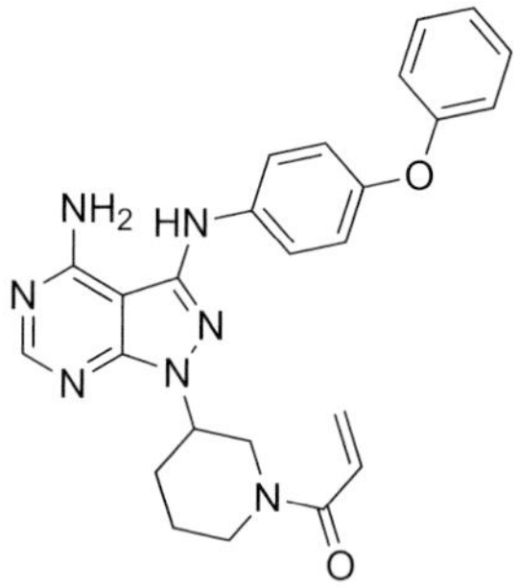

PCI-32765
BTK Inhibitor

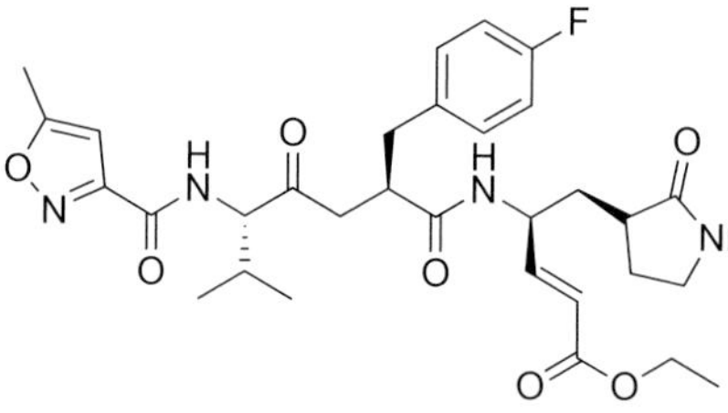

Rupintrivir (AG7088)

Figure 13.9 Structures of some other irreversible inhibitors that incorporate α,β-unsaturated Michael acceptors.

rhinovirus infections, is another example in which a combination of the specific binding of a small molecule with a moderately active Michael acceptor functionality leads to a highly potent and specific enzyme inhibitor [32].

Acylating agents, monocyclic β-lactams, cephalosporins or penems, β-lactones, carbamates, or esters, have also been incorporated into compounds to yield selective covalent modifiers (Figure 13.10).

Monocyclic
lactams

Cephalosporins
(bicyclic lactams)

Penems

β-lactones

Carbamates

Esters

Figure 13.10 Commonly used acylating agents as warheads.

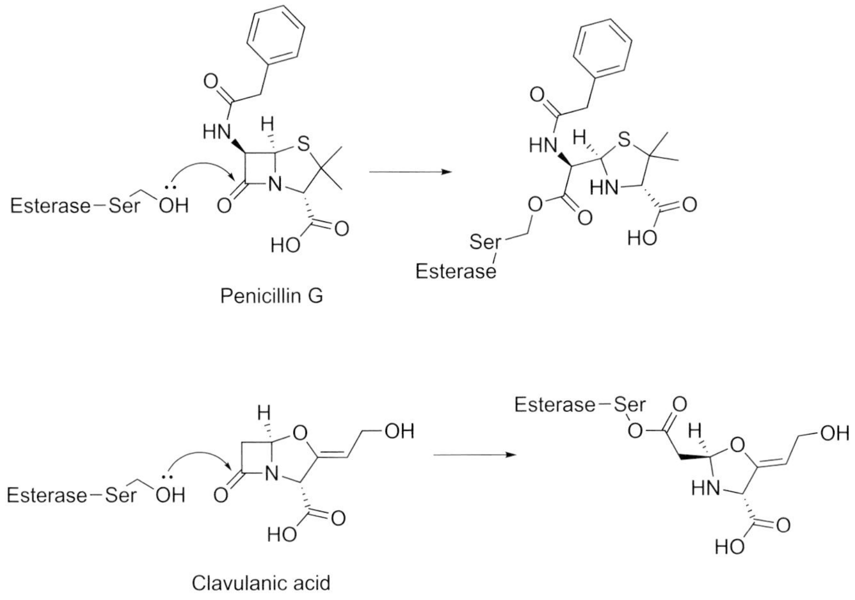

Figure 13.11 Acylation of serine residue of D-ala-D-ala carboxypeptidase and β-lactamase enzymes by penicillin G and clavulanic acid.

Several antibiotics containing a β-lactam nucleus are selective, mechanism-based covalent modifiers of serine-type D-ala-D-ala carboxypeptidase and β-lactamase enzymes. Some examples in this class include amoxicillin, ampicillin, penicillin, and clavulanic acid (Figure 13.11). All β-lactam antibiotics irreversibly acylate the active site serine to form kinetically stable serine ester–linked irreversible adducts, functionally inactivating the bacterial resistance mechanism (Figure 13.11) [2, 33–35].

This class of compounds has served as a particularly rich source of marketed drugs and has opened new areas of target-based drug discovery. Since its discovery nearly 80 years ago, this class of drugs is still in widespread use and continues to yield new agents for the treatment of bacterial infections. Although this class of drugs is generally well tolerated, the rate of allergic reaction can occur in as high as 18% of patients, at least for penicillin [36]. The acute nature of the treatment most likely aids the tolerability, considering that the daily doses of β-lactam antibiotics are very high. The adverse drug reactions associated with β-lactam antibacterial agents such as penicillin have been attributed to indiscriminant acylation of free amino and sulfhydryl groups on proteins via a nonenzymatic β-lactam ring scission. In fact, one of the principal metabolites of amoxicillin in humans is derived from the hydrolysis of the β-lactam ring.

The tempered electrophilicity and hydrolytic stability following carbamoylation has also made carbamate chemotype a privileged scaffold in the design of potent and selective serine hydrolase inhibitors. For example, rivastigmine (Figure 13.1), used to treat Alzheimer's disease, is an inhibitor of acetylcholinesterase that contains a carbamoyloxy group. The group is only activated for cleavage by the active site serine residue when the drug binds to the binding pocket of the enzyme (Figure 13.12a) [37]. Recently, several groups have reported piperazine/piperidine aryl ureas as an emerging class of very selective carbamoylating agents for a serine hydrolase, fatty acid amide hydrolase (FAAH) [38–40]. The enzyme degrades fatty acid amide family of signaling lipids. Inhibition of this enzyme leads to analgesic and anti-inflammatory response in rodents [40]. Covalent inhibition is a result of acylation of the serine residue (Ser241) in the active site of FAAH, through a carbamate linkage (Figure 13.12b) [41]. The exquisite selectivity of this class of compounds can be explained by a specific binding event that activates the urea motif in the FAAH active site, which then renders the chemical reactivity of the urea similar to that of an amide functionality.

The β-lactam bioisosteres, β-lactones, have also been used in leads that covalently modify enzymes after binding to the active site. Orlistat blocks the intestinal absorption of fats by selectively acylating the active site serine of a number of gastric and pancreatic lipases whose natural function is to hydrolyze dietary glyceryl triesters (Figure 13.12c) [42, 43]. This drug has served as a proof-of-principle lead for β-lactones as covalent inhibitors. Similarly, aspirin is a cyclooxygenase (COX) inhibitor, widely used for pain management, which irreversibly acylates a serine residue selectively in the active site of COX-1 (Ser530) and COX-2 (Ser516) (Figure 13.12d) [44].

13.2.2
Reversible Covalent Modification

The concept of reversible covalent modification has been put forth in the recent years to overcome the potential toxicological liabilities due to indiscriminate covalent binding. These inhibitors combine strong reversible binding to the target protein with very low reactivity toward macromolecular nucleophiles. Furthermore, the adducts formed with these nucleophiles are reversible in nature and revert to the parent drug. Although the esters and carbamate functionalities discussed above could theoretically form a reversible adduct (due to hydrolysis of the acyl moiety), functionalities that modulate the targets via this mechanism include aldehyde, ketone, and nitrile derivatives. Aldehyde- and ketone-containing compounds generally bind to the cysteine or serine residue via thiohemiacetal/thiohemiketal or hemiacetal/hemiketal bond formation (Figure 13.13a). On the other hand, nitriles react with the cysteine or serine residues via formation of a reversible imidate or thioimidate adduct (Pinner-type reaction) (Figure 13.13b) [45].

Several types of natural reversible cysteine protease inhibitors have been isolated from microorganisms, the most common being the peptidyl aldehydes. Among those isolated from *Streptomyces* and *Actinomycete* are the leupeptin, chymostatins, antipain, and elastinal (Figure 13.14). Some representatives containing the aldehyde/ketone have reached late stages of clinical trials, for example, telaprevir and boceprevir (Figure 13.14). Both these compounds are NS3 protease inhibitors that interact by forming a hemiketal intermediate with the serine residue in the binding pocket [46, 47].

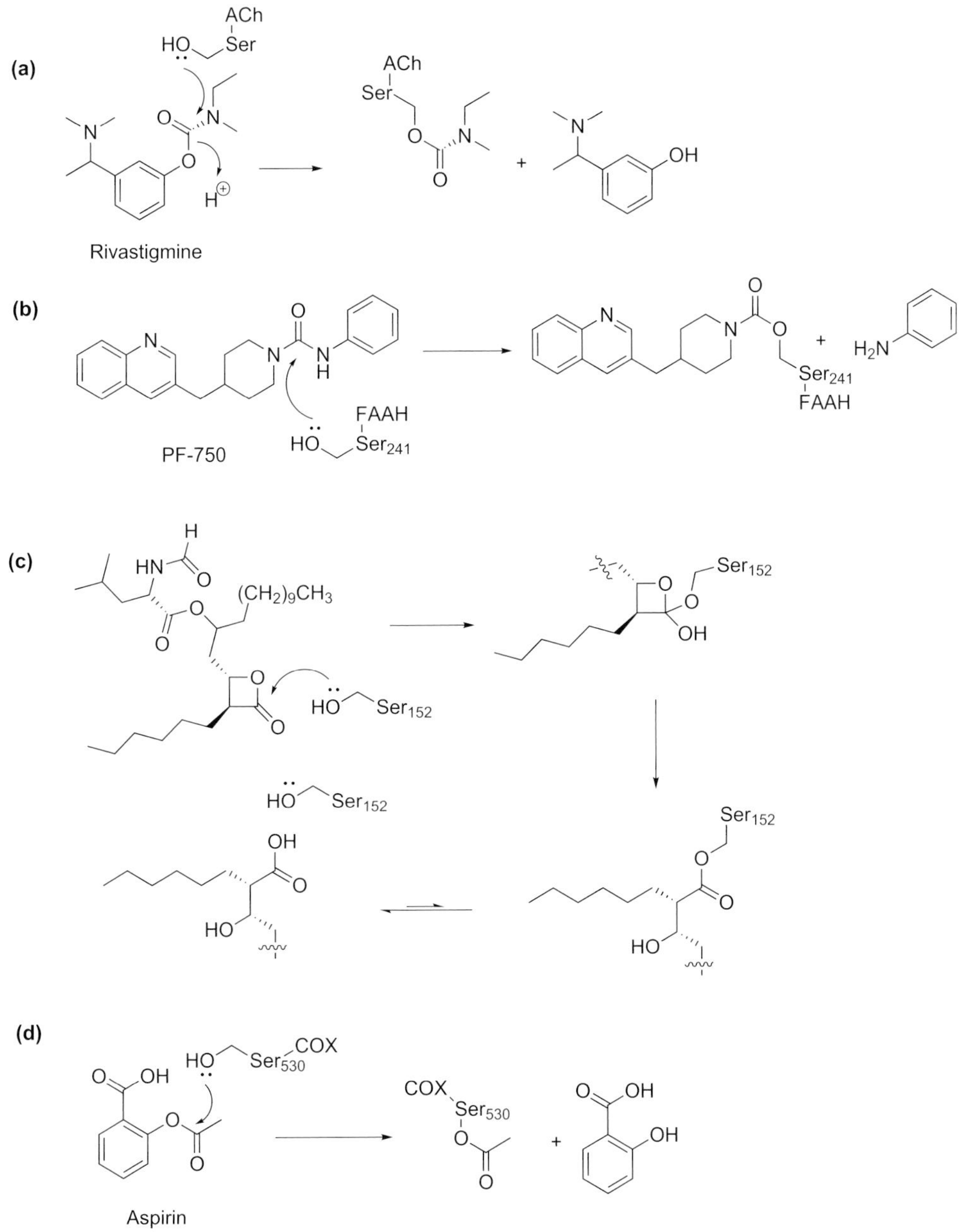

Figure 13.12 Acylation of serine residues by (a) rivastigmine, (b) FAAH inhibitor (PF-750), (c) orlistat, and (d) aspirin.

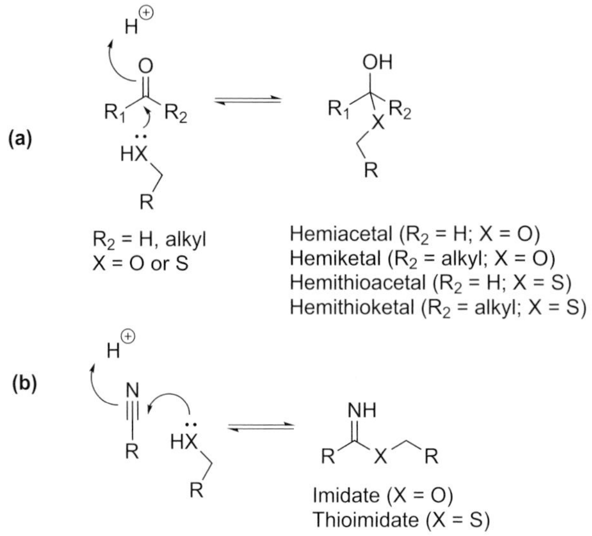

Figure 13.13 Reaction of aldehyde/ketones (a) and nitriles (b) with serine and cysteine of enzymes.

Use of nitrile group as an electrophilic warhead has gained importance in the recent years. This is because nitriles are chemically less reactive when compared to aldehydes [48, 49]. Nitrile-containing molecules have been known to inhibit cysteine proteases since 1960s when benzamidoacetonitrile was shown to be an inhibitor of papain [50]. Three chemical classes of nitrile-containing inhibitors are known: heteroaromatic nitriles, cyanamides, and α-amidoacetonitriles (Figure 13.15) [51–55]. Although all three classes of inhibitors react with enzymes in a reversible manner, there are profound differences in the electrophilicities of the nitrile moieties. Cyanamides and heteroaromatic nitriles are fairly reactive and impact the reaction with cellular nucleophiles [54], while amidoacetonitrile derivatives appear to have optimal level of electrophilicity [56]. Assessment of electrophilicity of the three functionalities using a cysteine reactivity assay [56] indicated that the cyanamide and cyanopyrimidine derivatives showed 71 and 79% conversion to the cysteine adduct, while balicatib, an amidoacetonitrile derivative, forms only 9% of the cysteine adduct.

Several amidoacetonitrile derivatives have been developed as reversible covalent modifiers of serine and/or cysteine proteases such as the dipeptidyl peptidase (DPP IV) or cathepsin inhibitors for treating diabetes and osteoporosis [49, 56, 57]. These candidates either have entered late-stage clinical trials or have been approved for commercial use. For instance, the cyanopyrrolidine derivative saxagliptin, a DPP IV inhibitor (Figure 13.16), was recently launched under the name of Onglyza [58], while the structurally related compound vildagliptin (Figure 13.16) was licensed in Europe [59]. Similarly, a search for cathepsin K inhibitors led to discovery of odanacatib (Figure 13.16) [55]. All these inhibitors are prone to nucleophilic attack on the nitrile group by an active site serine or cysteine residue resulting in a strong reversible imidate or thioimidate adduct formation with a slow off-rate (Figure 13.16) [60, 61].

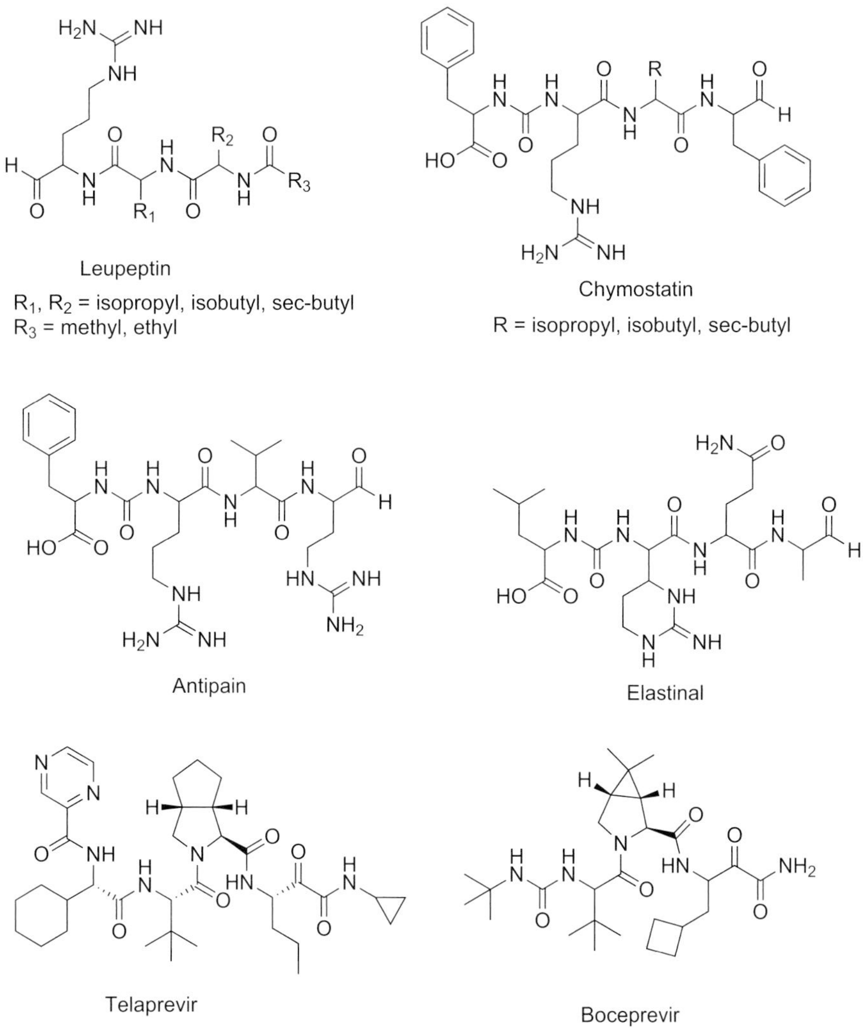

Leupeptin

R$_1$, R$_2$ = isopropyl, isobutyl, sec-butyl
R$_3$ = methyl, ethyl

Chymostatin

R = isopropyl, isobutyl, sec-butyl

Antipain

Elastinal

Telaprevir

Boceprevir

Figure 13.14 Natural cysteine protease inhibitors, which have been isolated from microorganisms. These contain aldehyde and/or ketone motif that form reversible covalent bond with their enzyme targets.

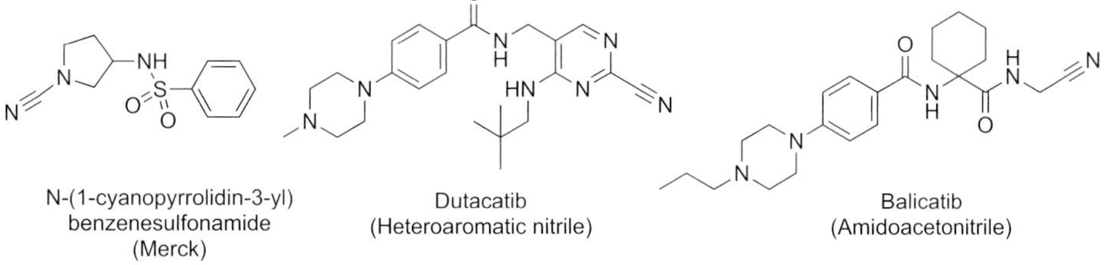

N-(1-cyanopyrrolidin-3-yl)
benzenesulfonamide
(Merck)

Dutacatib
(Heteroaromatic nitrile)

Balicatib
(Amidoacetonitrile)

Figure 13.15 Classes of nitrile-containing reversible covalent modifiers.

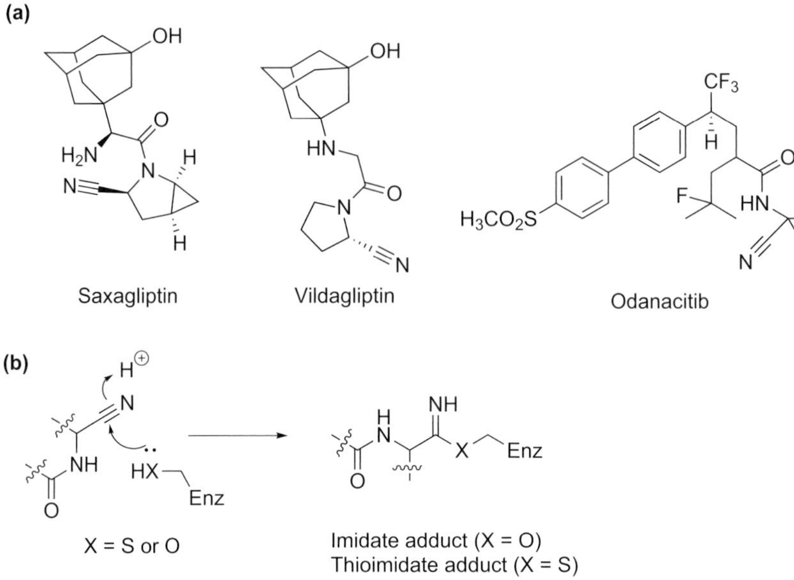

(a)

| Saxagliptin | Vildagliptin | Odanacitib |

(b)

X = S or O

Imidate adduct (X = O)
Thioimidate adduct (X = S)

Figure 13.16 Structures of reversible covalent inhibitors containing nitrile functionalities (a). Reaction of nitriles with cysteine and serine residue to the corresponding thioimidate or imidate adducts (b).

13.3
Optimization of Chemical Reactivity of the Warhead Moiety

Regardless of the nature of the warhead used in the design of a covalent modifier, introduction of an electrophilic moiety in a molecule increases the risk of indiscriminant covalent binding to macromolecules resulting in toxicity. Achieving high selectivity against off-target covalent interactions clearly requires that the intrinsic reactivity of the electrophilic warhead on the inhibitor must be sufficiently low so that no appreciable irreversible reaction occurs with other amino acid residues on proteins and GSH, even when these nucleophiles are present in a high concentration *in vivo* [20]. Hence, it is essential to understand the degree of reactivity of the warhead. Both experimental and *in silico* methods have been used for predicting reactivity of electrophiles.

13.3.1
Experimental Approaches

Experimental approach entails a simple *in vitro* experiment in which the chemical reactivity of a warhead within the potential irreversible inhibitor is determined by measuring the reaction rate with a model nucleophile that acts as a protein surrogate. The nucleophile can range from a small chemical entity such as *n*-butylamine (a lysine equivalent) to sulfhydryl derivatives such as GSH or *N*-acetylcysteine

[15–17, 62, 63]. The reactions are initiated by addition of the test compound to a solution of a nucleophile in phosphate buffer (pH 7.4) containing ethylene diamine tetraacetic acid. 4-(*p*-Nitrobenzyl)pyridine, a trap for alkylating agents with nucleophilic characteristics similar to those of DNA bases, has also been used to measure the alkylating potential and the mechanism of the reaction [64, 65]. The rates are estimated by monitoring the loss of the parent compound or the nucleophilic moiety by liquid chromatography tandem mass spectrometry (LC/MS–MS) or ultraviolet spectroscopy. Alternatively, the resulting adduct formed can be quantified by LC/MS–MS if the authentic adduct standard is available. These so-called *in chemico* approaches allow for a high control of the experimental conditions and a high reproducibility. The approach also provides a relatively easy means of screening chemicals, determining their chemical reactivity potential and therefore their potential to lead to nonspecific irreversible covalent binding. The main source of error of *in chemico* reactivity experiments is the degree of mismatch between the behavior of the exogenous nucleophile and the one present on a protein. A small chemical cannot completely represent the behavior of a protein nucleophile(s). However, the consequence of these effects is reduced if the chemical reactivity potency is treated on a relative scale since the chemical measurements will be systematically biased, but they will keep their relative potencies for rank ordering chemical reactivity.

Although these results aid in rank ordering compounds with respect to their chemical reactivity, the risks that are associated due to their reactivity cannot be assessed from these data. To assess the potential liability of chemical reactivity with other thiol-containing proteins, a compound can be identified to act as a point of reference to determine an acceptable level of chemical reactivity. Such a benchmark compound can be a marketed covalent modifier. The reactivity (in terms of half-life) of the test compound can then be compared to this reference to determine relative degree of chemical reactivity of the inhibitor. For instance, MacFaul *et al.*, in their risk assessment of a series of nitrile-containing covalent modifiers, identified nilvadipine as a benchmark (Figure 13.17) [66]. The compound is a calcium channel antagonist that has been on the market since 1991 and has a good safety record. It possesses a half-life of 40 h for the reaction with GSH and 2 h with cysteine [66]. Based on the reactivity of nilvadipine, the authors proposed a target half-life of 40 h, or greater, as a safe guideline for nitriles.

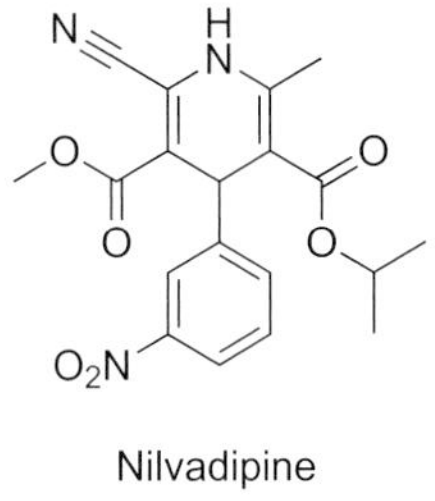

Nilvadipine

Figure 13.17 Structure of the calcium channel antagonist nilvadipine, a marketed drug that is used as a reference for assessing chemical reactivity with GSH.

Radiolabeled material is generally used for detailed risk assessment of covalent binding by irreversible enzyme inhibitors. Nonspecific binding assays performed using a radiolabeled compound are advantageous since they allow for quantification of the amount of drug–protein adduct formed. Incubation of the radiolabeled compound with liver proteins in the absence of NADPH, followed by radiometric analysis, can give an estimate of the amount of material bound to proteins based on the biochemical reactivity of the warhead in the parent compound. The level of binding is typically expressed in terms of pmol drug equivalents bound per mg protein after 1 h incubation [6]. The reactivity is considered acceptable if the amount of covalently bound radioactivity is less than the proposed target value. The "acceptable" range of protein covalent binding will always be defined differently throughout the industry. It has been proposed previously that a target value of less than 50 pmol adduct/mg protein should be considered an acceptable level [6]. The primary drawback of this approach is that it is tedious and not suitable to run routinely in the early stages of discovery. This technique has been used to assess the reactivity of nitrile-based inhibitors of cathepsin K by Oballa *et al.* and MacFaul *et al.* [54, 66].

Other experimental approaches such ^{1}H or ^{13}C NMR studies have also been used in determining the relative electrophilicity of the β-carbons of α,β-unsaturated carbonyl compounds [67]. For instance, Fujisawa and Kadoma have reported the prediction of GSH reactivity of dental methacrylate monomers, and hence their toxicity, using the ^{13}C NMR chemical shifts of β-carbon and the ^{1}H NMR shifts of the protons attached to β-carbon [68].

13.3.2
In Silico Approaches

Although chemical reactivity assays have the potential to provide information to assist in the identification of highly reactive electrophiles, there is current interest to move away from reliance on experimentation and use computational techniques to predict chemical reactivity. This is an attractive approach, especially where experimental measurements are not possible or restricted, for example, because of low solubility. Oballa *et al.* used a computational approach to calculate the theoretical reactivities of diverse nitriles [54]. The method assessed the electrophilicity of nitrile-containing compounds by calculating the energy difference between the thioimidate adduct, the precursor methanethiol, and the nitrile molecule. The calculated reactive index for the compounds was found to correlate well with the experimentally (using cysteine as a nucleophile) determined reactivity data. More recently, Schwöbel *et al.* have examined Michael addition reactivity toward GSH by transition state calculations. In this study, kinetic rate constants (k_{GSH}) for reaction of compounds acting as Michael acceptors with GSH were modeled by quantum chemical transition state calculations. These predicted k_{GSH} values were found to be in good agreement with experimental k_{GSH} values [69, 70]. In another approach, E_{LUMO} and E_{HOMO} values were computed for compounds containing α,β-unsaturated carbonyl motifs as electrophiles and were related to their biological activities [71]. This study demonstrated that Michael acceptor reactivity correlates to lower E_{LUMO} values. Parameters such as E_{LUMO} and partial charge on the β-carbon have also been used in other instances to assess the reactivity of Michael acceptors such as α,β-unsaturated aldehydes, ketones, and esters [15–17]. These results suggest that magnitudes of these coefficients correlate well with hepatocyte toxicity measurements with these compounds.

Although the above approaches are useful in optimizing the reactivity of the warheads used in designing covalent modifiers, achieving selectivity and avoiding nonspecific binding can still be challenging (even if the electrophile has very low intrinsic reactivity) if the compound targets a nucleophilic residue that is highly conserved across a protein family, because even relatively weak binding to the active site of an off-target protease within the same family could result in a covalent interaction with the conserved catalytic nucleophile and lead to irreversible inhibition resulting in loss of selectivity against enzyme isoforms [72].

13.3.3
Additional Derisking Factors

Other derisking factors that are in line with those that are applicable to risk assessment of reactive metabolites should also be considered for covalent modifiers. For example, the risk of idiosyncratic adverse drug reactions from reactive metabolites can be mitigated if a low dose of the drug can be used [73]. Similarly, it could be inferred that the risk associated with developing a covalent inhibitor could be minimized if the dose was less than 10 mg/day [20]. Second, it is questionable if one needs to optimize the pharmacokinetics of these compounds to achieve a once-a-day or twice-a-day dosing. Generally, the pharmacodynamic action of covalent inhibitors outlasts measurable plasma drug levels. Once covalently inactivated, the target is neutralized and the activity can only be recovered by synthesis of new protein. As long as resynthesis of the protein is not too fast, only enough drug exposure to inactivate the target is necessary and sustained systemic exposure of the drug (long half-life) may not be required. This can potentially deprioritize the need for high and prolonged systemic drug load and could therefore mitigate off-target activity and nonspecific covalent binding. In fact, after the target protein has been inactivated by the irreversible reaction, the drug should preferably be cleared rapidly to minimize off-target interactions (both covalent and noncovalent), which could conceivably reduce nonmechanism-based toxicity.

13.4
Concluding Remarks

Despite the many examples of successful covalent drugs, general interest in covalent modifiers as drug candidates has emerged only recently. Although these drugs possess the capability to elicit adverse effects due to the inherent electrophilic group in them, these can be developed into safe and effective drugs if proper derisking strategies are applied. The temperament of an electrophile can be monitored by assessing reactivity relative to other marketed covalent modifiers. A proper balance between the reactivity and selectivity of the compound can be achieved by combination of a tempered electrophile with a selective noncovalent binder. Ongoing clinical studies with an emerging cadre of highly selective covalent inhibitors will continue to offer insight into this drug discovery strategy and should further clarify their therapeutic utility and possible risks.

References

1 Robertson, J.G. (2005) Mechanistic basis of enzyme-targeted drugs. *Biochemistry*, **44**, 5561–5571.

2 Potashman, M.H. and Duggan, M.E. (2009) Covalent modifiers: an orthogonal approach to drug design. *Journal of Medicinal Chemistry*, **52**, 1231–1246.

3 Powers, J.C., Asgian, J.L., Ekici, O.D., and James, K.E. (2002) Irreversible inhibitors of serine, cysteine, and threonine proteases. *Chemical Reviews*, **102**, 4639–4750.

4 Uetrecht, J. (2008) Idiosyncratic drug reactions: past, present, and future. *Chemical Research in Toxicology*, **21**, 84–92.

5 Uetrecht, J. (2009) Immune-mediated adverse drug reactions. *Chemical Research in Toxicology*, **22**, 24–34.

6 Evans, D.C., Watt, A.P., Nicoll-Griffith, D.A., and Baillie, T.A. (2004) Drug–protein adducts: an industry perspective on minimizing the potential for drug bioactivation in drug discovery and development. *Chemical Research in Toxicology*, **17**, 3–16.

7 Zhou, S., Chan, E., Duan, W., Huang, M., and Chen, Y.Z. (2005) Drug bioactivation, covalent binding to target proteins and toxicity relevance. *Drug Metabolism Reviews*, **37**, 41–213.

8 Kumar, S., Kassahun, K., Tschirret-Guth, R.A., Mitra, K., and Baillie, T.A. (2008) Minimizing metabolic activation during pharmaceutical lead optimization: progress, knowledge gaps and future directions. *Current Opinion in Drug Discovery & Development*, **11**, 43–52.

9 Baillie, T.A. (2008) Metabolism and toxicity of drugs. Two decades of progress in industrial drug metabolism. *Chemical Research in Toxicology*, **21**, 129–137.

10 Swinney, D.C. (2004) Biochemical mechanisms of drug action: what does it take for success? *Nature Reviews. Drug Discovery*, **3**, 801–808.

11 Swinney, D.C. (2009) The role of binding kinetics in therapeutically useful drug action. *Current Opinion in Drug Discovery & Development*, **12**, 31–39.

12 Amslinger, S. (2010) The tunable functionality of alpha,beta-unsaturated carbonyl compounds enables their differential application in biological systems. *ChemMedChem*, **5**, 351–356.

13 Way, J.C. (2000) Covalent modification as a strategy to block protein–protein interactions with small-molecule drugs. *Current Opinion in Chemical Biology*, **4**, 40–46.

14 Jencks, W.P. (1975) Binding energy, specificity, and enzymic catalysis: the circe effect. *Advances in Enzymology and Related Areas of Molecular Biology*, **43**, 219–410.

15 Chan, K., Jensen, N., and O'Brien, P.J. (2008) Structure–activity relationships for thiol reactivity and rat or human hepatocyte toxicity induced by substituted *p*-benzoquinone compounds. *Journal of Applied Toxicology*, **28**, 608–620.

16 Chan, K. and O'Brien, P.J. (2008) Structure–activity relationships for hepatocyte toxicity and electrophilic reactivity of alpha,beta-unsaturated esters, acrylates and methacrylates. *Journal of Applied Toxicology*, **28**, 1004–1015.

17 Chan, K., Poon, R., and O'Brien, P.J. (2008) Application of structure–activity relationships to investigate the molecular mechanisms of hepatocyte toxicity and electrophilic reactivity of alpha,beta-

unsaturated aldehydes. *Journal of Applied Toxicology*, **28**, 1027–1039.

18 Ahn, B.Z. and Sok, D.E. (1996) Michael acceptors as a tool for anticancer drug design. *Current Pharmaceutical Design*, **2**, 247–262.

19 Cohen, M.S., Zhang, C., Shokat, K.M., and Taunton, J. (2005) Structural bioinformatics-based design of selective, irreversible kinase inhibitors. *Science*, **308**, 1318–1321.

20 Singh, J., Petter, R.C., Baillie, T.A., and Whitty, A. (2011) The resurgence of covalent drugs. *Nature Reviews. Drug Discovery*, **10**, 307–317.

21 Singh, J., Petter, R.C., and Kluge, A.F. (2010) Targeted covalent drugs of the kinase family. *Current Opinion in Chemical Biology*, **14**, 475–480.

22 Fry, D.W. (2000) Site-directed irreversible inhibitors of the erbB family of receptor tyrosine kinases as novel chemotherapeutic agents for cancer. *Anti-Cancer Drug Design*, **15**, 3–16.

23 Zhang, J., Yang, P.L., and Gray, N.S. (2009) Targeting cancer with small molecule kinase inhibitors. *Nature Reviews. Cancer*, **9**, 28–39.

24 Kwak, E.L., Sordella, R., Bell, D.W., Godin-Heymann, N., Okimoto, R.A., Brannigan, B.W., Harris, P.L., Driscoll, D.R., Fidias, P., Lynch, T.J., Rabindran, S.K., McGinnis, J.P., Wissner, A., Sharma, S.V., Isselbacher, K.J., Settleman, J., and Haber, D.A. (2005) Irreversible inhibitors of the EGF receptor may circumvent acquired resistance to gefitinib. *Proceedings of the National Academy of Sciences of the United States of America*, **102**, 7665–7670.

25 Heymach, J.V., Nilsson, M., Blumenschein, G., Papadimitrakopoulou, V., and Herbst, R. (2006) Epidermal growth factor receptor inhibitors in development for the treatment of non-small cell lung cancer. *Clinical Cancer Research*, **12**, 4441s–4445s.

26 Felip, E., Santarpia, M., and Rosell, R. (2007) Emerging drugs for non-small-cell lung cancer. *Expert Opinion on Emerging Drugs*, **12**, 449–460.

27 Wissner, A. and Mansour, T.S. (2008) The development of HKI-272 and related compounds for the treatment of cancer. *Archiv der Pharmazie*, **341**, 465–477.

28 Mukherji, D. and Spicer, J. (2009) Second-generation epidermal growth factor tyrosine kinase inhibitors in non-small cell lung cancer. *Expert Opinion on Investigational Drugs*, **18**, 293–301.

29 Cohen, M.S., Hadjivassiliou, H., and Taunton, J. (2007) A clickable inhibitor reveals context-dependent autoactivation of p90 RSK. *Nature Chemical Biology*, **3**, 156–160.

30 Wissner, A., Fraser, H.L., Ingalls, C.L., Dushin, R.G., Floyd, M.B., Cheung, K., Nittoli, T., Ravi, M.R., Tan, X., and Loganzo, F. (2007) Dual irreversible kinase inhibitors: quinazoline-based inhibitors incorporating two independent reactive centers with each targeting different cysteine residues in the kinase domains of EGFR and VEGFR-2. *Bioorganic and Medicinal Chemistry*, **15**, 3635–3648.

31 Pan, Z., Scheerens, H., Li, S.J., Schultz, B.E., Sprengeler, P.A., Burrill, L.C., Mendonca, R.V., Sweeney, M.D., Scott, K.C., Grothaus, P.G., Jeffery, D.A., Spoerke, J.M., Honigberg, L.A., Young, P.R., Dalrymple, S.A., and Palmer, J.T. (2007) Discovery of selective irreversible inhibitors for Bruton's tyrosine kinase. *ChemMedChem*, **2**, 58–61.

32 Binford, S.L., Maldonado, F., Brothers, M.A., Weady, P.T., Zalman, L.S., Meador, J.W. 3rd, Matthews, D.A., and Patick, A.K. (2005) Conservation of amino acids in human rhinovirus 3C protease correlates with broad-spectrum antiviral activity of rupintrivir, a novel human rhinovirus 3C protease inhibitor. *Antimicrobial Agents and Chemotherapy*, **49**, 619–626.

33 Lu, W.P., Kincaid, E., Sun, Y., and Bauer, M.D. (2001) Kinetics of beta-lactam interactions with penicillin-susceptible and -resistant penicillin-binding protein $2\times$ proteins from *Streptococcus pneumoniae*. Involvement of acylation and deacylation in beta-lactam resistance. *The Journal of Biological Chemistry*, **276**, 31494–31501.

34 Yocum, R.R., Rasmussen, J.R., and Strominger, J.L. (1980) The mechanism of action of penicillin. Penicillin acylates the active site of *Bacillus stearothermophilus* D-alanine carboxypeptidase. *The Journal of Biological Chemistry*, **255**, 3977–3986.

35 Waxman, D.J., Yocum, R.R., and Strominger, J.L. (1980) Penicillins and cephalosporins are active site-directed acylating agents: evidence in support of the substrate analogue hypothesis. *Philosophical Transactions of the Royal Society of London. Series B, Biological Sciences*, **289**, 257–271.

36 Bigby, M., Jick, S., Jick, H., and Arndt, K. (1986) Drug-induced cutaneous reactions. A report from the Boston Collaborative Drug Surveillance Program on 15,438 consecutive inpatients, 1975 to 1982. *JAMA: the Journal of the American Medical Association*, **256**, 3358–3363.

37 Bar-On, P., Millard, C.B., Harel, M., Dvir, H., Enz, A., Sussman, J.L., and Silman, I. (2002) Kinetic and structural studies on the interaction of cholinesterases with the anti-Alzheimer drug rivastigmine. *Biochemistry*, **41**, 3555–3564.

38 Ahn, K., Johnson, D.S., Mileni, M., Beidler, D., Long, J.Z., McKinney, M.K., Weerapana, E., Sadagopan, N., Liimatta, M., Smith, S.E., Lazerwith, S., Stiff, C., Kamtekar, S., Bhattacharya, K., Zhang, Y., Swaney, S., Van Becelaere, K., Stevens, R.C., and Cravatt, B.F. (2009) Discovery and characterization of a highly selective FAAH inhibitor that reduces inflammatory pain. *Chemistry & Biology*, **16**, 411–420.

39 Johnson, D.S., Ahn, K., Kesten, S., Lazerwith, S.E., Song, Y., Morris, M., Fay, L., Gregory, T., Stiff, C., Dunbar, J.B. Jr., Liimatta, M., Beidler, D., Smith, S., Nomanbhoy, T.K., and Cravatt, B.F. (2009) Benzothiophene piperazine and piperidine urea inhibitors of fatty acid amide hydrolase (FAAH). *Bioorganic & Medicinal Chemistry Letters*, **19**, 2865–2869.

40 Johnson, D.S., Weerapana, E., and Cravatt, B.F. (2010) Strategies for discovering and derisking covalent, irreversible enzyme inhibitors. *Future Medicinal Chemistry*, **2**, 949–964.

41 Mileni, M., Johnson, D.S., Wang, Z., Everdeen, D.S., Liimatta, M., Pabst, B., Bhattacharya, K., Nugent, R.A., Kamtekar,

S., Cravatt, B.F., Ahn, K., and Stevens, R.C. (2008) Structure-guided inhibitor design for human FAAH by interspecies active site conversion. *Proceedings of the National Academy of Sciences of the United States of America*, **105**, 12820–12824.

42 Hadvary, P., Sidler, W., Meister, W., Vetter, W., and Wolfer, H. (1991) The lipase inhibitor tetrahydrolipstatin binds covalently to the putative active site serine of pancreatic lipase. *The Journal of Biological Chemistry*, **266**, 2021–2027.

43 Guerciolini, R. (1997) Mode of action of orlistat. *International Journal of Obesity and Related Metabolic Disorders*, **21** (Suppl. 3), S12–S23.

44 Roth, G.J., Stanford, N., and Majerus, P.W. (1975) Acetylation of prostaglandin synthase by aspirin. *Proceedings of the National Academy of Sciences of the United States of America*, **72**, 3073–3076.

45 Dufour, E., Storer, A.C., and Menard, R. (1995) Peptide aldehydes and nitriles as transition state analog inhibitors of cysteine proteases. *Biochemistry*, **34**, 9136–9143.

46 Lin, C., Kwong, A.D., and Perni, R.B. (2006) Discovery and development of VX-950, a novel, covalent, and reversible inhibitor of hepatitis C virus NS3.4A serine protease. *Infectious Disorders – Drug Targets*, **6**, 3–16.

47 Kwo, P.Y., Lawitz, E.J., McCone, J., Schiff, E.R., Vierling, J.M., Pound, D., Davis, M. N., Galati, J.S., Gordon, S.C., Ravendhran, N., Rossaro, L., Anderson, F.H., Jacobson, I.M., Rubin, R., Koury, K., Pedicone, L.D., Brass, C.A., Chaudhri, E., and Albrecht, J.K. (2010) Efficacy of boceprevir, an NS3 protease inhibitor, in combination with peginterferon alfa-2b and ribavirin in treatment-naive patients with genotype 1 hepatitis C infection (SPRINT-1): an open-label, randomised, multicentre phase 2 trial. *Lancet*, **376**, 705–716.

48 Frizler, M., Lohr, F., Furtmann, N., Klas, J., and Gutschow, M. (2011) Structural optimization of azadipeptide nitriles strongly increases association rates and allows the development of selective cathepsin inhibitors. *Journal of Medicinal Chemistry*, **54**, 396–400.

49 Frizler, M., Stirnberg, M., Sisay, M.T., and Gutschow, M. (2010) Development of

nitrile-based peptidic inhibitors of cysteine cathepsins. *Current Topics in Medicinal Chemistry*, **10**, 294–322.

50 Lucas, E.C. and Williams, A. (1969) The pH dependencies of individual rate constants in papain-catalyzed reactions. *Biochemistry*, **8**, 5125–5135.

51 Deaton, D.N., Hassell, A.M., McFadyen, R.B., Miller, A.B., Miller, L.R., Shewchuk, L.M., Tavares, F.X., Willard, D.H. Jr., and Wright, L.L. (2005) Novel and potent cyclic cyanamide-based cathepsin K inhibitors. *Bioorganic & Medicinal Chemistry Letters*, **15**, 1815–1819.

52 Grabowskal, U., Chambers, T.J., and Shiroo, M. (2005) Recent developments in cathepsin K inhibitor design. *Current Opinion in Drug Discovery & Development*, **8**, 619–630.

53 Altmann, E., Cowan-Jacob, S.W., and Missbach, M. (2004) Novel purine nitrile derived inhibitors of the cysteine protease cathepsin K. *Journal of Medicinal Chemistry*, **47**, 5833–5836.

54 Oballa, R.M., Truchon, J.F., Bayly, C.I., Chauret, N., Day, S., Crane, S., and Berthelette, C. (2007) A generally applicable method for assessing the electrophilicity and reactivity of diverse nitrile-containing compounds. *Bioorganic & Medicinal Chemistry Letters*, **17**, 998–1002.

55 Gauthier, J.Y., Chauret, N., Cromlish, W., Desmarais, S., Duong le, T., Falgueyret, J.P., Kimmel, D.B., Lamontagne, S., Leger, S., LeRiche, T., Li, C.S., Masse, F., McKay, D.J., Nicoll-Griffith, D.A., Oballa, R.M., Palmer, J.T., Percival, M.D., Riendeau, D., Robichaud, J., Rodan, G.A., Rodan, S.B., Seto, C., Therien, M., Truong, V.L., Venuti, M.C., Wesolowski, G., Young, R.N., Zamboni, R., and Black, W.C. (2008) The discovery of odanacatib (MK-0822), a selective inhibitor of cathepsin K. *Bioorganic & Medicinal Chemistry Letters*, **18**, 923–928.

56 Black, W.C. and Percival, M.D. (2006) The consequences of lysosomotropism on the design of selective cathepsin K inhibitors. *Chembiochem: A European Journal of Chemical Biology*, **7**, 1525–1535.

57 Fleming, F.F., Yao, L., Ravikumar, P.C., Funk, L., and Shook, B.C. (2010) Nitrile-

containing pharmaceuticals: efficacious roles of the nitrile pharmacophore. *Journal of Medicinal Chemistry*, **53**, 7902–7917.

58 Dhillon, S. and Weber, J. (2009) Saxagliptin. *Drugs*, **69**, 2103–2114.

59 Mathieu, C. and Degrande, E. (2008) Vildagliptin: a new oral treatment for type 2 diabetes mellitus. *Journal of Vascular Health and Risk Management*, **4**, 1349–1360.

60 Li, C.S., Deschenes, D., Desmarais, S., Falgueyret, J.P., Gauthier, J.Y., Kimmel, D.B., Leger, S., Masse, F., McGrath, M.E., McKay, D.J., Percival, M.D., Riendeau, D., Rodan, S.B., Therien, M., Truong, V.L., Wesolowski, G., Zamboni, R., and Black, W.C. (2006) Identification of a potent and selective non-basic cathepsin K inhibitor. *Bioorganic & Medicinal Chemistry Letters*, **16**, 1985–1989.

61 Metzler, W.J., Yanchunas, J., Weigelt, C., Kish, K., Klei, H.E., Xie, D., Zhang, Y., Corbett, M., Tamura, J.K., He, B., Hamann, L.G., Kirby, M.S., and Marcinkeviciene, J. (2008) Involvement of DPP-IV catalytic residues in enzyme–saxagliptin complex formation. *Protein Science: A Publication of the Protein Society*, **17**, 240–250.

62 Aptula, A.O., Patlewicz, G., Roberts, D.W., and Schultz, T.W. (2006) Non-enzymatic glutathione reactivity and in vitro toxicity: a non-animal approach to skin sensitization. *Toxicology In Vitro: An International Journal Published in Association with BIBRA*, **20**, 239–247.

63 Schultz, T.W., Yarbrough, J.W., and Johnson, E.L. (2005) Structure–activity relationships for reactivity of carbonyl-containing compounds with glutathione. *SAR and QSAR in Environmental Research*, **16**, 313–322.

64 Cespedes-Camacho, I.F., Manso, J.A., Perez-Prior, M.T., Gomez-Bombarelli, R., Gonzalez-Perez, M., Calle, E., and Casado, J. (2010) Reactivity of acrylamide as an alylating agent: a kinetic approach. *Journal of Physical Organic Chemistry*, **23**, 171–175.

65 Bardos, T.J., Datta-Gupta, N., Hebborn, P., and Triggle, D.J. (1965) A study of comparative chemical and biological

activities of alkylating agents. *Journal of Medicinal Chemistry*, **8**, 167–174.

66 MacFaul, P.A., Morley, A.D., and Crawford, J.J. (2009) A simple in vitro assay for assessing the reactivity of nitrile containing compounds. *Bioorganic & Medicinal Chemistry Letters*, **19**, 1136–1138.

67 Dinkova-Kostova, A.T., Massiah, M.A., Bozak, R.E., Hicks, R.J., and Talalay, P. (2001) Potency of Michael reaction acceptors as inducers of enzymes that protect against carcinogenesis depends on their reactivity with sulfhydryl groups. *Proceedings of the National Academy of Sciences of the United States of America*, **98**, 3404–3409.

68 Fujisawa, S. and Kadoma, Y. (2009) Prediction of the reduced glutathione (GSH) reactivity of dental methacrylate monomers using NMR spectra – relationship between toxicity and GSH reactivity. *Dental Materials Journal*, **28**, 722–729.

69 Schwöbel, J.A., Madden, J.C., and Cronin, M.T. (2010) Examination of Michael

addition reactivity towards glutathione by transition-state calculations. *SAR and QSAR in Environmental Research*, **21**, 693–710.

70 Schwöbel, J.A., Wondrousch, D., Koleva, Y.K., Madden, J.C., Cronin, M.T., and Schuurmann, G. (2010) Prediction of Michael-type acceptor reactivity toward glutathione. *Chemical Research in Toxicology*, **23**, 1576–1585.

71 Zoete, V., Rougee, M., Dinkova-Kostova, A.T., Talalay, P., and Bensasson, R.V. (2004) Redox ranking of inducers of a cancer-protective enzyme via the energy of their highest occupied molecular orbital. *Free Radical Biology & Medicine*, **36**, 1418–1423.

72 Turk, B. (2006) Targeting proteases: successes, failures and future prospects. *Nature Reviews. Drug Discovery*, **5**, 785–799.

73 Uetrecht, J.P. (2000) Is it possible to more accurately predict which drug candidates will cause idiosyncratic drug reactions? *Current Drug Metabolism*, **1**, 133–141.

14
Dealing with Reactive Metabolite–Positive Compounds in Drug Discovery

Abbreviations

BSEP   Bile salt export pump
CaSR   Human calcium sensing receptor
CYP   Cytochrome P450
FIH   First-in-human
GSH   Glutathione
HLM   Human liver microsomes
IADRs   Idiosyncratic adverse drug reactions
PK/PD   Pharmacokinetic/pharmacodynamic
UGT   Uridine diphospho glucuronosyltransferase

14.1
Introduction

The availability of methodology to assess reactive metabolite formation has clearly aided to replace a vague perception of a chemical class effect with a sharper picture of individual molecular peculiarity with respect to occurrence of idiosyncratic adverse drug reactions (IADRs) with drugs. Under the basic premise that a reactive metabolite–negative compound could potentially mitigate immune-mediated IADR risks, screens have been implemented to assess reactive metabolite formation from new compounds with the ultimate goal of minimizing or eliminating this liability through iterative medicinal chemistry efforts (see Chapters 10 and 11). General avoidance of structural alerts (Chapter 5) is almost a norm in drug design, particularly at the lead optimization/candidate selection stage. While these approaches appear reasonable in the quest for safer medicines, there is a growing concern that the perceived safety hazards associated with incorporation of a structural alert may be overexaggerated. For instance, as examined in Chapter 12, almost half of all new small molecule drugs launched in the past five years possess at least one structural alert. Moreover, as discussed in Chapter 5, the vast majority of drugs possess a phenyl ring, which is a structural alert in its own right, since phenyl ring

Reactive Drug Metabolites, First Edition. Amit S. Kalgutkar, Deepak Dalvie, R. Scott Obach, and Dennis A. Smith.
© 2012 Wiley-VCH Verlag GmbH & Co. KGaA. Published 2012 by Wiley-VCH Verlag GmbH & Co. KGaA.

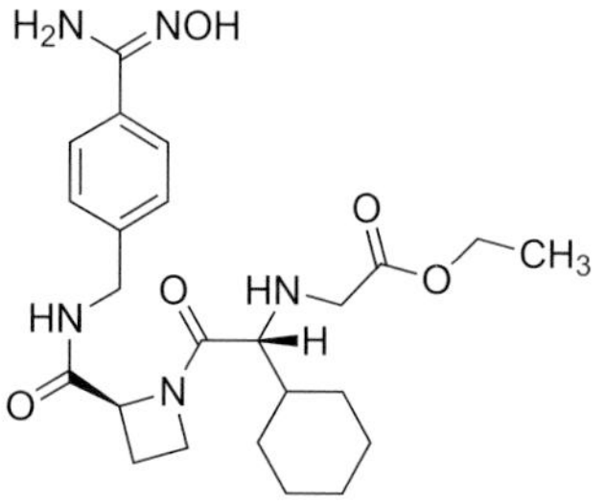

Figure 14.1 Structure of the thrombin inhibitor ximelagatran, which was withdrawn from commercial use due to cases of idiosyncratic hepatotoxicity.

metabolism to the corresponding phenol can proceed through a reactive epoxide intermediate. Aromatic ring epoxidation also represents the rate-limiting step in the carcinogenic and/or hepatotoxic effects of organic solvents such as benzene and bromobenzene. In addition, there are real concerns that simple reactive metabolite screening tools detailed in Chapter 10, such as glutathione (GSH) trapping and covalent binding assays, may be too stringent and could halt the development of useful new medicines. These concerns stem from the fact that several blockbuster drugs contain structural alerts and are subject to reactive metabolite formation and/or covalent binding to cellular proteins but are devoid of idiosyncratic toxicity. In addition to these challenges, the simplistic notion that the absence of reactive metabolite formation from a drug candidate serves as a guarantee of its safety is not necessarily true. For example, there is no evidence that the idiosyncratic hepatotoxicity associated with the recalled thrombin inhibitor ximelagatran (Figure 14.1) is associated with reactive metabolite formation and, as such, the drug does not exhibit any alerts in its chemical structure [1].

14.2
Avoiding the Use of Structural Alerts in Drug Design

The concept of structural alerts as defined in modern medicinal chemistry originated from bioactivation studies with many of the drugs associated with idiosyncratic toxicity (withdrawn from commercial use or associated with a black box warning) [2]. Thus, it is not surprising that a strong relationship exists between reactive metabolite formation, protein covalent binding, and idiosyncratic toxicity with these agents. However, as discussed in Chapter 12, a compelling argument for chemotype-specific toxicity is evident from structure–activity analyses as shown in Figure 14.2 with toxic/nontoxic drug pairs such as alpidem/zolpidem, trovafloxacin/levofloxacin, clozapine/quetiapine, and nefazodone/buspirone, wherein absence of reactive metabolite liability is associated with the improved safety profile of successor drugs. Although anecdotal for the most part, the structure–toxicity relationships support the notion that avoiding structural alerts in drug design

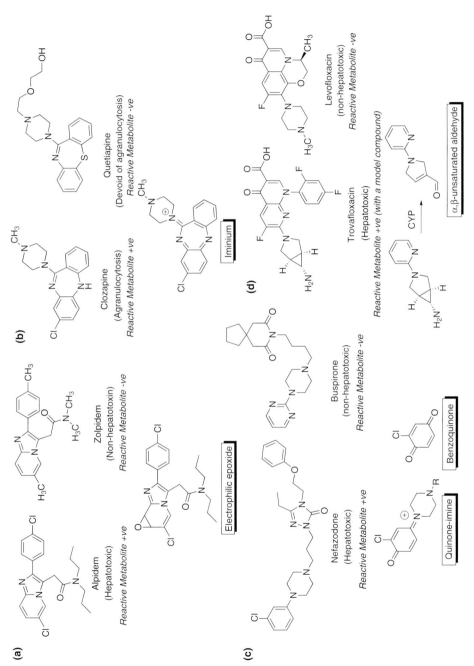

Figure 14.2 (a–d) Structure–toxicity relationships.

would lead to therapeutic agents devoid of idiosyncratic toxicities. Furthermore, as outlined in Chapter 12, approximately half of the top 200 drugs for 2009 (based on dispensed prescriptions) contain one or more alerts in their chemical architecture [2]. With the exception of acetaminophen, furosemide, lamotrigine, sulfamethoxazole/trimethoprim, trazodone, amitriptyline, and the β-lactam antibiotics, the vast majority of the structural alert–containing drugs are rarely associated with significant IADR incidences, despite years of use.

14.3
Structural Alert and Reactive Metabolite Formation

From a drug discovery perspective, it is imperative to demonstrate experimentally whether structural alerts, if present in a candidate of interest, actually are prone to reactive metabolite formation. As novel (and proprietary) functional groups are continuously sought in drug design, it is possible that unanticipated bioactivation pathways leading to reactive metabolites will emerge as illustrated in Chapter 11. With molecules that contain structural alerts, it is possible that metabolism can occur at a site other than the structural alert, and lead to non-reactive metabolites. For example, both sudoxicam and meloxicam contain the 2-aminothiazole structural alert, but only sudoxicam forms the reactive acylthiourea [3]. With meloxicam, the C-5 methyl group functions as a metabolic soft spot for oxidative metabolism leading to the primary alcohol metabolite, its principal metabolite fate in humans. [3].

Likewise, entacapone contains the nitrocatechol motif present in tolcapone, but does not generate electrophilic quinone imine species detected with tolcapone (Figure 14.3) [4, 5]. Although catechol glucuronidation is the major metabolic fate of tolcapone in humans, the corresponding reduction products of the nitrocatechol group, namely, the aniline and *N*-acetylaniline derivatives, have been detected as minor metabolites in human excreta [6]. The two metabolites undergo a facile two-electron oxidation to an electrophilic quinone imine species that can be trapped by GSH in human liver microsomes (HLM) [4]. A close association between hepatotoxicity and mutations in the uridine diphospho glucuronosyltransferase (UGT) 1A9 gene (which encodes the UGT isozyme responsible for tolcapone glucuronidation) has been observed in tolcapone-treated patients, suggesting that reactive metabolite formation through the redox bioactivation pathway may be more pronounced in UGT1A9 poor metabolizer genotype(s) [7]. From a structural standpoint, entacapone also possesses the nitrocatechol moiety and, despite administration at a high daily dose of 1600 mg, the drug is not associated with the IADRs observed with tolcapone. Metabolic profiling of entacapone in humans indicates that the analogous aniline and *N*-acetylaniline metabolites are not formed; primary metabolic routes in human involve isomerization of the double bond to the cis isomer followed by catechol glucuronidation, and hydroxylation on the *N*-diethyl substituent [5].

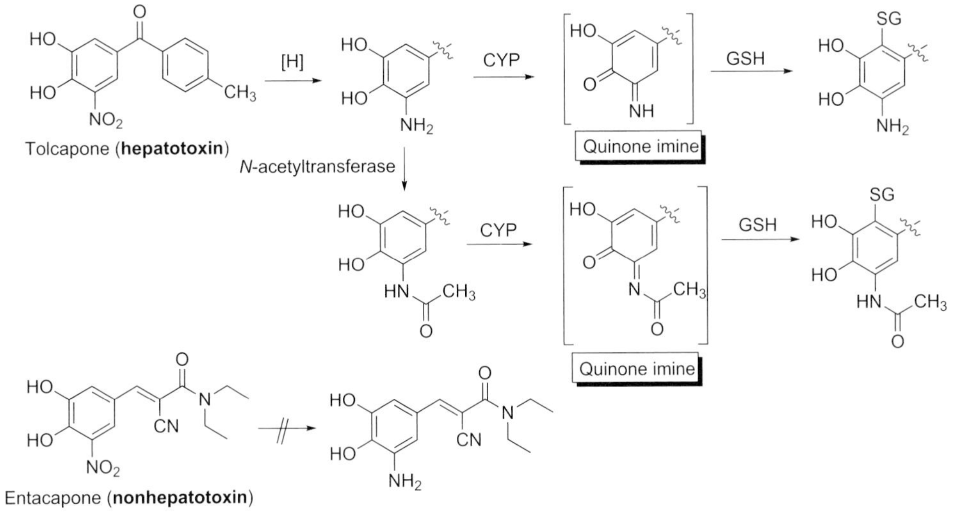

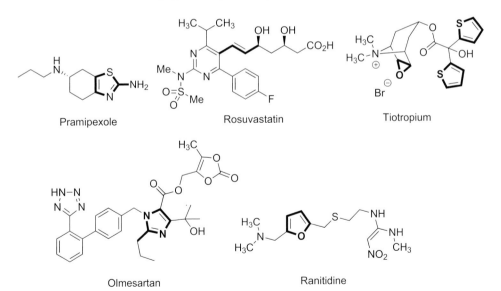

Figure 14.3 A scenario where metabolic soft spots circumvent reactive metabolite formation on a structural alert.

Studies that examine nonmetabolic routes of clearance (e.g., biliary and/or renal excretion of parent drug), which can supersede metabolism (including reactive metabolite formation), should also be taken into consideration. For instance, drugs that feature structural alerts such as pramipexole, rosuvastatin, tiotropium, olmesartan, and ranitidine (Figure 14.4) are subject to extensive renal excretion

Pramipexole

Rosuvastatin

Tiotropium

Olmesartan

Ranitidine

Figure 14.4 Illustrations of structural alert–containing drugs whose clearance in humans does not require metabolism. Structural alerts are highlighted in bold.

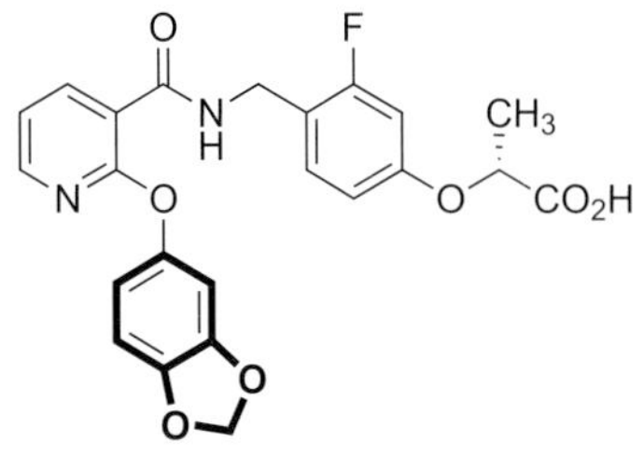

Figure 14.5 Chemical structure of a clinical candidate (CP-671,305) for the treatment of asthma. The methylenedioxyphenyl structural alert is highlighted in bold.

in humans (often mediated by transport proteins), and are resistant to metabolism/bioactivation. In the case of the nonergot dopamine receptor agonist pramipexole, used in the treatment of Parkinson's disease, urinary excretion in unchanged form is the major route ($\sim$90% of the daily dose of 4.5 mg) of elimination in humans. Metabolite formation (including cleavage products of the 2-aminothiazole structural alert) has not been observed in circulation and/or urine (pramipexole package insert). The observation that the renal clearance of pramipexole is $\sim$3 times greater than the glomerular filtration rate is consistent with the involvement of the organic cation transport system in its renal excretion [8].

An illustration of applying such considerations in the selection of drug candidates is shown with the phosphodiesterase 4 inhibitor, CP-671,305 (Figure 14.5), nominated for the potential treatment of asthma and chronic obstructive pulmonary disease. While the presence of the methylenedioxyphenyl alert in the structure of CP-671,305 raised significant concern from a toxicity standpoint, subsequent metabolism studies revealed that CP-671,305 was generally resistant to metabolism (including the formation of reactive catechol/quinone species) in animals and humans. Consistent with this observation, CP-671,305 did not inactivate any of the major human cytochrome P450 (CYP) isozymes via ring scission of the methylenedioxyphenyl motif. CP-671,305 was primarily cleared via renal and biliary excretion (in the unchanged form) through active transport, which alleviated toxicity concerns and supported its nomination for clinical development [9, 10].

14.4
Should Reactive Metabolite–Positive Compounds be Nominated as Drug Candidates?

While the weight of evidence suggests that reactive metabolites are responsible for many IADRs, it is important to note that virtually any functional group, including a phenyl ring, can generate a reactive metabolite and/or covalently bind to protein in *in vitro* systems (e.g., HLM) when measured with sensitive bioanalytical methodology. In fact, as illustrated in Chapter 12, numerous blockbuster drugs such as atorvastatin, esomeprazole, clopidogrel, ethinylestradiol, losartan, paroxetine, raloxifene, aripiprazole, pioglitazone, duloxetine, olanzapine, and so on, form reactive metabolites and/or covalently bind to proteins [2] but are not associated with significant incidences of IADRs. Furthermore, as noted in Chapters 6, 7 and 12, reactive metabolite formation by CYP2C19 is essential for the antiplatelet effects of clopidogrel. Clearly, these drugs challenge the notion of structural alert and/or *in vitro/in vivo* reactive metabolite analysis as stand-alone predictors of toxicity.

14.4.1
Impact of Competing, Detoxification Pathways

Overall, the observations on reactive metabolite–positive drugs with impeccable safety records raise a fundamental question – why are some reactive metabolite–positive drugs safe, while others are not? A limitation of the *in vitro* reactive metabolite screens is that they are typically conducted in HLM (in the presence and absence of NADPH cofactor), which only examines CYP-catalyzed bioactivation processes. In some instances, reactive metabolite formation may be observed in HLM in a CYP-dependent fashion, but, *in vivo*, the compound may undergo a distinctly different and perhaps more facile metabolic fate that reduces and/or completely circumvents CYP catalysis. An important illustration is the clopidogrel case, where the majority (>70%) of its daily dose is rapidly hydrolyzed by carboxylesterases to the inactive carboxylic acid metabolite (~80–85% of circulating metabolite (s)), which suggests that only a small percentage of the parent drug (20 mg or less) is theoretically available for conversion to the "active" reactive species. Indeed, covalent binding to platelets accounts for only 2% of radiolabeled clopidogrel in human mass balance studies (Plavix package insert).

Additional examples of this behavior, which were apparent in Chapter 12, include the widely prescribed drugs paroxetine and raloxifene. Both drugs also form GSH conjugates and covalently bind to HLM in a CYP-dependent fashion [11, 12]; however, *in vivo*, the quinone precursors of these compounds are principally metabolized via competing glucuronidation and/or O-methylation pathways [13, 14]. As such, paroxetine and raloxifene fulfill all the obligatory requirements of a molecule prone to reactive metabolite formation and, in the absence of additional metabolism data (examining detoxification/competing elimination routes), such isolated findings could be interpreted as being a harbinger of a potential toxicological outcome in the clinic. It is tempting to speculate that in the modern drug discovery paradigm, paroxetine and raloxifene would unlikely be considered as candidates for clinical development because of the high degree of microsomal covalent binding and GSH adduct formation.

As such, it can be concluded that reactive metabolite detection assays (exogenous trapping with nucleophiles and/or covalent binding to proteins) are not intended to predict toxicity, but rather to detect the formation of reactive metabolites, some of which may carry a toxic liability. Reducing exposure to such potential toxins can be viewed as one approach to minimize risk during drug development. The detection of a reactive metabolite for a drug candidate does not warrant an instant demise of the compound *per se*, but it does trigger additional due diligence, including the examination of competing detoxification pathways. Initial reactive metabolite assessments in HLM (reactive metabolite trapping with nucleophiles and/or protein covalent binding) should be followed by more detailed studies in fully integrated *in vitro* biological matrices such as hepatocytes and S9 fractions from both human and animal species. Establishing a clear understanding of the *in vivo* clearance mechanisms in animals and how that relates to reactive metabolite formation *in vitro* matrices would lead to data-driven decision making with regards to compound selection. Against this backdrop, it is noteworthy to point out that adduction of GSH to reactive metabolites is not necessarily a bad attribute; instead, it confirms the ability of the endogenous thiol antioxidant to efficiently scavenge electrophilic intermediates. It is only in cases where the concentration of the reactive metabolite formed is so high that it depletes the endogenous antioxidant pool leading to toxicity, as observed with the anti-inflammatory agent acetaminophen.

14.4.2
The Impact of Dose Size

Perhaps the most striking observation (albeit empirical for the most part) is that high-dose drugs (>100 mg) tend to be the ones that most frequently cause IADRs, while low-dose drugs (<10 mg) rarely are problematic in this regard (whether or not these agents are prone to reactive metabolite formation leading to protein covalent binding). Examples of this phenomenon are readily apparent with the amineptine/tianeptine, clozapine/olanzapine, troglitazone/pioglitazone, nefazodone/aripiprazole, and amitriptyline/cyclobenzaprine pairs of drugs shown in Figure 14.6.

In the case of the tricyclic antidepressant and hepatotoxicant amineptine, NADPH-dependent microsomal covalent binding is believed to arise via an electrophilic epoxide intermediate, since addition of an epoxide hydrolase inhibitor increases microsomal covalent binding [15, 16]. In contrast to amineptine, the structural analogue tianeptine appears to be relatively safe in the clinic despite sharing amineptine's liabilities involving bioactivation by CYP into a reactive arene oxide [17]. It is likely that the improved tolerance of tianeptine in the clinic arises from the approximately fivefold to sixfold lower recommended dose relative to amineptine.

The high incidence of immune-mediated agranulocytosis associated with the antipsychotic agent clozapine is thought to occur via a myeloperoxidase-mediated oxidation of the dibenzodiazepine ring to a reactive iminium ion, which covalently binds to the target tissues and also reacts with GSH [18, 19]. Olanzapine forms a reactive iminium metabolite very similar to the one observed with clozapine, yet olanzapine is not associated with a significant incidence of blood dyscrasias [20]. The key difference between the two drugs is the daily dose – the maximum recommended daily doses of clozapine and olanzapine are 900 and 10 mg, respectively.

With troglitazone, both the chromane and the thiazolidinedione ring systems are bioactivated to form reactive metabolites (quinone methide and thiazolidinedione ring scission products) by CYP3A4 [21, 22]. Interestingly, the idiosyncratic hepatotoxicity with troglitazone has not been discerned with the blockbuster antidiabetic

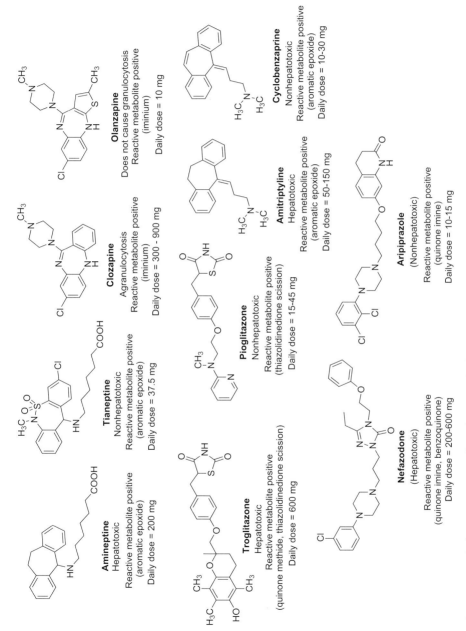

Figure 14.6 Daily dose as a mitigating factor for IADR risks for reactive metabolite–positive drugs.

agent pioglitazone. Pioglitazone contains the thiazolidinedione scaffold, which is metabolized to yield reactive metabolites similar to those detected with troglitazone [23]. While oxidation of the thiazolidinedione ring is a common theme in these drugs, a key difference lies in their daily doses – troglitazone (200–400 mg/day) versus pioglitazone (<10 mg/day).

The antidepressant nefazodone has been associated with numerous cases of idiosyncratic hepatotoxicity at therapeutic doses in the range of 200–400 mg/day, many of which required liver transplantation and/or resulted in fatalities. Evidence linking nefazodone hepatotoxicity with reactive metabolite formation has been established; the *para*-hydroxyaniline architecture in *para*-hydroxynefazodone, a circulating metabolite of nefazodone in humans, is metabolized by CYP3A4 to electrophilic quinonoid species, which are trapped as GSH adducts [24, 25]. The bioactivation pathway is analogous to the one deciphered with the closely related derivative trazodone, which is also associated with rare incidences of hepatotoxicity (see Chapter 12). The nefazodone bioactivation pathway catalyzed by CYP3A4 is also accompanied by mechanism-based inactivation of the enzyme [24]. This *in vitro* observation is consistent with nefazodone's nonlinear pharmacokinetics (due to autoinactivation) and clinical drug–drug interactions with CYP3A4 substrates. Like nefazodone, CYP3A4-mediated aromatic hydroxylation on the 2,3-dichlorophenylpiperazine ring in aripiprazole results in the formation of the *para*-hydroxyaripiprazole circulating metabolite, which can form a reactive quinone imine species similar to nefazodone. Absence of GSH adducts derived from conjugation with the *para*-hydroxyaripiprazole metabolite in HLM incubations, however, suggests that the bioactivation pathway does not occur with aripiprazole [25]. Besides the arylpiperazine/aniline alert, aripiprazole also contains an acetanilide alert that has been shown to form a reactive quinone imine intermediate in HLM [25]. A likely explanation for the markedly improved safety profile of aripiprazole (versus nefazodone), despite the accompanying reactive metabolite liability, is the vastly improved human pharmacokinetics of aripiprazole (aripiprazole: oral bioavailability = 87%, clearance = 0.8 ml/(min kg), half-life = 75 h; nefazodone: oral bioavailability = 20%, clearance = 7.5 ml/(min kg), half-life = 1 h) due to reduced CYP3A4-mediated metabolism/bioactivation, which translates to a significantly lower daily dose (10–15 mg) compared with nefazodone (200–600 mg).

Among the many biotransformation pathways of the idiosyncratic hepatotoxin amitriptyline, the characterization of a dihydrodiol metabolite in human urine has been an area of focus with regards to its possible association with reactive metabolite formation [26]. Wen *et al.* [27] have intercepted the intermediate aromatic ring epoxide via GSH trapping studies in HLM. A similar bioactivation pathway has been noted with nortriptyline, an antidepressant that is also associated with idiosyncratic hepatotoxicity [27]. Nortriptyline is the *N*-dealkylated metabolite of amitriptyline. While the principal metabolic fate of the skeletal muscle relaxant cyclobenzaprine in humans involves *N*-glucuronidation, a significant proportion (~7–10% of the administered dose) of a dihydrodiol (10,11-dihydroxynortriptyline) metabolite has been detected in human urine [28]. The formation of the dihydrodiol metabolite is consistent with olefin epoxidation as a rate-limiting step. Despite the potential reactive metabolite liability, no IADRs have been reported with cyclo-benzaprine at its low daily dose range of 10–30 mg. It is possible that the manifestation of idiosyncratic toxicity due to reactive metabolite formation with amitriptyline may be related to its higher daily dose of 50–150 mg.

As examined in Chapter 12, the vast majority of structural alert–positive drugs in the top 200 list (prescription) are low-dose drugs. The improved safety of low-dose drugs (atorvastatin, olanzapine, pioglitazone, and aripipra-zole) could arise from a marked reduction in the total body burden to reactive metabolite exposure via efficient scavenging by GSH (and other competing metabolic pathways), such that the reactive species are unlikely to exceed the safety threshold needed for toxicity. This may well be the case for clopidogrel whose principal clearance mechanism proceeds via ester bond hydrolysis; consequently, the amount of reactive metabolite produced must not exceed the threshold for toxicity. A similar "low-dose" argument may be applicable for atorvastatin, which is susceptible to bioactivation leading to protein covalent binding in HLM in a NADPH-dependent fashion [29, 30].

Given this general trend, optimization of lead compounds in drug discovery programs should focus on improving pharmacokinetics and intrinsic potency as a means of decreasing the projected clinically efficacious plasma concentrations (and hence the dose) and the associated "body burden" of parent drug and its metabolites as a strategy for mitigating IADR risks. However, it is clear that there will be classes of drugs (e.g., antibacterials, antiretrovirals, etc.) where this will be difficult to achieve. Recent advances in risk assessment methodologies, such as by the estimate of total daily body burden of covalent binding in hepatocytes or by zone classification taking the clinical dose into consideration [30], are positive steps toward quantitative prediction of IADR risks with drug candidates associated with reactive metabolite formation.

14.4.3
Consideration of the Medical Need/Urgency

An additional consideration of much importance is the clinical indication. The level of risk that would be deemed acceptable for drug candidates intended to treat major unmet medical need and/or a life-threatening disease is likely to be significantly higher relative to treatment of chronic nondebilitating conditions where alternate treatment options are already available. An excellent illustration of this phenomenon is evident with the tyrosine kinase inhibitor sunitinib (Figure 14.7), which is associated with a black box warning for hepatotoxicity, but is widely used in cancer treatment.

14.4.4
Consideration of the Duration of Treatment

Drugs used to treat chronic illnesses are more frequently associated with IADRs than ones used for acute treatment periods. An example of this phenomenon is

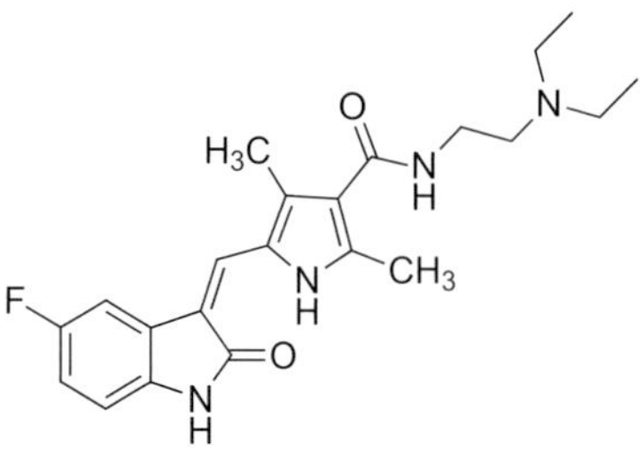

Figure 14.7 Structure of the tyrosine kinase inhibitor and anticancer drug sunitinib.

evident with the widely prescribed β-lactam class of antibacterial agents (e.g., amoxicillin), which derive their pharmacology through irreversible covalent binding of the β-lactam ring with an active site serine residue in their pharmacological target (serine-type D-ala-D-ala carboxypeptidase) [31]. Although β-lactam drugs are generally well tolerated, they are also frequently associated with IADRs (e.g., drug allergy and anaphylaxis) [32]. The IADRs have been linked to indiscriminant acylation of free amino and sulfydryl groups on proteins via a nonenzymatic β-lactam ring scission, which leads to an immune response against the penicillin–protein adduct, and if the antibody response generates sufficient IgE antibodies, a severe allergic reaction such as anaphylaxis can occur [33–35]. The acute nature of antibiotic treatment most likely aids the tolerability, considering that the daily doses of β-lactam antibiotics are very high (>1000 mg/day).

14.4.5
Consideration of Novel Pharmacological Targets

While elimination of reactive metabolite formation may be a fruitful endeavor for drug development in the "best-in-class" segment, from a drug discovery standpoint, there needs to be some balance prior to embarking on a lengthy effort toward "fixing" reactive metabolite issues in discovery programs dealing with novel, unprecedented pharmacological targets and/or uncertainty around predicted human pharmacokinetics. Our recent experience with human calcium sensing receptor (CaSR) antagonists for the potential treatment of osteoporosis provides an excellent example of this theme. On the basis of its potency against CaSR and disposition attributes, (R)-2-(2-hydroxyphenyl)-3-(1-phenylpropan-2-yl)-5-(trifluoromethyl)pyrido[4,3-d]pyrimidin-4(3H)-one (compound A, Figure 14.8) was considered for rapid advancement to first-in-human (FIH) trials to mitigate uncertainty surrounding the pharmacokinetic/pharmacodynamic (PK/PD) predictions for a short-acting bone anabolic agent [36]. During the course of metabolic profiling, however, GSH conjugates of compound A were detected in HLM in an NADPH-dependent fashion. Characterization of the GSH conjugate structures allowed insight(s) into the bioactivation pathway, which involved CYP3A4-mediated phenol ring oxidation to the catechol, followed by further oxidation to the electrophilic *ortho*-quinone species (Figure 14.8). While the reactive metabolite liability

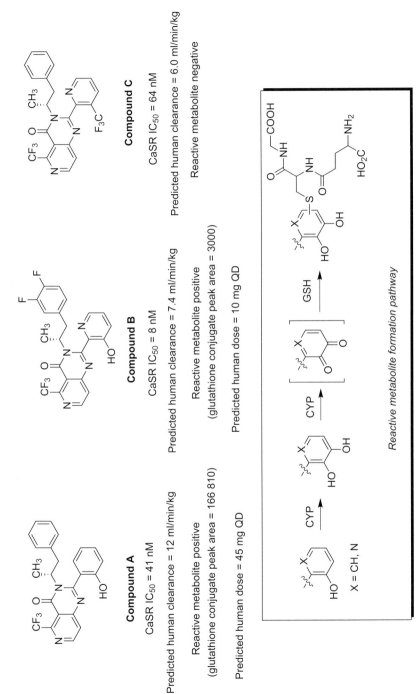

Figure 14.8 Discovery tactics to mitigate IADR risks with antagonists of the human calcium receptor.

raised concerns around the likelihood of a potential toxicological outcome, a more immediate program goal was establishing confidence in human PK predictions in the FIH study. Furthermore, the availability of a clinical biomarker (serum parathyroid hormone) meant that PD could be assessed side by side with PK, an ideal scenario for a relatively unprecedented pharmacological target. Consequently, progressing compound A into the clinic was given a high priority, provided the compound demonstrated an adequate safety profile to support FIH studies. Despite forming the identical reactive metabolite in rat liver microsomes, no clinical or histopathological signs prototypical of target organ toxicity were observed with compound A in *in vivo* safety assessments in rats. Compound A was also devoid of metabolism-based mutagenicity in *in vitro* (e.g., *Salmonella* Ames) and *in vivo* assessments (micronuclei induction in bone marrow) in rats. Likewise, metabolism-based studies (e.g., evaluation of detoxifying routes of clearance and exhaustive PK/PD studies in animals to prospectively predict the likelihood of a low human efficacious dose) were also conducted, which mitigated the risks of idiosyncratic toxicity to a large degree. In parallel, medicinal chemistry efforts were initiated to identify additional compounds with a complementary range of human PK predictions, which would maximize the likelihood of achieving the desired PD effect in the clinic. The backup strategy also incorporated an overarching goal of reducing/eliminating reactive metabolite formation observed with compound A, which led to compounds B and C as backup clinical candidates with CaSR potency comparable to compound A. Compound B (which contained a 3-pyridinylphenol motif instead of the phenol) demonstrated reduced propensity toward reactive *ortho*-quinone formation and compound C (which contained a 3-pyridinyltrifluoromethyl substituent) was devoid of reactive metabolite formation.

14.5
The Multifactorial Nature of IADRs

While necessary diligence is observed toward the discovery of a "reactive metabolite–negative" candidate with the optimal balance of pharmacology and pharmacokinetics, it is noteworthy to point out that a negative finding in the reactive metabolite and/or covalent binding assays is not a guarantee of safety as noted earlier with ximelagatran. Overall, the risk of reactive metabolite formation is only part of a multifaceted, integrated risk–benefit assessment of a drug candidate and should not serve as a stand-alone criterion to suspend the development of a clinical candidate. It is well recognized that IADRs can be multifactorial in nature. Mechanisms other than or in addition to reactive metabolite formation can individually or collectively account for idiosyncratic liver injury. For instance, hepatotoxicity associated with the antidiabetic agent troglitazone has been attributed to: (a) RM formation, (b) inhibition of bile salt export pump (BSEP) by the parent drug and its sulfate metabolite, and (c) mitochondrial dysfunction and cell death [37]. BSEP is critically involved in the secretion of bile salts into bile; its impairment may lead to cholestasis and accumulation of cytotoxic bile salts in hepatocytes and, consequently, to liver disease [38]. Genetic studies have shown that polymorphism(s) in the gene coding for BSEP and/or inherited mutations lead to progressive familial intrahepatic cholestasis and severe liver disease [39]. Mitochondrial dysfunction induced by drugs can originate from several different mechanisms, including the inhibition of fatty acid β-oxidation, the uncoupling of electron transport from ATP synthesis, and the opening of the mitochondrial permeability transition pore leading to irreversible collapse of the transmembrane potential and release of proapoptotic factors [40].

Besides troglitazone, amineptine, tolcapone, alpidem, ketoconazole, and nefazodone are examples of drugs that form reactive metabolites and also demonstrate mitochondrial toxicity. An interesting structure–activity relationship also emerges with tolcapone, alpidem, and nefazodone, based on the findings that structurally related drugs with improved safety (entacapone, zolpidem, and buspirone) do not form reactive species, and do not impair mitochondrial function [2]. Equally provocative is the emergence of BSEP inhibition as a contributor to cholestatic injury observed with several drugs including troglitazone, ketoconazole, nefazodone, glyburide, and so on [41]. Despite a lower daily dose (2.5–20 mg), glyburide (Figure 14.9) is associated with much greater incidence and severity of hepatic injury than any of the sulfonyl ureas. Compared with the older hydrophilic sulfonyl ureas such as chlorpropamide (Figure 14.9), which are mainly excreted renally, glyburide is more lipophilic and undergoes significant biliary excretion, possibly mediated through active hepatobiliary transport. While glyburide is devoid of structural alerts, the drug is a potent inhibitor of BSEP ($IC_{50} \sim 6~\mu M$) compared with related sulfonyl ureas such as chlorpropamide ($IC_{50} \sim 135~\mu M$) [42]. All evidence thus points to the greater inhibitory potency of glyburide against hepatobiliary transporters as a key determinant of its cholestatic potential.

Overall, the observations with troglitazone and the other drugs imply that both metabolism-dependent and -independent mechanisms may need to be considered when truly attempting to derisk IADR potential of new drug candidates. Screens for mitochondrial toxicity and BSEP inhibition are routinely available in a drug discovery setting, and can prove useful toward establishing structure–activity relationships as evident with the potent mitochondrial toxicity and BSEP inhibitory effects of nefazodone but not buspirone [43, 44]. However, as in the case of reactive

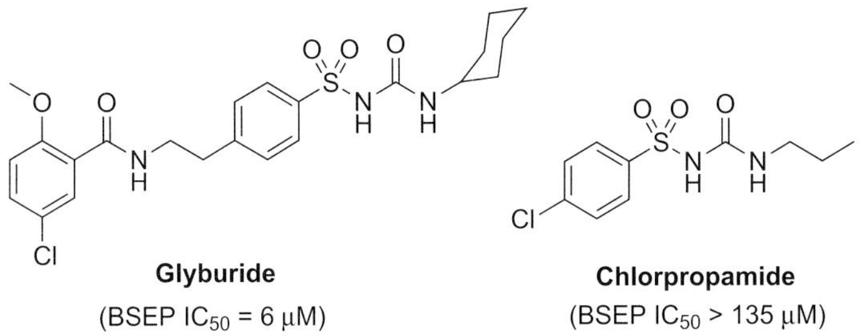

Glyburide
(BSEP IC_{50} = 6 μM)

Chlorpropamide
(BSEP IC_{50} > 135 μM)

Figure 14.9 Structure–activity relationship for BSEP inhibition by sulfonyl urea-based antidiabetic agents glyburide and chlorpropamide.

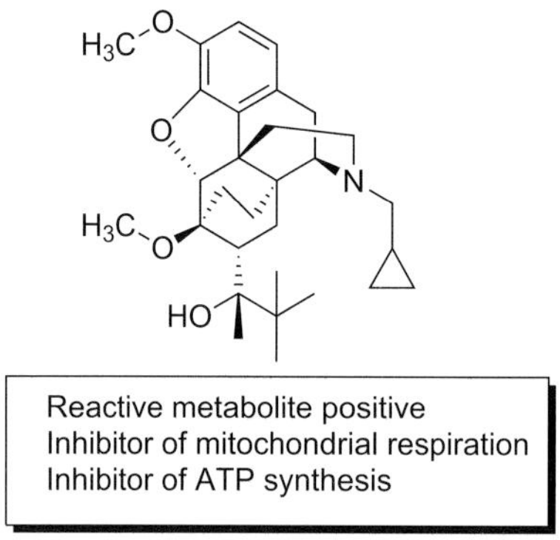

Figure 14.10 Structure of analgesic buprenorphine.

metabolite–positive compounds, interpretation of mitochondrial toxicity and BSEP inhibition data requires additional scrutiny. For example, buprenorphine (Figure 14.10) impairs mitochondrial respiration and ATP formation [45], but does not cause hepatotoxicity at its recommended doses of 2–8 mg. Similarly, *in vitro* BSEP inhibition seen with troglitazone has also been noted with rosiglitazone and pioglitazone [41], which are not hepatotoxic. Furthermore, simvastatin and ethinylestradiol also exhibit potent BSEP inhibition [41], but are not associated with cholestatic injury in humans. It is likely that the therapeutic concentrations of these drugs in the liver are significantly below the IC_{50} values for inhibition of BSEP activity in the liver. This brings up the question of whether a low-dose drug (leading to low hepatic and systemic concentrations) would mitigate idiosyncratic hepatotoxicity risks due to BSEP inhibition and mitochondrial toxicity (in a similar manner as reactive metabolite formation). From a drug discovery viewpoint, determination of the BSEP IC_{50}/projected portal inlet drug concentration (surrogate of liver concentrations) ratio could provide a therapeutic index to derisk cholestatic potential due to BSEP inhibition. However, such derisking strategies will need validation prior to introduction in a drug discovery setting for risk mitigation of cholestatic injury due to BSEP inhibition.

14.6
Concluding Remarks

Experiments that define the relationship between drug bioactivation (e.g., the *in vivo* demonstration of protein covalent binding and/or GSH conjugate formation) and toxicity in humans are extremely rare [46, 47]. Furthermore, whether covalent binding measures *in vivo* are likely to be more informative of the *in vivo* safety risk than covalent binding studies *in vitro* remains to be established. This is because of a lack of data on absolute levels of *in vivo* covalent binding that could lead to a toxic outcome versus levels of binding that are safe. As such, next to dosimetry and quantitative considerations of reactive metabolite exposure, identifying toxicologically relevant protein targets of reactive metabolites is an important challenge to a better understanding of the links between covalent binding to critical proteins and organ toxicity [48]. Which protein targets are "critical" for toxicity is, of course, a key question, and one to which we do not currently have answers. However, methodology to identify the proteins that are subject to covalent modification by electrophilic drug metabolites is now available, thanks to advances in proteomics mass spectrometry, and databases of the type established by Hanzlik *et al.* at the University of Kansas ultimately will reveal which protein targets are critical to cell survival following alkylation [49]. Perhaps the biggest gap in the field is the lack of knowledge about the nature of the antigenic determinants that trigger an immunological response to drug–protein covalent adducts. Without this information, it will not be possible to predict the potential for a given compound that undergoes metabolic activation to cause "idiosyncratic" toxicity in humans through haptenization of key proteins.

Animals are poor predictors of IADRs in humans, and because reactive metabolites have been implicated in the etiology of many IADRs, screens to examine bioactivation also have been implemented to assist in compound design. While this is a useful and pragmatic starting point toward eliminating potential IADR risks, in order to truly mitigate *covert* toxicity risks (particularly idiosyncratic hepatotoxicity) there is a need for a more integrated *in vitro* screening paradigm that involves examination of bioactivation potential as well as cellular effects mediated by the parent compound (and its metabolites). Consistent with this viewpoint, many companies have advocated the use of cell-based (e.g., ATP depletion in transformed human liver epithelial cells) cytotoxicity measures, BSEP inhibition, mitochondrial toxicity, and RM assessments in a drug discovery paradigm [50]. With the plethora of new *in vitro* safety screens available, it is likely that drug discovery teams will tend to overinterpret the output from these assays, the primary purpose of which is merely to identify chemotype hazard risks and not predict idiosyncratic toxicity. Consequently, how such a collective output would be used in the holistic assessment of IADR risks will ultimately rest with the individual companies. Until we gain a better understanding of the biochemical mechanisms that underline IADRs in the clinic, such *in vitro* safety predictors will remain a critical issue for further investigation and debate.

References

1 Testa, L., Bhindi, R., Agostoni, P., Abbate, A., Zoccai, G.G., and van Gaal, W.J. (2007) The direct thrombin inhibitor ximelagatran/melagatran: a systematic review on clinical applications and an evidence based assessment of risk benefit profile. *Expert Opinion in Drug Safety*, **6** (4), 397–406.

2 Stepan, A.F., Walker, D.P., Bauman, J., Price, D.A., Baillie, T.A., Kalgutkar, A.S., and Aleo, M.D. (2011) Structural alert/reactive metabolite concept as applied in medicinal chemistry to mitigate the risk of idiosyncratic drug toxicity: a perspective based on the critical examination of trends in the top 200 drugs

marketed in the United States. *Chemical Research in Toxicology*, **24** (9), 1345–1410.

3 Obach, R.S., Kalgutkar, A.S., Ryder, T.F., and Walker, G.S. (2008) In vitro metabolism and covalent binding of enol-carboxamide derivatives and anti-inflammatory agents sudoxicam and meloxicam: insights into the hepatotoxicity of sudoxicam. *Chemical Research in Toxicology*, **21** (9), 1890–1899.

4 Smith, K.S., Smith, P.L., Heady, T.N., Trugman, J.M., Harman, W.D., and Macdonald, T.L. (2003) In vitro metabolism of tolcapone to reactive intermediates: relevance to tolcapone liver toxicity. *Chemical Research in Toxicology*, **16** (2), 123–128.

5 Wikberg, T., Vuorela, A., Ottoila, P., and Taskinen, J. (1993) Identification of the major metabolites of the catechol-*O*-methyl transferase inhibitor entacapone in rats and humans. *Drug Metabolism and Disposition*, **21** (1), 81–92.

6 Jorga, K., Fotteler, B., Heizmann, P., and Gasser, R. (1999) Metabolism and excretion of tolcapone, a novel inhibitor of catechol-*O*-methyltransferase. *British Journal of Clinical Pharmacology*, **48** (4), 513–520.

7 Martignoni, E., Cosentino, M., Ferrari, M., Porta, G., Mattarucchi, E., Marino, F., Lecchini, S., and Nappi, G. (2005) Two patients with COMT inhibitor-induced hepatic dysfunction and UGT1A9 genetic polymorphism. *Neurology*, **65** (11), 1820–1822.

8 Diao, L., Shu, Y., and Polli, J.E. (2010) Uptake of pramipexole by human organic cation transporters. *Molecular Pharmacology*, **7** (4), 1342–1347.

9 Kalgutkar, A.S., Choo, E., Taylor, T.J., and Marfat, A. (2004) Disposition of CP-671,305, a selective phosphodiesterase 4 inhibitor in preclinical species. *Xenobiotica*, **34** (8), 755–770.

10 Kalgutkar, A.S., Feng, B., Nguyen, H.T., Frederick, K.S., Campbell, S.D., Hatch, H. L., Bi, Y.A., Kazolias, D.C., Davidson, R.E., Mireles, R.J., Duignan, D.B., Choo, E.F., and Zhao, S.X. (2007) Role of transporters in the disposition of the selective phosphodiesterase-4 inhibitor (+)-2-[4-({[2-benzo[1,3]dioxol-5-yloxy)-pyridine-3-carbonyl]-amino}-methyl)-3-fluoro-phenoxy]-propionic acid in rat and human. *Drug Metabolism and Disposition*, **35** (11), 2111–2118.

11 Zhao, S.X., Dalvie, D.K., Kelly, J.M., Soglia, J.R., Frederick, K.S., Smith, E.B., Obach, R.S., and Kalgutkar, A.S. (2007) NADPH-dependent covalent binding of [3H]paroxetine to human liver microsomes and S-9 fractions: identification of an electrophilic quinone metabolite of paroxetine. *Chemical Research in Toxicology*, **20** (11), 1649–1657.

12 Chen, Q., Ngui, J.S., Doss, G.A., Wang, R. W., Cai, X., DiNinno, F.P., Blizzard, T.A., Hammond, M.L., Stearns, R.A., Evans, D. C., Baillie, T.A., and Tang, W. (2002) Cytochrome P450 3A4-mediated bioactivation of raloxifene: irreversible enzyme inhibition and thiol adduct formation. *Chemical Research in Toxicology*, **15** (7), 907–914.

13 Haddock, R.E., Johnson, A.M., Langley, P. F., Nelson, D.R., Pope, J.A., Thomas, D. R., and Woods, F.R. (1989) Metabolic pathways of paroxetine in animals and man and the comparative pharmacological properties of the metabolites. *Acta Psychiatrica Scandinavica Supplement*, **350**, 24–26.

14 Dalvie, D., Kang, P., Zientek, M., Xiang, C., Zhou, S., and Obach, R.S. (2008) Effect of intestinal glucuronidation in limiting hepatic exposure and bioactivation of raloxifene in humans and rats. *Chemical Research in Toxicology*, **21** (12), 2260–2271.

15 Genève, J., Larrey, D., Letteron, P., Descatoire, V., Tinel, M., Amouyal, G., and Pessayre, D. (1987) Metabolic activation of the tricyclic antidepressant amineptine – I. Cytochrome P-450-mediated *in vitro* covalent binding. *Biochemical Pharmacology*, **36** (3), 323–329.

16 Genève, J., Degott, C., Letteron, P., Tinel, M., Descatoire, V., Larrey, D., Amouyal, G., and Pessayre, D. (1987) Metabolic activation of the tricyclic antidepressant amineptine – II. Protective role of GSH against in vitro and in vivo covalent binding. *Biochemical Pharmacology*, **36** (3), 331–337.

17 Fromenty, B. and Pessayre, D. (1995) Inhibition of mitochondrial beta-oxidation

as a mechanism of hepatotoxicity. *Pharmacology and Therapeutics*, **67** (1), 101–154.

18 Liu, Z.C. and Uetrecht, J.P. (1995) Clozapine is oxidized by activated human neutrophils to a reactive nitrenium ion that irreversibly binds to the cells. *Journal of Pharmacology and Experimental Therapeutics*, **275** (3), 1476–1483.

19 Maggs, J.L., Williams, D., Pirmohamed, M., and Park, B.K. (1995) The metabolic formation of reactive intermediates from clozapine, a drug associated with agranulocytosis in man. *Journal of Pharmacology and Experimental Therapeutics*, **275** (3), 1463–1475.

20 Uetrecht, J.P., Zahid, N., Tehim, A., Fu, J. M., and Rakhit, S. (1997) Structural features associated with reactive metabolite formation in clozapine analogues. *Chemico-Biological Interactions*, **104** (2–3), 117–129.

21 Kassahun, K., Pearson, P.G., Tang, W., McIntosh, I., Leung, K., Elmore, C., Dean, D., Wang, R., Doss, G., and Baillie, T.A. (2001) Studies on the metabolism of troglitazone to reactive intermediates in vitro and in vivo. Evidence for novel biotransformation pathways involving quinone methide formation and thiazolidinedione ring scission. *Chemical Research in Toxicology*, **14** (1), 62–70.

22 He, K., Talaat, R.E., Pool, W.F., Reilly, M. D., Reed, J.E., Bridges, A.J., and Woolf, T. F. (2004) Metabolic activation of troglitazone: identification of a reactive metabolite and mechanisms involved. *Drug Metabolism and Disposition*, **32** (6), 639–646.

23 Alvarez-Sanchez, R., Montavon, F., Hartung, T., and Pahler, A. (2006) Thiazolidinedione bioactivation: a comparison of the bioactivation potentials of troglitazone, rosiglitazone, and pioglitazone using stable isotope-labeled analogues and liquid chromatography tandem mass spectrometry. *Chemical Research in Toxicology*, **19** (8), 1106–1116.

24 Kalgutkar, A.S., Vaz, A.D., Lame, M.E., Henne, K.R., Soglia, J., Zhao, S.X., Abramov, Y.A., Lombardo, F., Collin, C., Hendsch, Z.S., and Hop, C.E. (2005) Bioactivation of the nontricyclic

antidepressant nefazodone to a reactive quinone-imine species in human liver microsomes and recombinant cytochrome P450 3A4. *Drug Metabolism and Disposition*, **33** (2), 243–253.

25 Bauman, J.S., Frederick, K.S., Sawant, A., Walsky, R.L., Cox, L.M., Obach, R.S., and Kalgutkar, A.S. (2008) Comparison of the bioactivation potential of the antidepressant and hepatotoxin nefazodone with aripiprazole, a structural analog and marketed drug. *Drug Metabolism and Disposition*, **36** (6), 1016–1029.

26 Prox, A. and Breyer-Pfaff, U. (1987) Amitriptyline metabolites in human urine. Identification of phenols, dihydrodiols, glycols, and ketones. *Drug Metabolism and Disposition*, **15** (6), 890–896.

27 Wen, B., Ma, L., and Zhu, M. (2008) Bioactivation of the tricyclic antidepressant amitriptyline and its metabolite nortriptyline to arene oxide intermediates in human liver microsomes and recombinant P450s. *Chemico-Biological Interactions*, **173** (1), 59–67.

28 Breyer-Pfaff, U. (2004) The metabolic fate of amitriptyline, nortriptyline and amitriptylinoxide in man. *Drug Metabolism Reviews*, **36** (3–4), 723–746.

29 Lennernas, H. (2003) Clinical pharmacokinetics of atorvastatin. *Clinical Pharmacokinetics*, **42** (13), 1141–1160.

30 Nakayama, S., Atsumi, R., Takakusa, H., Kobayashi, Y., Kurihara, A., Nagai, Y., Nakai, D., and Okazaki, O. (2009) A zone classification system for risk assessment of idiosyncratic drug toxicity using daily dose and covalent binding. *Drug Metabolism and Disposition*, **37** (9), 1970–1977.

31 Lu, W.P., Kincaid, E., Sun, Y., and Bauer, M.D. (2001) Kinetics of beta-lactam interactions with penicillin-susceptible and -resistant penicillin-binding protein 2x proteins from *Streptococcus pneumoniae*. Involvement of acylation and deacylation in beta-lactam resistance. *Journal of Biological Chemistry*, **276** (34), 31494–31501.

32 Fontana, R.J., Shakil, A.O., Greenson, J.K., Boyd, I., and Lee, W.M. (2005) Acute liver failure due to amoxicillin and amoxicillin clavulanate. *Digestive Diseases and Sciences*, **50** (10), 1785–1790.

33 Zhao, Z., Baldo, B.A., and Rimmer, J. (2002) beta-Lactam allergenic determinants: fine structural recognition of a cross-reacting determinant on benzylpenicillin and cephalothin. *Clinical and Experimental Allergy*, **32** (11), 1644–1650.

34 Levine, B.B. (1960) Formation of D-penicillamine–cysteine mixed disulfide by reaction of D-benzylpenicilloic acid with cysteine. *Nature*, **187**, 940–941.

35 Levine, B.B. and Ovary, Z. (1961) Studies on the mechanism of the formation of the penicillin antigen. III. The *N*-(D-alpha-benzylpenicilloyl) group as an antigenic determinant responsible for hypersensitivity to penicillin G. *Journal of Experimental Medicine*, **114**, 875–904.

36 Kalgutkar, A.S., Griffith, D.A., Ryder, T., Sun, H., Miao, Z., Bauman, J.N., Didiuk, M.T., Frederick, K.S., Zhao, S.X., Prakash, C., Soglia, J.R., Bagley, S.W., Bechle, B.M., Kelley, R.M., Dirico, K., Zawistoski, M., Li, J., Oliver, R., Guzman-Perez, A., Liu, K.K., Walker, D.P., Benbow, J.W., and Morris, J. (2010) Discovery tactics to mitigate toxicity risks due to reactive metabolite formation with 2-(2-hydroxyaryl)-5-(trifluoromethyl) pyrido[4,3-d]pyrimidin-4(3h)-one derivatives, potent calcium-sensing receptor antagonists and clinical candidate (s) for the treatment of osteoporosis. *Chemical Research in Toxicology*, **23** (6), 1115–1126.

37 Yokoi, T. (2010) Troglitazone. *Handbook of Experimental Pharmacology*, **196**, 419–435.

38 Stieger, B. (2010) Role of the bile salt export pump, BSEP, in acquired forms of cholestasis. *Drug Metabolism Reviews*, **42** (3), 437–445.

39 Lang, C., Meier, Y., Stieger, B., Beuers, U., Lang, T., Kerb, R., Kullack-Ublick, G.A., Meier, P.J., and Pauli-Magnus, C. (2007) Mutations and polymorphisms in the bile salt export pump and the multidrug resistance protein 3 associated with drug-induced liver injury. *Pharmacogenetics and Genomics*, **17** (1), 47–60.

40 Nadanaciva, S. and Will, Y. (2009) The role of mitochondrial dysfunction and drug

safety. *IDrugs: the Investigational Drugs Journal*, **12** (11), 706–771.

41 Morgan, R.E., Trauner, M., van Staden, C. J., Lee, P.H., Ramachandran, B., Eschenberg, M., Afshari, C.A., Qualls, C. W. Jr., Lightfoot-Dunn, R., and Hamadeh, H.K. (2010) Interference with bile salt export pump function is a susceptibility factor for human liver injury in drug development. *Toxicological Sciences*, **118** (2), 485–500.

42 Smith, D.A., Harrison, A., and Morgan, P. (2011) Multiple factors govern the association between pharmacology and toxicity in a class of drugs: toward a unification of class effect terminology. *Chemical Research in Toxicology*, **24** (4), 463–474.

43 Kostrubsky, S.E., Strom, S.C., Kalgutkar, A.S., Kulkarni, S., Atherton, J., Mireles, R., Feng, B., Kubik, R., Hanson, J., Urda, E., and Mutlib, A. (2006) Inhibition of hepatobiliary transport as a predictive method for clinical hepatotoxicity of nefazodone. *Toxicological Sciences*, **90** (2), 451–459.

44 Dykens, J.A., Jamieson, J.D., Marroquin, L.D., Nadanaciva, S., Xu, J.J., Dunn, M.C., Smith, A.R., and Will, Y. (2008) In vitro assessment of mitochondrial dysfunction and cytotoxicity of nefazodone, trazodone, and buspirone. *Toxicological Sciences*, **103** (2), 335–345.

45 Berson, A., Fau, D., Fornacciari, R., Degove-Goddard, P., Sutton, A., Descatoire, V., Haouzi, D., Letteron, P., Moreau, A., Feldmann, G., and Pessayre, D. (2001) Mechanisms for experimental buprenorphine hepatotoxicity: major role of mitochondrial dysfunction versus metabolic activation. *Journal of Hepatology*, **34** (2), 261–269.

46 Park, B.K., Boobis, A., Clarke, S., Goldring, C.E., Jones, D., Kenna, J.G., Lambert, C., Laverty, H.G., Naisbitt, D.J., Nelson, S., Nicoll-Griffith, D.A., Obach, R.S., Routledge, P., Smith, D.A., Tweedie, D.J., Vermeulen, N., Williams, D.P., Wilson, I.D., and Baillie, T.A. (2011) Managing the challenge of chemically reactive metabolites in drug development. *Nature Reviews in Drug Discovery*, **10** (4), 292–306.

47 Tingle, M.D., Mahmud, R., Maggs, J.L., Pirmohamed, M., and Park, B.K. (1997) Comparison of the metabolism and toxicity of dapsone in rat, mouse and man. *Journal of Pharmacology and Experimental Therapeutics*, **283** (2), 817–823.

48 Liebler, D.C. (2008) Protein damage by reactive electrophiles: targets and consequences. *Chemical Research in Toxicology*, **21** (1), 117–128.

49 Hanzlik, R.P., Fang, J., and Koen, Y.M. (2009) Filling and mining the reactive metabolite target protein database. *Chemico-Biological Interactions*, **179** (1), 38–44.

50 Thompson, R.A., Isin, E.M., Li, Y., Weaver, R., Weidolf, L., Wilson, I., Claesson, A., Page, K., Dolgos, H., and Gerry Kenna, J. (2011) Risk assessment and mitigation strategies for reactive metabolites in drug discovery and development. *Chemico-Biological Interactions*, **192** (1–2), 65–71.

15
Managing IADRs – a Risk–Benefit Analysis

Abbreviations

ALF	Acute liver failure
ALT	Alanine transaminase
AST	Aspartate transaminase
CCR5	Chemokine receptor type 5
FDA	US Food and Drug Administration
HLA	Human leukocyte antigen
NSAIDs	Nonsteroidal anti-inflammatory drugs
ULN	Upper limit of normal

15.1
Risk–Benefit Analysis

Risk–benefit analysis is performed at all stages in the discovery and development of a drug. Although complex at the early stages, the process becomes more difficult throughout the course of a drug's lifetime. The benefit of a new drug may seem obvious, but even for a new drug target with an unprecedented mechanism the efficacy observed is often incremental to existing established therapies. Short-term efficacy benefit has to be balanced with long-term outcomes that may vary across different drug classes used in a single indication. The risk is also variable and graded, the crudest gradation being the severity of injury against the number of patients affected. But this risk has to set against benefit. The source of the data moves through the drug life cycle from existing information on the drug target (perhaps gained from null expressers of a receptor) and compound structure at the early discovery stage to adverse event reports submitted by prescribers concerning individual patients at the postmarketing stage.

Table 15.1 illustrates the supply of data throughout the drug life cycle. As the drug is developed, a continual assessment of benefit risk is performed to

Reactive Drug Metabolites, First Edition. Amit S. Kalgutkar, Deepak Dalvie, R. Scott Obach, and Dennis A. Smith.
© 2012 Wiley-VCH Verlag GmbH & Co. KGaA. Published 2012 by Wiley-VCH Verlag GmbH & Co. KGaA.

Table 15.1 Sources of drug safety data and its potential limitations.

Discovery	Null expression of receptor in patient population – gene polymorphism	High-quality data, amenable to further investigation. Limited extrapolation beyond direct effects of the target
	Gene knockout animals	
Preclinical	*In vitro* and *in vivo* testing in animals	High-quality data, but interpreted usually against gross effects on systems
Phase I	Volunteers' toleration of pharmacological effects. Exaggeration of side effects by con meds, disease, and so on, normally evaluated by pharmacokinetic surrogate	High-quality data. Tightly controlled and objective, highly instrumented and numerical output
		Patient numbers – about 100
Phase II	Patient side effects due to primary and secondary pharmacology	High-quality data. Tightly controlled and objective, relatively small patient numbers, about 1000
Phase III	Some indication of low-incidence effects	High-quality data. Well controlled and objective. Patient numbers of up to 10 000 treated. Incidents of low-frequency adverse events highly variable due to control background, con meds, and protocol variations
Postmarketing	Clarification of low-incidence events	Patient numbers of upwards of 100 000. Lower quality data unless part of phase 4 studies with specific end points. Reporting highly subjective and depending on prescriber vigilance and awareness. Highly influenced by patient compliance, known or unknown con meds, patient health, and other nontreated disease states

determine its suitability for further progression (and substantial investment). This means that the largest impact occurs when an unobserved serious adverse event(s) occurs postmarketing. By definition, this effect is not predicted by the existing data and the event is of low frequency related to the number of subjects studied previously. Importantly, it is worth clarifying that these findings do not disqualify the preceding work. Many compounds are halted early due to questionable benefit risk. Moreover, the systems have been sufficiently robust and "accurate" to ensure drug safety in the vast majority of individuals (29 999 out of 30 000 for a 1 in 30 000 incidence).

15.2
How Common is Clinical Drug Toxicity?

As much as drugs improve life expectancy and quality of life for billions of patients, adverse drug reactions can be so severe as to cause death in thousands of patients each week. At the extreme, one meta-analysis estimates that 106 000 deaths in the United States in 1994 might have been due to adverse drug reactions [1]. This would make drug side effects the sixth leading cause of death in the United States (4.6% of all deaths). In other studies using death certificates and/or the US MedWatch data, the death rate is much lower with between 0.1 and 0.3% of all deaths attributed to adverse drug reactions. The assumption made is that these deaths involve dangerous drugs that can be withdrawn from the market making drug use "safer." Table 15.2 looks at examples of drug withdrawals to illustrate the benefit and risk associated with these decisions.

A retrospective analysis of hospitals in Liverpool [2] of fatal drug reactions per hospital admission gave a similar figure to the higher rate above. This showed 28 drug deaths out of 18 820 admissions with 1225 admissions due to adverse drug reactions. In considering reactive metabolites and idiosyncratic reactions, *it is important to understand that almost all of the adverse reactions stemmed from their primary pharmacology.* The "most dangerous drug" was aspirin that was the sole medicine or in combination (particularly with other non-steroidal anti-inflammatory drugs (NSAIDs) and warfarin) in 17 of the 28 deaths. The figures somewhat reflect the huge numbers of treated patients: 30 million people take NSAIDs against an estimated 16 500 deaths each year in the United States that are caused by NSAIDs [3]. The detailed studies allowed conclusions around the cause of the toxicities and prescription errors (e.g., combining warfarin with an NSAID and resultant gastrointestinal bleeding) account for a substantial proportion of those deaths. For example, more than 7000 deaths/year in the United States are thought to be a result of medication errors [4].

When considering adverse drug reactions and serious side effects, it is important to understand the relative risks of an event. Many of the effects seen can occur due to "natural" causes and are part of a background incidence. The types of serious side effect caused by reactive metabolites are low incidence, although in certain cases the actual proportion of events triggered by drugs and reactive metabolites can be high. Other serious events can have much higher background incidence, with drugs a minor causality factor; however, the overall numbers of drug-induced cases may exceed the high-causality, low-incidence events. High-incidence events tend to have less association with perceived drug risks in public perception. This is illustrated in Figure 15.1, which contrasts low-incidence events often triggered by reactive metabolites such as toxic epidermal necrolysis, aplastic anemia, agranulocytosis, and anaphylaxis with high-incidence events such as road accidents [5].

Table 15.2 Selected drug withdrawals, the cause, and their estimated risk/benefit profile.

Drug Name	Year Withdrawn	Reason for Withdrawal	Cause of Withdrawal	Number of Deaths due to Drug	Number of Patients	Other Drugs of the Same Class Remain Available After Withdrawal?	Health Benefits	Medical Need of Health Condition Treated by Withdrawn Drugs
Fen-phen	1997	Damage to heart valves and pulmonary artery interstitial cells – fibromyxoid plaques	Second pharmacology. Activation of 5HT2B receptors in addition to 5HT2C	113	1.2–4.7 million	Limited effective alternatives to treat obesity exist	Reduces weight and improves morbidity/mortality	>100 000 estimated excess deaths in the United States p.a. through obesity
Cisapride	2000	Fatal arrythmias	Second pharmacology. Inhibition of Ikr potassium channel	80	30 million prescriptions	Alternative therapies involve decreasing acid production or neutralizing stomach acidity	Reduces acid reflux (and thereby avoids some esophageal cancer)	Estimated 8000 esophageal cancers in the United States p.a. caused by acid reflux
Troglitazone	2000	Hepatotoxicity	Reactive metabolites together with second pharmacology. Inhibition of BSEP	63	Approximately 1 million	Yes, several options in the same class emerged at the time of withdrawal	Avoids potentially lethal diabetes complications	Estimated >70 000 deaths in the United States p.a. through diabetes

Cerivastatin	2001	Rhabdomyolysis	Higher systemic concentrations than other statins (HMG-CoA reductase inhibitors)	100	6 million	Yes, several statins provide options postcerivastatin withdrawal	Avoids heart attacks and stroke	Estimated >900 000 cardiovascular disease deaths in the United States p.a. through hypertension and high blood lipids
Rofecoxib	2004	Increased risk of thrombotic cardiovascular events	Primary pharmacology. Suppression of endothelial vascular PG12 while not inhibiting platelet-derived TXA2 production	10 000 court cases filed	90 million prescriptions	Yes, other COX-2 inhibitors provide options, although actual cardiovascular events may reflect dose response	Improves quality of life	GI side effects associated with the use of nonselective NSAID pain killers (estimated 16 500 deaths from NSAIDs in arthritis patients in the United States in 1997)

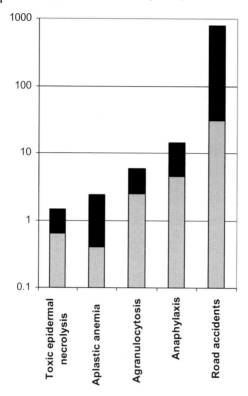

Figure 15.1 Comparison of incidence of diseases and serious drug side effects causing hospital admission/10^6 patients, contrasting total incidence (black) and proportion drug related (gray). Note the logarithmic scale. The road accidents shown are severe and result in hospital admission [5].

A large impact has been made over the last four decades by the improvement in monitoring of drug safety. Serious adverse event reporting has increased year on year based on US Food and Drug Administration (FDA) published data. In response to better monitoring more warnings, black box warnings and even marketing withdrawals are made. Considering just marketing withdrawals, in the period 1970–1979 there were no withdrawals, between 1980 and 1989 there were 5 withdrawals, between 1990 and 1999 there were 10 withdrawals, and in the five-year period between 2000 and 2005 there were 9 withdrawals for safety reasons. This does not imply that more recent drugs are showing more adverse events. When year of approval, rather than year of withdrawal, is considered, there is a steady or declining rate. For instance, of the 488 drugs approved between 1971 and 1992, there were 14 safety-based withdrawals (2.9%). For the 325 drugs approved between 1992 and 2005, there were corresponding 10 withdrawals (3.1%). When divided into five-year cohorts, the rate of subsequent withdrawals was 3.2% (1979–1983), 3.5% (1984–1988), 1.6% (1989–1993), and 1.2% (1994–1998).

15.3
Rules and Laws of Drug Toxicity

Drug hepatotoxicity is a major concern and was highlighted by the withdrawal of a series of drugs including bromfenac and troglitazone. Examination of all available data has led to the need to interpret possible drug hepatotoxicity from the clinical chemistry findings during drug development rather than in the postmarketing phase. The most important signals are alanine transaminase (ALT) and bilirubin. Increases above background of $3\times$ of these liver function markers are seen as indicative of potential hepatotoxicity. A pragmatic rule termed Hy's law or modified Hy's law is applied when ALT $>3\times$ *and* bilirubin $>2\times$ or $3\times$ upper limit of normal (ULN). The predictability that incidences of patients with these liver function results will lead to acute liver failure (ALF) in larger patient numbers is unknown, being based on retrospective studies [6, 7]. Recently decisions to not approve the thrombin inhibitor ximelagatran were based on a number of unequivocal cases of elevations in ALT and bilirubin during phase 3 trials [6, 7]. Experience with these rules shows that these risk factors are present in most seriously hepatotoxic drugs. Moreover, the combination of bilirubin and ALT elevations can be understood conceptually to be more serious than elevations in ALT alone.

Many agents, including those that eventually cause ALF, give elevations in hepatic markers (ALT and aspartate transaminase (AST)) in a large number of patients. These elevations do not progress and often return to baseline values. Among these drugs are the HMG-CoA reductase inhibitors [7]. These examples make extrapolation very difficult since the comparatively "large" early signal is not reflected in actual hepatotoxicity. It is clear though that some perturbation of liver function is taking place: due to either local effects on lipids (HMG-CoA reductase inhibitors) or the generation of reactive metabolites and frank cell injury (e.g., tacrine and isoniazid). The incidence of liver toxicity for statins is very low, but ALT and AST elevations exceeding three times ULN are dependent on dose and occur in up to 2% of treated patients [8, 9]. A dose relationship was demonstrated for lovastatin and appears to exist for the other statins as well. It has been proposed that the ALT increases and the accompanying centrizonal necrosis seen in rabbit livers might be the result of an exaggerated pharmacological action that depletes mevalonic acid synthesis. This hepatotoxicity triggered by lovastatin could be prevented (or reversed) in animals given mevalonate before (or after) hepatotoxicity developed. The development of hepatotoxicity in patients, in the few cases observed, usually occurs in the first few weeks to months of treatment [8, 9]. In general, all patients requiring lipid-lowering medication should have baseline ALT and AST levels. Follow-up levels should be obtained at six weeks, three months, six months, and one year. Unless the dose is increased, pravastatin and simvastatin do not require further liver enzyme monitoring if no enzyme elevations are detected during the first year of therapy. The newer statins – cerivastatin, fluvastatin, and atorvastatin – require periodic liver enzyme monitoring.

Tacrine's (a centrally active, reversible acetylcholinesterase inhibitor) major biotransformation product is 1-hydroxytacrine. In human liver microsomes

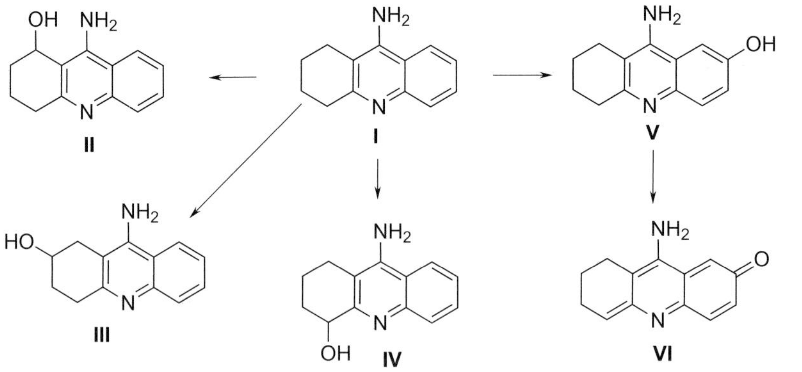

Figure 15.2 Structures of (I) tacrine and its (II) 1-OH, (III) 2-OH, and (IV) 4-OH metabolites. Oxidation of the phenyl ring yields the (V) 7-OH metabolite that can undergo further oxidation to the reactive (VI) quinone methide species.

irreversible covalent binding is observed in tacrine incubations in the presence of NADPH. Addition of glutathione inhibits the irreversible binding of tacrine metabolites, whereas human epoxide hydrolase inhibitors had a relatively minor effect. A mechanism has been proposed involving a quinone methide intermediate (Figure 15.2) in the bioactivation and irreversible binding of the drug [10, 11].

More than 190 000 patients in the United States received tacrine during the first two years following marketing approval [12]. The most common tacrine-associated adverse events were elevated liver transaminase levels (ALT) and, to a lesser degree, AST and peripheral cholinergic events. ALT elevations greater than 3× ULN occurred in 25% of patients, necessitating routine monitoring early in treatment. The elevations were almost always asymptomatic, rarely accompanied by significant increases in bilirubin, and related to time on drug rather than to dose (90% occurred within the first 12 weeks of treatment). ALT elevations were reversible and after cessation of the drug and rechallenge, patients were able to resume drug therapy in many cases. Guidelines when tacrine had no alternatives in treating Alzheimer's disease focused on treating the maximum number of patients with the minimum morbidity within sensible economic constraints [13]. Within this ALT monitoring was considered the best practical approach. The upper limit of rises in 3× ULN was used pragmatically to withdraw treatment, but rechallenge was encouraged. Thus, 25% of patients would be withdrawn but could be rechallenged. Rechallenge was favored with a small dose of drug and exclusion was warranted by ALT 20× ULN, suggestive of substantial hepatocyte necrosis or other symptoms of immune-based reactions such as fever, eosinophilia, or rash together with 3× ULN. It was expected that 12% of patients would have to be excluded following rechallenge. The standard dosage recommendation of 40 mg/day increasing every six weeks to a maximum of 160 mg/day must be adhered to and rechallenge should never exceed 40 mg/day. Regular weekly or biweekly monitoring of ALT levels was regarded as compulsory until the patients were stabilized on dose for long terms and then more relaxed monitoring was allowed. The success of

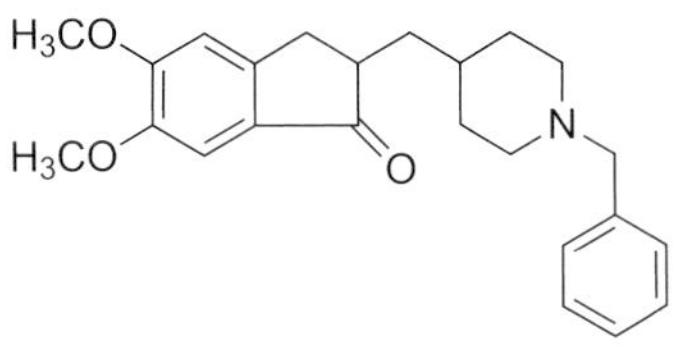

Figure 15.3 Structure of donepezil.

monitoring programs has been very mixed and was placed into context by the case of troglitazone outlined in Section 15.5. The use of tacrine has been super-seded by second-generation agents with improved efficacy and safety. Donepezil (Figure 15.3) as the next approved cholinesterase inhibitor demonstrated only adverse events associated with its primary pharmacology: nausea, diarrhea, head-ache, insomnia, dizziness, rhinitis, vomiting, asthenia/fatigue, and anorexia [14]. Donepezil use has not been associated with hepatotoxicity [14]. Importantly, done-pezil is administered as once-daily doses of 5 and 10 mg (compared to 160 mg for tacrine).

15.4
Difficulties in Defining Cause and Black Box Warnings

Maraviroc (Selzentry ^{R}), a chemokine receptor type 5 (CCR5) inhibitor, illustrates the multiple factors that can contribute to a black box warning. For a novel drug there is considerable caution. Maraviroc labeling carries the following warning on hepatotoxicity:

Warning: Hepatotoxicity

Hepatotoxicity has been reported with SELZENTRY use. Evidence of a systemic allergic reaction (e.g., pruritic rash, eosinophilia or elevated IgE) prior to the development of hepatotoxicity may occur. Patients with signs or symptoms of hepatitis or allergic reaction following use of SELZENTRY should be evaluated immediately.

The history behind this warning is one or two events in the course of maraviroc development. Analysis of the hepatotoxic potential has been conducted [15] across all Pfizer-sponsored maraviroc clinical trials, in which 2350 volunteers received the drug. Sporadic hepatic enzyme abnormalities were reported in 34 phase 1/2a stud-ies of up to 28-day duration with no dose relationship or association with hyper-bilirubinemia. In the four phase 2b/3 studies in antiretroviral-naive and -experienced patients, there was no significant imbalance in hepatic enzyme abnor-malities or hepatobiliary adverse events in maraviroc versus comparator arms. In patients coinfected with hepatitis B and/or C virus a similar balance of findings was observed. In these trails a female volunteer reported a sore throat and

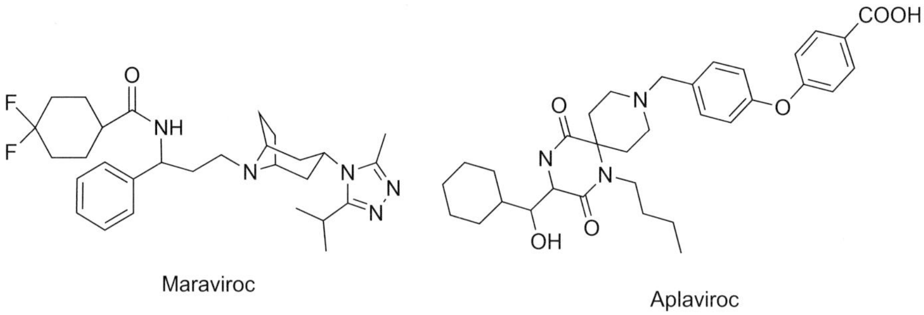

Figure 15.4 Structures of CCR5 antagonists maraviroc and aplaviroc.

developed flu-like symptoms and cervical/submaxillary lymphadenopathy. The pharangeal culture was positive for group A streptococcus. The volunteer received over 4 g of acetaminophen. All symptoms resolved after discontinuing the drug, although detectable concentrations of maraviroc were present. The more serious event occurred in a patient who was receiving trimethoprim–sulfamethoxazole and isoniazid at the screening visit approximately seven weeks before maraviroc treatment. After five days of maraviroc treatment, pyrexia, rash, and abnormal liver function tests were noted. Maraviroc was discontinued, but acetaminophen, lopinavir/ritonavir, zidovudine/lamivudine, and trimethoprim–sulfamethoxazole were still prescribed. The hepatic function continued to decline and a liver transplant was required. The most likely explanation of these events is co-trimoxazole or isoniazid hepatotoxicity, but the role of maraviroc cannot be ruled out, leading to the black box wording. Another factor that was considered was the possibility of class effects [15] implicating the CCR5 receptor. Aplaviroc, a structurally and physicochemically different CCR5 receptor antagonist, was halted in development due to hepatotoxicity. Four subjects in the course of development trials with aplaviroc had raised serum ALT (up to 70× ULN) and bilirubin (up to 5× ULN) after taking the drug. The zwitterionic nature of aplaviroc, compared to the basic maraviroc (Figure 15.4), potentially changes the permeability and transporter protein interactions of the drugs.

Aplaviroc has been characterized as a substrate and inhibitor of the organic anion-transporting polypeptide 1B1 and concentrations of radioactivity after ^{14}C-labeled aplaviroc are 70- to 100-fold greater in liver than in blood. The evidence for a possible class effect is limited to CCR5 knockout mice that are more sensitive in certain experiments to concanavalin A–induced, immune-mediated hepatic toxicity [16], although these experiments have been difficult to replicate [15]. The human polymorphism of CCR5 (the finding that led to the rationale for CCR5 antagonists and HIV treatment) does not convey increased risk of hepatic injury and additionally shows no influence on the severity of hepatitis C virus cirrhosis. Aplaviroc [17] shows no hepatic effects in macaque monkeys treated with 2000 mg/(kg day), a species in which aplaviroc inhibits the CCR5 receptor in contrast to hepatic findings (raised ALT and bilirubin levels) in rats at 500 mg/(kg day), a species whose CCR5 receptor does not bind aplaviroc. The black box warning for maraviroc taken in isolation may be seen as a positive reference to the drug being hepatotoxic, but the available evidence to this is largely contradictory. It certainly should not be used to characterize the drug into comparative *in vitro* tests. It also indicates the difficult task of assessing risk/benefit with the available data on a new drug.

15.5
Labeling Changes, Contraindications, and Warnings: the Effectiveness of Side Effect Monitoring

As reports of adverse events are processed, boxed or black box labeling is introduced as soon as a credible link to safety issues arises. This can affect drugs for which are there are few or no switching alternatives, or in some cases may affect the whole class of drugs. In response to this, prescribers should adapt their prescribing and monitoring behavior to the specific risks associated with the black box–labeled drug. In addition, they should communicate the meaning of such a label for a particular drug to their patients by contrasting the relative risk of taking the medicine compared to not taking the medicine, or by presenting some other relevant comparator of risk. In particular, early symptoms of the side effect may be noticed by an informed patient or the prescriber conducts regular monitoring of patients for the side effect. The effectiveness of contraindications, warnings, and black box warnings is highly variable.

Soon after marketing in 1997 the diabetes drug troglitazone was found to have potentially serious effects on the liver. The cause of this may be due to reactive metabolite formation and/or inhibition of the bile salt export pump. The US FDA put in place a comprehensive risk management program, including repeated labeling changes and "Dear Healthcare Professional" letters, on the requirement for liver enzyme monitoring of patients taking troglitazone [18]. The program consisted of four progressively more stringent liver monitoring recommendations. Although baseline testing increased from 15% before any FDA monitoring recommendations to 45% following the most severe warnings, the monitoring was highest following one month of therapy and had fallen back to the baseline value after three months. The risk management efforts, therefore, did not achieve the sustained improvement in liver enzyme testing necessary for the safe prescribing of troglitazone. Because of the failure of the program, the drug was withdrawn after 63 deaths from ALF (out of over 1 million users). One important point is that pioglitazone and rosiglitazone were available with better risk profiles in terms of the hepatic effects and less complications with drug interactions. Troglitazone was a clinical CYP3A4 inducer. Neither pioglitazone nor rosiglitazone showed these effects even though they had similar *in vitro* potencies with human hepatocytes. Again, the low doses due to primary target affinity mitigated these effects from appearing clinically.

In contrast, clozapine is an atypical antipsychotic agent that has several advantages over conventional antipsychotics. Clozapine has demonstrated superior

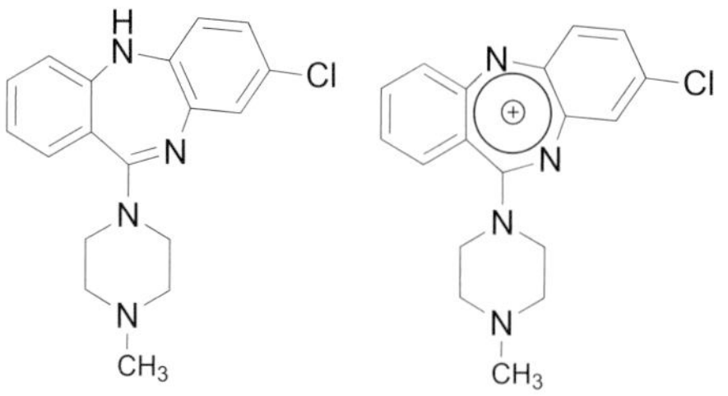

Figure 15.5 Structures of clozapine (I) and its reactive nitrenium ion (II), generated by oxidation.

efficacy in relieving positive and negative symptoms in treatment-resistant schizophrenic patients [19]. Unlike other antipsychotics, it causes minimal extrapyramidal side effects and has little effect on serum prolactin. Although other alternatives are available, each of the drugs has a discrete receptor profile that means each agent exhibits different responses in patients. In comparison trials in patients with schizophrenia who failed to improve with an atypical antipsychotic, clozapine was more effective than switching to other atypical antipsychotics such as olanzapine, quetiapine, and risperidone [20]. However, agranulocytosis [21] is seen in 0.8% of patients. The target cells affected are the myeloid precursors and possibly the mature neutrophil. The parent drug and its stable metabolites, desmethylclozapine and clozapine-*N*-oxide, are not implicated in the toxicity. Clozapine is metabolized by human liver microsomes, peripheral blood neutrophils, and their bone marrow precursors to a reactive intermediate that has been postulated to be a nitrenium ion (Figure 15.5).

The reactive nitrenium metabolite covalently binds to neutrophil proteins, suggesting that it may be a key element in the toxicological outcome. Mechanisms include binding and perturbing the structure of essential cellular proteins, thus disrupting neutrophil function, or acting as a hapten to initiate immune-mediated destruction of the neutrophil. In recent years mandatory blood monitoring in patients receiving clozapine has significantly reduced both the incidence of agranulocytosis and its associated mortality. The monitoring follows detailed analysis of the timing of side effects and is reported in the labeling of the drug. "The hematologic risk analysis was conducted based upon the available information in the Clozapine National Registry for U.S. patients. Based upon a cut-off date of April 30, 1995, the incidence rates of agranulocytosis based upon a weekly monitoring schedule rose steeply during the first two months of therapy, peaking in the third month. For patients who continued the drug beyond the third month, the weekly incidence of agranulocytosis fell to a substantial degree. After 6 months, the weekly incidence of agranulocytosis declines still further, however, it never reached zero. It should be noted that any type of reduction in the frequency of monitoring white blood cell counts may result in an increased incidence of agranulocytosis." The actual labeling describing the monitoring is reproduced below. Importantly, this is a firm contract between manufacturer, pharmacy, prescriber, and regulatory authority.

CLOZARIL^R (clozapine) IS AVAILABLE ONLY THROUGH A DISTRIBUTION SYSTEM THAT ENSURES MONITORING OF WHITE BLOOD CELL (WBC) COUNT AND ABSOLUTE NEUTROPHIL COUNT (ANC) ACCORDING TO THE SCHEDULE DESCRIBED BELOW PRIOR TO DELIVERY OF THE NEXT SUP-PLY OF MEDICATION.

PATIENTS WHO ARE BEING TREATED WITH CLOZARIL^R (clozapine) MUST HAVE A BASELINE WBC COUNT AND ANC BEFORE INITIATION OF TREAT-MENT, AND A WBC COUNT AND ANC EVERY WEEK FOR THE FIRST 6 MONTHS. THEREAFTER, IF ACCEPTABLE WBC COUNTS AND ANC (WBC $\geq$3500/mm^3 and ANC $\geq$2000/mm^3) HAVE BEEN MAINTAINED DURING THE FIRST 6 MONTHS OF CONTINUOUS THERAPY, WBC COUNTS AND ANC CAN BE MONITORED EVERY 2 WEEKS FOR THE NEXT 6 MONTHS. THERE-AFTER, IF ACCEPTABLE WBC COUNTS AND ANC (WBC $\geq$3500/mm^3 and ANC $\geq$2000/mm^3) HAVE BEEN MAINTAINED DURING THE SECOND 6 MONTHS OF CONTINUOUS THERAPY, WBC COUNT AND ANC CAN BE MONITORED EVERY 4 WEEKS.

WHEN TREATMENT WITH CLOZARIL^R (clozapine) IS DISCONTINUED (REGARDLESS OF THE REASON), WBC COUNT AND ANC MUST BE MONI-TORED WEEKLY FOR AT LEAST 4 WEEKS FROM THE DAY OF DIS-CONTINUATION OR UNTIL WBC $\geq$3500/mm^3 AND ANC $\geq$2000/mm^3.

Such a monitoring allows the drug to be used as potentially serious side effects are observed early and the drug discontinued. Clearly, the burden of monitoring is high with weekly tests for the first six months, falling to fort-nightly for patients without side effects until after a year when the monitoring is monthly. Ultimately, monitoring for a side effect is not ideal, since patients will need to be stabilized on a different drug if side effects are observed and the patients will also experience the toxicity of the drug, albeit in an abbreviated and hopefully milder form.

15.6
Allele Association with Hypersensitivity Induced by Abacavir: Toward a Biomarker for Toxicity

HIV patients treated with antiretroviral drugs show a high frequency of cuta-neous adverse drug reactions, including toxic epidermal necrolysis, Stevens–Johnson syndrome, and hypersensitivity syndrome. Abacavir is a guanosine analogue nucleoside reverse transcriptase inhibitor used for treatment of HIV infection. Hypersensitivity to abacavir occurs in approximately 5–8% of patients within one to six weeks of the initial dose. The hypersensitivity syn-drome is associated with fever, rash, and gastrointestinal symptoms. The ori-gin of these side effects is immunological and probably involving reactive

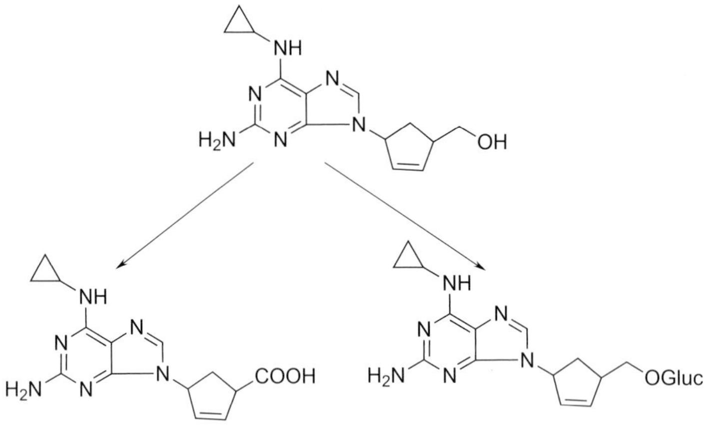

Figure 15.6 Metabolism of abacavir to a glucuronide and carboxylic metabolite. The metabolism to the acid proceeds via an aldehyde intermediate. Migration of the double bond of the cyclopentene ring is observed to yield an α,β-unsaturated aldehyde that can be trapped with an amine nucleophile.

metabolites. Abacavir is metabolized to glucuronide and carboxylic acid metabolites (Figure 15.6).

The metabolism of the alcohol to the carboxylic acid metabolite is via an aldehyde intermediate [22]. The aldehyde can undergo isomerization by migration of the double bond in the cyclopentene ring and further oxidation or reduction by aldehyde oxidase isoenzymes. The double bond migrated isomer is an α,β-unsaturated aldehyde, a well-known Michael acceptor, and a reactive metabolite that has been trapped with methoxylamine to yield the corresponding Schiff base. Metabolism of abacavir *in vitro* leads to covalent binding to proteins. The abacavir analogue with a cyclopentane ring (dihydro abacavir) undergoes metabolism to an acid but does not form covalently bound protein adducts, supporting the role of the α,β-unsaturated aldehyde in covalent binding [22].

The role of human leukocyte antigen (HLA) class I alleles in processing the reactive metabolite adducts is now more clear [22]. The drug antigen (e.g., drug–peptide complex) is presented by the specific HLA molecule on the antigen-presenting cells and recognized by effector T cells through the T cell receptor for HLA-restricted T cell activation. HLA class I–restricted CD8[+] T cells and HLA class II–restricted CD4[+] T cells are thought to induce an immune response, including hypersensitivity and cutaneous toxicities. The initial association between abacavir-induced hypersensitivity and HLA-B∗5701 was reported in Australian and British populations. To examine the universality of the sensitivity and specificity of HLA-B∗5701 association with abacavir hypersensitivity the Study of Hypersensitivity to Abacavir and Pharmacogenetic Evaluation (SHAPE) was performed. Caucasians have a significantly higher carriage of HLA-B∗5701. This study showed that 100% of both white and black patch test–positive patients carried HLA-B∗5701, and therefore HLA-B∗5701 was predictive for abacavir-induced hypersensitivity.

In Caucasians, around 8% of patients carry HLA-B*5701. Although all current studies show the requirement for HLA-B*5701 for development of abacavir-induced hypersensitivity syndrome, 45% of patients who carry HLA-B*5701 do not develop the hypersensitivity syndrome. Therefore, it is likely that HLA-B*5701 is necessary but not sufficient for development of abacavir-induced hypersensitivity syndrome [23].

Because this screening is potentially a future direction, it is worth further examination. The accuracy of the screening is defined by false positives and false negatives. The probability that a patient will be correctly identified, by the screen, as someone who will suffer a side effect to the drug is termed sensitivity. The probability that a patient who will not suffer a side effect is correctly identified is termed specificity. The screens for abacavir hypersensitivity referred to above have a sensitivity of 100% for immunologically confirmed abacavir hypersensitivity reactions. Against suspected hypersensitivity reactions the sensitivity of HLA-B*5701 falls to 14 and 44% for black and white patients, respectively, which is explained by the problem of correctly diagnosing and assigning hypersensitivity to a particular drug. The specificities of HLA-B*5701 among white and black patients are 96 and 99%, respectively. With a 2% carriage frequency of HLA-B*5701 among black patients, 98% would be identified as HLA-B*5701 negative and could confidently initiate therapy with very low risk of developing an immunologically confirmed hypersensitivity reaction. Two percent of HLA-B*5701-positive black patients would not be treated, but only one would have been expected to develop a hypersensitivity reaction. The other patient would have tolerated the drug and so would have benefited from therapy.

A number of cost-effective analyses [24, 25] have been performed on HLA-B*5701 screening and concluded that successful implementation of pharmacogenetic screening requires that a range of criteria be adequately addressed: (a) lack of alternative treatments with similar or improved cost effectiveness, safety, and efficacy, (b) accurate diagnosis of the adverse event, in the case of abacavir provided by adjunctive epicutaneous patch testing, (c) objective evidence of the test's predictive value and generalizability (in the case of abacavir provided by the SHAPE trial), (d) availability of quality-assured laboratory services that provide targeted genetic screening, and (e) the cost of the screening (HLA-B*5701) testing and the prevalence of HLA-B*5701 in different populations.

Such screening can be made point of care and of lower initial cost by further refinements, but with loss of specificity. A monoclonal antibody specific for HLA-B57 and HLA-B58 has been produced [26] that provides an inexpensive and sensitive screen. Patients who test negative by mAb screening comprise 90–95% of all individuals in most human populations and require no further HLA typing. Patients who test positive by mAb screening proceed to specific assays to ascertain the definitive presence of HLA-B*5701 or HLA-B*5801. Such tests allow simple and inexpensive ways to identify low-risk patients who can begin immediate treatment. Although extremely promising for the development of diagnostics to predict patients at risk, the field is complicated, not surprisingly, by multiple genetic links. For instance, HLA-B*5801 has been strongly linked with allopurinol-induced cutaneous toxicity including Stevens–Johnson syndrome/toxic epidermal necrolysis in Caucasian and Asian patients (including the Japanese) [27, 28]. In contrast, the strong association between carbamazepine-induced Stevens–Johnson syndrome/toxic epidermal necrolysis and HLA-B*1502 found in Southeast Asian patients is not seen in Caucasian and Japanese patients [27, 28]. Whether such associations can be strengthened by further genetic analysis including the enzymes that metabolize (activate and detoxify) drugs and their metabolites remains to be seen. Preliminary studies have shown some promising correlations.

Hepatotoxicity is the most frequent adverse drug reaction in Japanese treated with ticlopidine. Combination of cytochrome P450 (CYP) 2B6 and HLA haplotypes revealed that individuals possessing CYP2B6*1H or *1J with HLA-A*3303 have the highest susceptibility to ticlopidine-induced hepatotoxicity [29]. It has been shown recently that loss-of-function alleles of some P450 genes, especially CYP2C19*2, are responsible for reduced reaction of platelets to clopidogrel and thereby increased cardiac risk, suggesting that CYP2C19 is the major enzyme catalyzing the conversion of clopidogrel to its active (reactive) metabolite [30]. Although some autoinhibition of this CYP occurs, by far the most potent effect is with CYP2B6. Inhibition of CYP2B6 [31] is dependent on time, concentration, and NADPH, and is irreversible, indicative of a mechanism-based mode of action. Inhibition was attenuated by the presence of alternative active site ligands but not by nucleophilic trapping agents or reactive oxygen scavengers, further supporting mechanism-based action. As noted in chapter 12 (Figure 12.6), reactive metabolites (e.g., sulfenic acid) have been characterized in in vitro human liver microsomal incubations of clopidogrel.

The association with CYP2B6*1H or *1J suggests that the alteration of these isoforms from the wild type is implicated in the CYP enzyme as a catalyst for drug hepatotoxicity and may have parallels to those described in Chapter 1 (Section 1.9) with drugs such as tienilic acid. Whether our understandings advance sufficiently to be able to screen rationally for diagnostic markers based on metabolism and toxicity pathways will be of interest over the next decade.

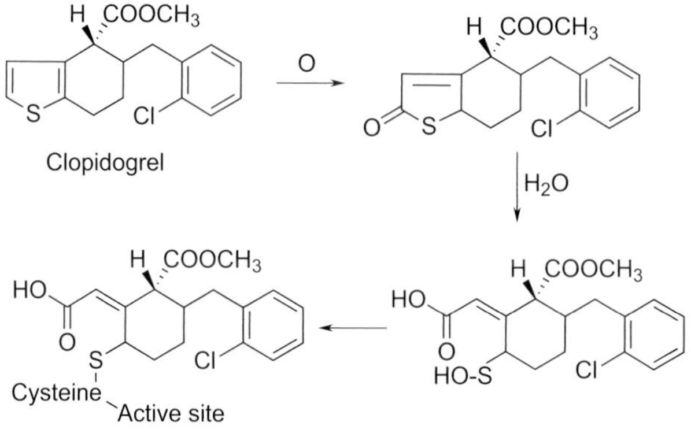

Figure 15.7 Oxidation of ticlopidine to a thiol metabolite, which can bind to the active site of the P2Y$_{12}$-ADP-receptor or the P450 isozyme(s) presumably via the electrophilic sulfenic acid metabolite.

15.7
More Questions than Answers: Benefit Risk for ADRs

Risk/benefit decisions are taken on the severity of the disease, the number of patients afflicted, the frequency and ease that those patients can be monitored, the adverse event profile in terms of severity and numbers, and the availability of other forms of treatment. These decisions are taken against a continually moving scenario of knowledge about the pros and cons of drug intervention in the disease process, together with the introduction of new drugs and other technologies. To illustrate the grayness of these decisions the case of benzbromarone is highlighted [32]. Benzbromarone, a potent uricosuric drug, was introduced in the 1970s in 20 countries throughout Asia, South America, and Europe. The drug was withdrawn by Sanofi-Synthelabo in 2003 due to serious hepatotoxicity. A major circulating metabolite, 6-hydroxybenzbromarone, with a long half-life ($\sim$30 h) is mainly responsible for the uricosuric activity of benzbromarone. The clearance of benzbromarone and the formation of 6-hydroxybenzbromarone are mediated by the polymorphically expressed CYP2C9. The drug is more effective as a standard dosage of 100 mg/day compared to allopurinol (300 mg/day) or probenecid (1000 mg/day). Four cases of benzbromarone-induced hepatotoxicity were identified from the literature by Lee *et al.* [32], although 11 cases were reported by Sanofi-Synthelabo. Only one of the four published cases demonstrated a clear relationship between the drug and liver injury as demonstrated by rechallenge. If all the reported cases were assumed to be due to benzbromarone, the risk of hepatotoxicity was 1 in 17 000 patients. The alternative, less effective drugs to benzbromarone are associated with adverse reactions. Rash occurs in 2% of patients taking allopurinol and usually leads to cessation of prescription of the drug. Allopurinol can also cause a life-threatening hypersensitivity syndrome in 1 in 56 000 patients. Probenecid has also been associated with similar life-threatening reactions but in much smaller number. Because of its efficacy, the authors concluded that the withdrawal of benzbromarone was not in the best interest of patients with gout. Since this report, febuxostat [33], a nonpurine selective inhibitor of xanthine oxidase, has been approved for the treatment of hyperuricemia in patients with gout. The drug is as effective as allopurinol with a different adverse effect profile. The skin effects of allopurinol are of much lower frequency compared with febuxostat, but there is an apparently greater incidence of cardiovascular events. Postapproval, the manufacturer of febuxostat has initiated a large, FDA-mandated study of cardiovascular safety of the drug. A final point to conclude this chapter is the structure of benzbromarone (Figure 15.7): was it a loaded gun (e.g., the bromobenzene structural alert)?

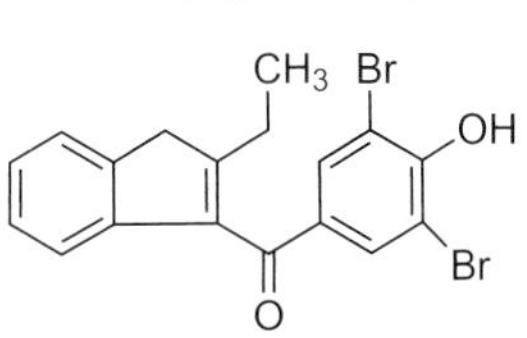

Figure 15.7 Structure of benzbromarone.

If so, drug design can alleviate some (not all) of the discussions and weigh the scales slightly more to benefit.

References

1 Lazarou, J., Pomeranz, B.H., and Corey, P.N. (1998) Incidence of adverse drug reactions in hospitalised patients. *JAMA: the Journal of the American Medical Association*, **279** (15), 1200–1205.

2 Pirmohamed, M., James, S., Meakin, S., Green, C., Scott, A.K., Walley, T.J., Farrar, K., Park, K.B., and Breckenridge, A.M. (2004) Adverse drug reactions as cause of admission to hospital: prospective analysis of 18,820 patients. *British Medical Journal*, **329** (7456), 15–19.

3 Hampton, T. (2006) Medication errors. *JAMA: the Journal of the American Medical Association*, **296** (4), 384.

4 Wolfe, M.M., Lichtenstein, D.R., and Singh, G. (1999) Gastrointestinal toxicity of nonsteroidal antiinflammatory drugs. *New England Journal of Medicine*, **340** (24), 1888–1899.

5 Edwards, I.R. (2001) The management of adverse drug reactions: from diagnosis to signal. *Therapie*, **56** (6), 727–733.

6 Lewis, J.H. (2006) "Hy's law", the "Rezulin Rule," and other predictors of severe drug-induced hepatotoxicity: putting risk–benefit into perspective. *Pharmacoepidemiology and Drug Safety*, **15** (2), 221–229.

7 Kaplowitz, N. (2006) Rules and laws of drug hepatotoxicity. *Pharmacoepidemiology and Drug Safety*, **15** (2), 231–233.

8 Diaczok, B.J. and Shali, R. (2003) Statins unmasking a mitochondrial myopathy: a case report and proposed mechanism of disease. *Southern Medical Journal*, **96** (3), 318–320.

9 Lewis, J.H., Mortensen, M.E., Zweig, S., Fusco, M.J., Medoff, J.R., and Belder, R. (2007) Efficacy and safety of high-dose pravastatin in hypercholesterolemic patients with well-compensated chronic liver disease: results of a prospective, randomized, double-blind, placebo-controlled, multicenter trial. *Hepatology*, **46** (5), 1453–1463.

10 He, K., Talaat, R.E., Pool, W.F., Reily, M.D., Reed, J.E., Bridges, A.J., and Wool, T.F. (1993) Bioactivation and irreversible binding of the cognition activator tacrine using human and rat liver microsomal preparations. Species difference. *Drug Metabolism and Disposition*, **21** (5), 874–882.

11 Patocka, J., Jun, D., and Kamil, K. (2008) Possible role of hydroxylated metabolites of tacrine in drug toxicity and therapy of Alzheimer's disease. *Current Drug Metabolism*, **9** (4), 332–335.

12 Watkins, P.B., Zimmerman, H.J., Knapp, M.J., Gracon, S.I., and Lewis, K.W. (1994) Hepatotoxic effects of tacrine administration in patients with Alzheimer's disease. *JAMA: the Journal of the American Medical Association*, **271** (13), 992–998.

13 Balson, R., Gibson, P.R., Ames, D., and Bhathal, P.S. (1995) Tacrine-induced hepatotoxicity: tolerability and management. *CNS Drugs*, **4** (3), 168–181.

14 Pratt, R.D., Perdomo, C.A., Surick, I.W., and Ieni, J.R. (2002) Donepezil: tolerability and safety in Alzheimer's disease. *International Journal of Clinical Practice*, **56** (9), 710–717.

15 Ayoub, A., Alston, S., Goodrich, J., Heera, J., Hoepelman, A.I., Lalezari, J., Mchale, M., Nelson, M., van der Ryst, E., and Mayer, H. (2010) Hepatic safety and tolerability in the maraviroc clinical development program. *AIDS*, **24** (17), 2743–2750.

16 Smith, D.A., Harrison, A., and Morgan, P. (2011) Multiple factors govern the association between pharmacology and toxicity in a class of drugs: toward a unification of class effect terminology. *Chemical Research in Toxicology*, **24** (4), 463–474.

17 Nichols, W.G., Steel, H.M., Bonny, T., Adkison, K., Curtis, L., Millard, J., Kabeya, K., and Clumeck, N. (2008) Hepatotoxicity

observed in clinical trials of aplaviroc (GW873140). *Antimicrobial Agents and Chemotherapy*, **52** (3), 858–865.

18 Graham, D.J., Drinkard, C.R., Shatin, D., Tsong, Y., and Burgess, M.J. (2001) Liver enzyme monitoring in patients treated with troglitazone. *JAMA: the Journal of the American Medical Association*, **286** (7), 831–833.

19 Miller, D.D. (2000) Review and management of clozapine side effects. *Journal of Clinical Psychiatry*, **61** (Suppl. 8), 14–19.

20 McEvoy, J.P., Lieberman, J.A., Stroup, T.S., Davis, S.M., Meltzer, H.Y., Rosenheck, R.A., Swartz, M.S., Perkins, D.O., Keefe, R.S.E., Davis, C.E., Severe, J., and Hsiao, J.K. (2006) Effectiveness of clozapine versus olanzapine, quetiapine, and risperidone in patients with chronic schizophrenia who did not respond to prior atypical antipsychotic treatment. *American Journal of Psychiatry*, **163** (4), 600–610.

21 Pirmohamed, M. and Park, K. (1997) Mechanism of clozapine-induced agranulocytosis. Current status of research and implications for drug development. *CNS Drugs*, **7** (2), 139–158.

22 Walsh, J.S., Reese, M.J., and Thurmond, L.M. (2002) The metabolic activation of abacavir by human liver cytosol and expressed human alcohol dehydrogenase isozymes. *Chemico-Biological Interactions*, **142** (1–2), 135–154.

23 Hetherington, S., Hughes, A. R., Mosteller, M., Shortino, D., Baker, K. L., Spreen, W., Lai, E., Davies, K., Handley, A., Dow, D. J., Fling, M. E., Stocum, M., Bowman, C., Thurmond, L. M., and Roses, A. D. (2002) Genetic variations in HLA-B region and hypersensitivity reactions to abacavir. Lancet, 359(9312), 1121–1122.

24 Schackman, B.R., Scott, C.A., Walensky, R.P., Losina, E., Freedberg, K.A., and Sax, P.E. (2008) The cost-effectiveness of HLA-B∗5701 genetic screening to guide initial antiretroviral therapy for HIV. *AIDS*, **22** (15), 2025–2037.

25 Nolan, D. (2009) HLA-B∗5701 screening prior to abacavir prescription: clinical and laboratory aspects. *Critical Reviews in Clinical Laboratory Sciences*, **46** (3), 153–165.

26 Kostenko, L., Kjer-Nielsen, L., Nicholson, I., Hudson, F., Lucas, A., Foley, B., Chen, K., Lynch, K., Nguyen, J., Wu, A.H., Tait, B.D., Holdsworth, R., Mallal, S., Rossjohn, J., Bharadwaj, M., and McCluskey, J. (2011) Rapid screening for the detection of HLA-B57 and HLA-B58 in prevention of drug hypersensitivity. *Tissue Antigens*, **78** (1), 11–20.

27 Aihara, M. (2011) Pharmacogenetics of cutaneous adverse drug reactions. *Journal of Dermatology*, **38** (3), 246–254.

28 Pichler, W.J., Naisbitt, D.J., and Park, B.K. (2011) Immune pathomechanism of drug hypersensitivity reactions. *Journal of Allergy and Clinical Immunology*, **127** (3S), S74–S81.

29 Ariyoshi, N., Iga, Y., Hirata, K., Sato, Y., Miura, G., Ishii, I., Nagamori, S., and Kitada, M. (2010) Enhanced susceptibility of HLA-mediated ticlopidine-induced idiosyncratic hepatotoxicity by CYP2B6 polymorphism in Japanese. *Drug Metabolism and Pharmacokinetics*, **25** (3), 298–306.

30 Momary, K.M. and Dorsch, M.P. (2010) Factors associated with clopidogrel nonresponsiveness. *Future Cardiology*, **6** (2), 195–210.

31 Richter, T., Muerdter, T.E., Heinkele, G., Pleiss, J., Tatzel, S., Schwab, M., Eichelbaum, M., and Zanger, U.M. (2004) Potent mechanism-based inhibition of human CYP2B6 by clopidogrel and ticlopidine. *Journal of Pharmacology and Experimental Therapeutics*, **308** (1), 189–197.

32 Lee, M.-H.H., Graham, G.G., Williams, K.M., and Day, R.O. (2008) A benefit–risk assessment of benzbromarone in the treatment of gout: was its withdrawal from the market in the best interest of patients? *Drug Safety*, **31** (8), 643–665.

33 Kelly, V.M. and Krishnan, E. (2011) Febuxostat for the treatment of hyperuricemia in patients with gout. *International Journal of Clinical Rheumatology*, **6** (5), 485–490.

Index

Reactive Drug Metabolites, First Edition. Amit S. Kalgutkar, Deepak Dalvie, R. Scott Obach, and Dennis A. Smith.
© 2012 Wiley-VCH Verlag GmbH & Co. KGaA. Published 2012 by Wiley-VCH Verlag GmbH & Co. KGaA.